Biopathology of the Liver
An Ultrastructural Approach

This book is dedicated to my beloved daughter, Cecilia,
on the occasion of her 8th birthday: May 28, 1988

Biopathology of the Liver
An Ultrastructural Approach

Edited by

Pietro M. Motta, MD, PhD

Chairman and Professor,
Department of Anatomy,
Faculty of Medicine,
University 'La Sapienza', Rome, Italy

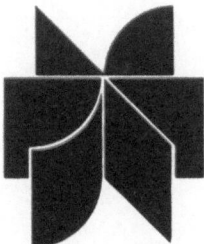

KLUWER ACADEMIC PUBLISHERS
DORDRECHT / BOSTON / LONDON

Distributors

for the United States and Canada: Kluwer Academic
Publishers, PO Box 358, Accord Station, Hingham, MA 02018-
0358, USA
for all other countries: Kluwer Academic Publishers Group,
Distribution Center, PO Box 322, 3300 AH Dordrecht, The
Netherlands

British Library Cataloguing in Publication Data

Biopathology of the liver.
  1. Man. Liver. Pathology
  I. Motta, P.M. (Pietro M.)
  616.3′6207

Library of Congress Cataloging in Publication Data

Biopathology of the liver.

  Includes bibliographies and index.
  1. Liver—Pathophysiology.   2. Liver—Ultrastructure.
I. Motta, Pietro M. [DNLM: 1. Liver—ultrastructure.
2. Liver Diseases—pathology.   3. Microscopy, Electron.
W1 700 B6105]
RC846.9.B56 1988   616.3′6207   88-9260
ISBN-13: 978-94-010-7049-2   e-ISBN-13: 978-94-009-1239-7
DOI: 10.1007/978-94-009-1239-7

CONTENTS

'... *La Natura per esercitare le mirabili operationi negli animali, e nei vegetabili, si è compiaciuta comporre il loro corpo organico con moltissime machine, le quali per necessita sono fatte di parti minutissime in tal maniera configurate, e situate, che formano un mirabile organo, la di cui struttura, e compositione con gli occhi nudi, e senza aiuto del microscopio per lo più non si arriva; anzi molte e molte di grande importanza sfuggono; onde non è da sprezzarsi la diligenza dell'arte nel procurar instrumenti, e praticarli per arrivare all'artificio mirabile delle parti, che sono principio dell'operazione sana e morbosa ...*'

'... Nature, in order to carry out its wonderful operations in animals and plants, has rejoiced in composing their organic body of many machines which, necessarily, are made up of tiny parts in such a way that, placed together, they form a marvelous organ whose structure and composition, to the naked eye and without the aid of the microscope, usually cannot be appreciated; indeed, many, many details of great importance escape us; therefore, the diligence of art in procuring and employing instruments in order to elucidate the wondrous artifice of the parts, which play the principal role in sickness and in health, should not be discounted ...'

Marcello Malpighi, *Risposta* to his work, *De Viscerum Structura*, Messina, 1665

Contributors

Bernaert, D.
Laboratoire de Cytologie et de Cancérologie
Expérimentale,
Free University of Brussels,
Faculty of Medicine,
1 rue Héger-Bordet,
B-1000 Brussels,
Belgium

Bouwens, L.
Laboratory for Cell Biology and Histology,
Free University of Brussels (VUB),
Laarbeeklaan 103,
B-1090 Brussels,
Belgium

Brühl, B.
Anatomisches Institut III,
Universität Heidelberg,
Im Neuenheimer Feld 307,
D-6900 Heidelberg,
Federal Republic of Germany

Caramia, F. G.
Dipartimento di Medicina Sperimentale,
University of Rome 'La Sapienza',
Viale Regina Elena 324,
00161 Roma,
Italy

Correr, S.
Department of Anatomy,
University of Rome 'La Sapienza',
Faculty of Medicine,
Viale Regina Elena 289,
00161 Rome,
Italy

DiDio, L. J. A.
Department of Anatomy,
Medical College of Ohio,
C.S. 10888 Toledo,
Ohio 43699
USA

Forssmann, W. G.
Anatomisches Institut III,
Universität Heidelberg,
Im Neuenheimer Feld 307,
D-6900 Heidelberg,
Federal Republic of Germany

Fujita, T.
Department of Anatomy,
Niigata University, School of Medicine,
Asahimachi 1,
Niigata 951,
Japan

Galand, P.
Laboratoire de Cytologie et de Cancérologie
Expérimentale,
Free University of Brussels,
Faculty of Medicine,
1 rue Héger-Bordet,
B-1000 Brussels,
Belgium

Gaudio, E.
Department of Anatomy,
University of L'Aquila,
Faculty of Medicine,
Collemaggio,
67100 L'Aquila,
Italy

Geerts, A.
Laboratory for Cell Biology and Histology,
Free University of Brussels (VUB),
Laarbeeklaan 103,
B-1090 Brussels,
Belgium

Goldblatt, P. J.
Department of Pathology,
Medical College of Ohio,
C.S. 10008 Toledo,
Ohio 43699,
USA

Hamlett, W. C.
Department of Anatomy,
Medical College of Ohio,
C.S. 10008 Toledo,
Ohio 43699,
USA

Hampton, J. A.
Department of Pathology,
Medical College of Ohio,
C.S. 10008 Toledo,
Ohio 43699,
USA

Ito, S.
Department of Anatomy,
Harvard Medical School,
25 Shattuck Street,
Boston,
Massachusetts 02115,
USA

Klaunig, J. E.
Department of Pathology,
Medical College of Ohio,
C.S. 10008 Toledo,
Ohio 43699,
USA

Macchiarelli, G.
Department of Anatomy,
University of Rome 'La Sapienza',
Faculty of Medicine,
Viale Regina Elena 289,
00161 Rome,
Italy

Metz, J.
Department of Anatomy,
Universität Heidelberg,
Im Neuenheimer Feld 307,
D-6900 Heidelberg,
Federal Republic of Germany

Modesti, A.
Dipartimento di Medicina Sperimentale,
University of Rome 'La Sapienza',
Faculty of Medicine,
Viale Regina Elena 289,
00161 Rome,
Italy

Mosselmans, R.
Laboratoire de Cytologie et de Cancérologie
Expérimentale,
Free University of Brussels,
Faculty of Medicine,
1 rue Héger-Bordet,
B-1000 Brussels,
Belgium

Motta, P. M.
Department of Anatomy,
University of Rome 'La Sapienza',
Faculty of Medicine,
Viale Regina Elena 289,
00161 Rome,
Italy

Ohtani, O.
Department of Anatomy,
Okayama University, School of Medicine,
2-5-1 Shikata-cho,
Okayama,
700 Japan

de Ridder, L.
Laboratory of Histology,
State University of Ghent,
2 Louis Pasteurlaan,
B-9000 Ghent,
Belgium

Robenek, H.
Department of Cell Biology,
University of Münster,
Faculty of Medicine,
Domagkstr. 3,
D-4400 Münster,
Federal Republic of Germany

Takahashi-Iwanaga, H.
Department of Anatomy,
Niigata University, School of Medicine,
Asahimachi 1,
Niigata 951,
Japan

Tanikawa, K.
Second Department of Medicine
Kurume University School of Medicine,
Asahimachi 67,
Kurume-shi,
Fukuoka-ken,
830 Japan

Torrisi, M. R.
Dipartimento di Medicina Sperimentale,
University of Rome 'La Sapienza',
Faculty of Medicine,
Viale Regina Elena 324,
00161 Rome,
Italy

Wake, K.
Department of Anatomy,
Faculty of Medicine,
Tokyo Medical and Dental University,
Yushima 1-5-45,
Bunkyo-ku,
Tokyo 113,
Japan

Wisse, E.
Laboratory for Cell Biology and Histology,
Free University of Brussels (VUB),
Laarbeeklaan 103,
B-1090 Brussels,
Belgium

Foreword

In the preface for the book on *The Liver by Scanning Electron Microscopy* that I prepared ten years ago in collaboration with Drs M. Muto and T. Fujita, it was concluded: 'We think what has recently been done on the liver – as well as on other organs – by SEM methods is fascinating, but we believe what will be done in the future, when more investigators are at work, will surely be even more fruitful.'

Since that pioneering work on the liver through the use of SEM, not only have these specific techniques been improved and employed by a great number of scientists, but, integrated with other new methods which use electrons for fine resolution, they are able to provide more complete and more easily interpretable views of cells, tissues and organs which are therefore routinely used for basic research as well as for diagnostic purposes.

The liver is a particularly strategic and multiform organ central to a variety of basic, experimental and clinical studies which nowadays are facilitated by highly sophisticated techniques. Among these, the enormous advances in electron microscopy have surely contributed much in furnishing a more complete and 'realistic' portrait of the hepatocytes and other liver tissues. When such structures are examined with high resolution microscopes at the macromolecular level, the information so obtained can be promptly and easily correlated with concurrent biochemical data, providing easily interpretable morphodynamic data useful under normal as well as altered conditions. As a result of such an approach, these ultrastructural observations can consistently help in the formulation of diagnoses (ultrastructural histopathology) and ultimately be of great benefit in the application of therapy. The idea of having a volume devoted to the ultrastructure of the liver in which basic information can be coupled with diagnostic and clinical aspects was the logical conclusion of a workshop on the subject that I was asked to organize on the occasion of the 7th International Symposium on Morphological Sciences, held in Brussels in September, 1986. In addition to the few colleagues who were invited to present their data at the meeting I later decided to invite some other scientists who are very active in the field to contribute to this volume in order to provide a more encompassing overview of the fine structure of the liver.

In addition, if one considers that important information on specific electron microscopic techniques and ultrastructural results on the liver is generally disseminated in a great variety of specialized biomedical journals, a further scope of this work is to present and review in a concise and simple manner in the light of an integrated methodical approach. Therefore each chapter offers a different 'ultrastructural' or 'microscopic' point of view of the liver which should ultimately converge towards the unitary 'structure' of the hepatocyte and other liver tissues. In each chapter the individual authors have not only summarized the results so far obtained in their laboratories – emphasizing these aspects with the generous use of micrographs – but have also tried to indicate new trends and possibilities in the application of the specific methods used to investigate the liver structually. The authors of the book have been selected as authoritative experts in their own field and the possibility that some of their indications might come true in the near future should not be overlooked.

Our hope is that, at least in a simple and mainly illustrative way (and this reflects the limitations of a pure morphologist, as essentially the editor of this volume is), the volume – in atlas format – will be of interest not only to morphologists but also to biochemists, cell biologists, physiologists, pathologists and all others – students and specialists – who still believe that structure is the easiest way by which our brain looks at the objects around us and tries to interpret the biological mechanics behind them.

It is our opinion that the more confidence we have in the ultrastructural approach, the more easy it will be to interpret the function and alteration of tissues. We also believe that future methodologies and progress in this area will greatly depend on integrating ultrastructural (even at a macromolecular anatomical level) events with more gross physiopathological aspects. To achieve this, the morphologist, in turn, closely depends on a continuous correlation of various structural and ultrastuctural methods. Ultimately, this integrative approach should render the most realistic image of tissues or organs at a certain stage of their life.

This volume should therefore be regarded as a modest tribute to such an integrative biopathological approach, to which, of course, more could be added as microscopical techniques continue to evolve.

April 15, 1988: Rome   PIETRO M. MOTTA.

Acknowledgments

I would like to express my sincere thanks to my colleagues for their contributions to this volume and for their special patience regarding my continuous requests. My appreciation also goes to Prof. A. Dhem, President of the 7th International Symposium on Morphological Sciences, in which the original workshop was organized and without which the subsequent work surely would never have been realized. Thanks are particularly due to David Finn and Dr Sharon Greene for having read and carefully checked the manuscripts. Furthermore, I would like to express my gratitude to Dr J. M. Brevis and Mr P. Johnstone at Kluwer Academic Publishers for their continuous kind and invaluable assistance in completing this endeavour. Finally, my special thanks go to my wife, Prof. S. Correr, and to the rest of my family, without whose incredible patience and tolerance during all the stages of 'gestation and release' this book would never have been possible.

1

The human hepatocyte: Ultrastructural features of adult and fetal liver

A. MODESTI, M. R. TORRISI and F. G. CARAMIA

INTRODUCTION

The liver is comprised of five different cell types, the most common of which is the hepatocyte which contributes 70% of the organ's total weight. Hepatocytes are polygonal in shape and their outer cell membranes may be divided schematically into several facets. Two or three facets are in contact with the space of Disse, while the remaining facets make contact with adjacent liver cells. Hepatocytes have a large, central nucleus and contain a great number of cellular organelles, such as ER, Golgi apparatus, mitochondria, lysosomes, peroxisomes, glycogen etc. Bile canaliculi run between adjacent hepatocytes, their lumen being generally surrounded by two, or occasionally three of these cells, whose lateral plasma membranes are joined by two bands of tight junctions, excluding the lumen of the bile canaliculum from the lateral extracellular space between the hepatocytes and that from the perisinusoidal space of Disse. The two free hepatocyte surfaces (that towards the lumen of the bile canaliculum and that facing the perisinusoidal space) are provided with numerous, small, fingerlike processes (microvilli) which are highly variable in number and size and which greatly increase the cell's surface area (see Figures 2–5).

In addition to the hepatocytes, various cell types have been recognized in the liver: the lining endothelial cells, the Kupffer cells and the fat-storing cells (Ito), or other Ito cells, which are vitamin A-storing cells. These will be discussed elsewhere in this volume (Chapters 2–5).

The hepatocytes perform a variety of complex functions using mechanisms similar to those of other cells. They elaborate bile pigments which are secreted into the bile canaliculi and, via the biliary ducts, into the duodenum. In addition, they regulate the catabolism and synthesis of fats, carbohydrates and proteins, maintaining their homeostasis in the organism. Hepatocytes also play a major role in the synthesis and catabolism of hormones, lipoproteins and plasma proteins.

In the embryonal age (Figure 1), the liver is considered the major haematopoietic organ. The hepatic haemopoiesis initiates around the 6th week of gestational age, increasing up to the 6th month, after which it declines during the terminal stages of pregnancy[1–3].

This chapter deals with our current information on the ultrastructural organization of the human liver cell, and is correlated with some relevant biochemical data.

HEPATOCYTES

Nucleus

The nuclei of liver cells are large and usually central. The nuclear envelope consists of a double membrane composed of two lipid bilayers separated by a gap of 20–40 nm known as a perinuclear space[4,5]. The membrane is mostly fenestrated, and nuclear pores, measuring 40–100 nm, provide for rapid exchanges between the nucleoplasm and the cytoplasm (Figures 2 and 3). Since the nuclear envelope is continuous with the endoplasmic reticulum, the nuclear membrane can grow, expanding and contracting rapidly, by direct exchange of material with the endoplasmic reticulum membrane. This can cause rapid changes in the area of the nuclear membrane, permitting its breakdown and reformation during mitosis. The region of the nuclear membrane also increases in volume when the formerly quiescent nucleus begins to rapidly synthesize RNA or DNA. Mitotic activity is rare in the intact normal adult liver (1 mitosis per 10 000–20 000 cells); in fact, the minimum average life span of a liver parenchymal cell is about 150 days. Large intranuclear glycogen bodies have been described in both diabetic and non-diabetic patients. Biopsied periportal hepatocytes show rounded glycogen bodies of the monoparticulate type and are without a limiting membrane[6].

Nucleolus

Unlike the cytoplasmic organelles, the nucleolus does not have any kind of membrane to keep it together. As in other cell types which synthesize high levels of proteins (Figure 3), three partially segregated regions of the nucleolus can be distinguished by electron microscopy:

(1) A pale-staining constituent containing DNA from the nuclear organizer region of a chromosome;

(2) A granular component containing particles having a diameter of 15 nm and representing the most mature of the ribosomal precursor particles; and

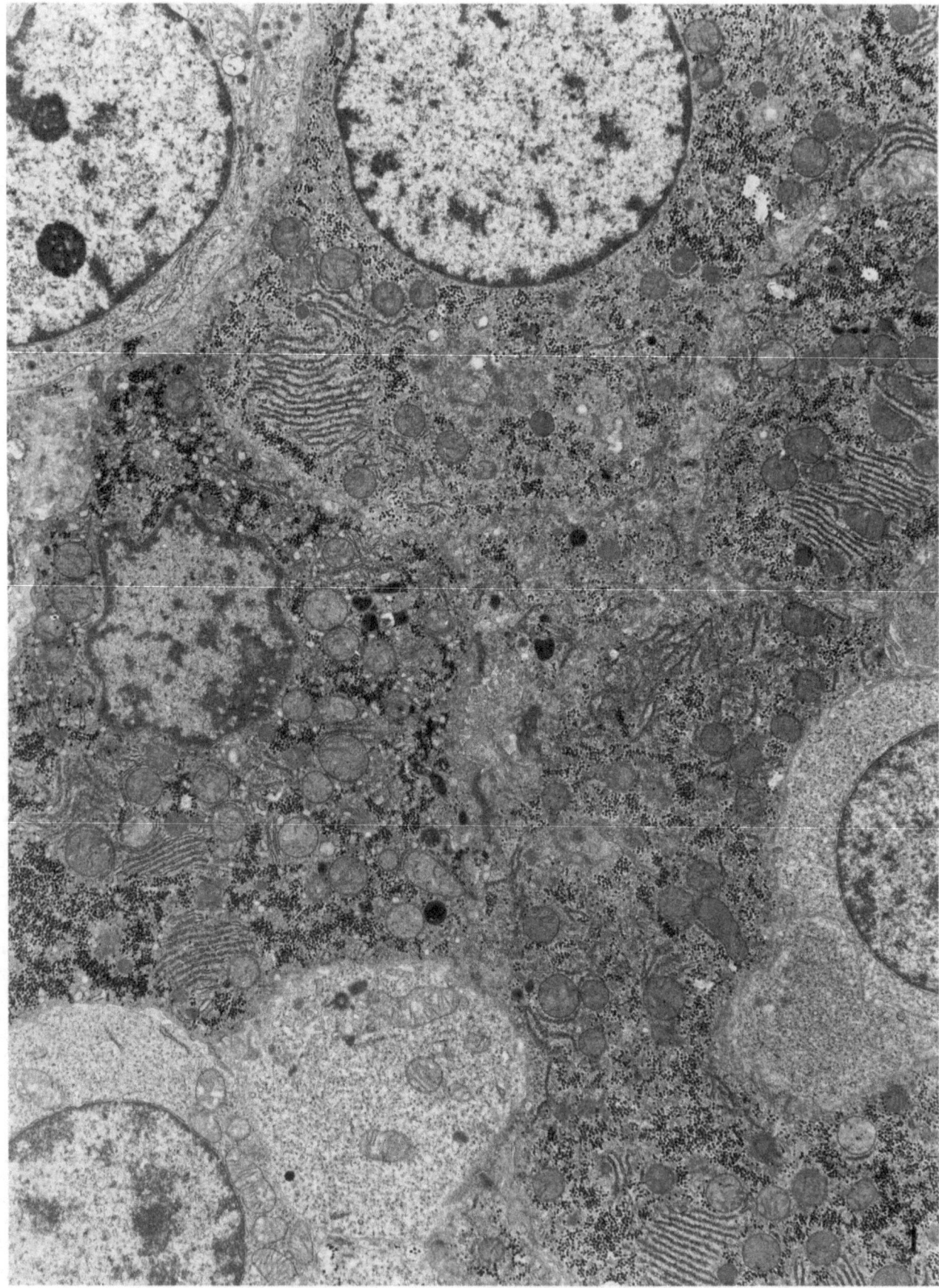

Figure 1 Liver of a 18–20-week-old human embryo. The micrograph shows an early myelocyte (upper part) with two prominent nucleoli and two erythroblasts (lower part) surrounded by hepatocytes. × 8000

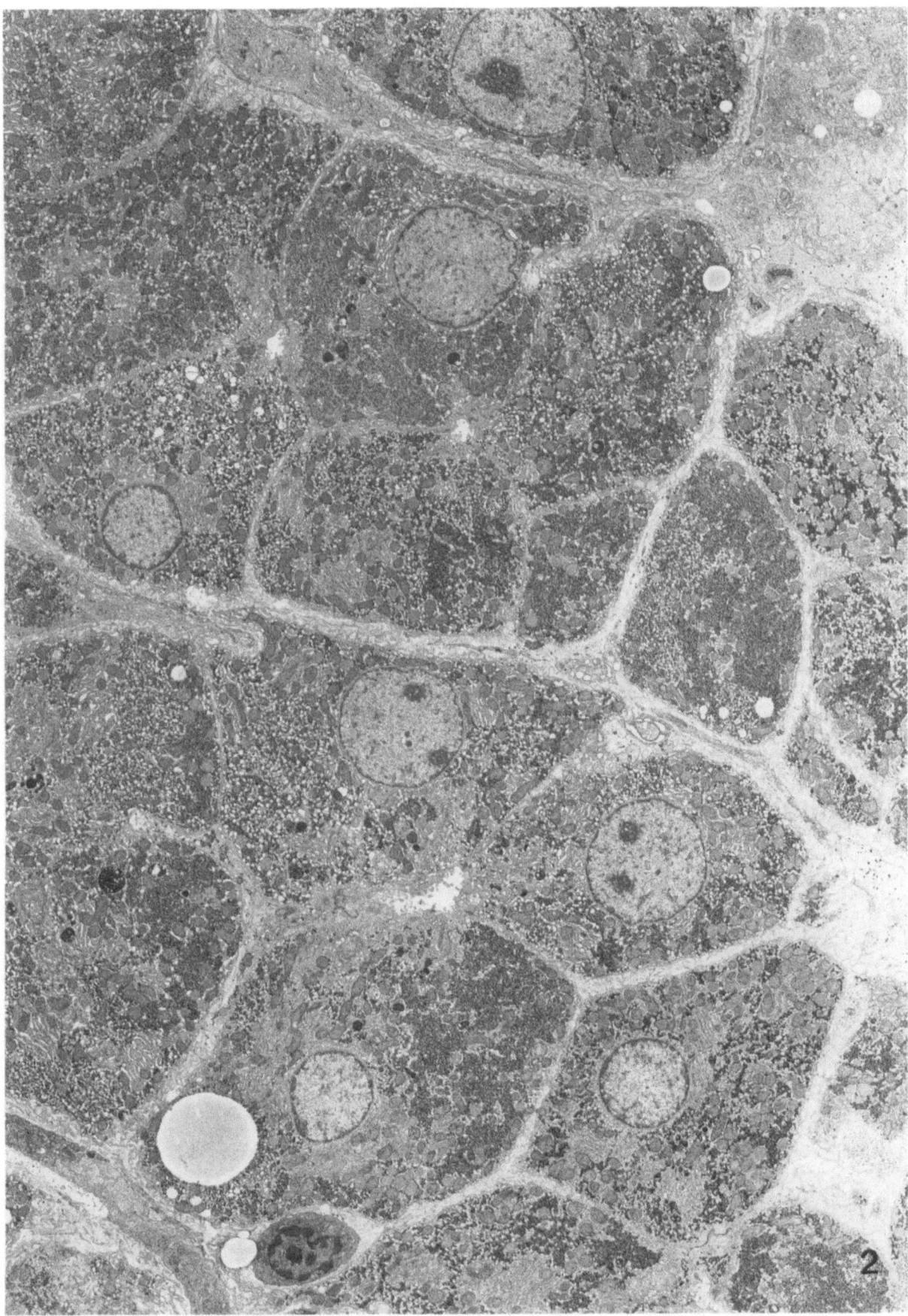

Figure 2 Liver of a two-year-old child. The micrograph shows, at low magnification, the arrangement of liver cells in plates, which, in young children, are for the most part two cells thick. The cells have a polygonal form with well-defined border and a round nucleus containing one or two nucleoli. The cytoplasm contains variable amounts of glycogen and few lipid droplets. × 2800

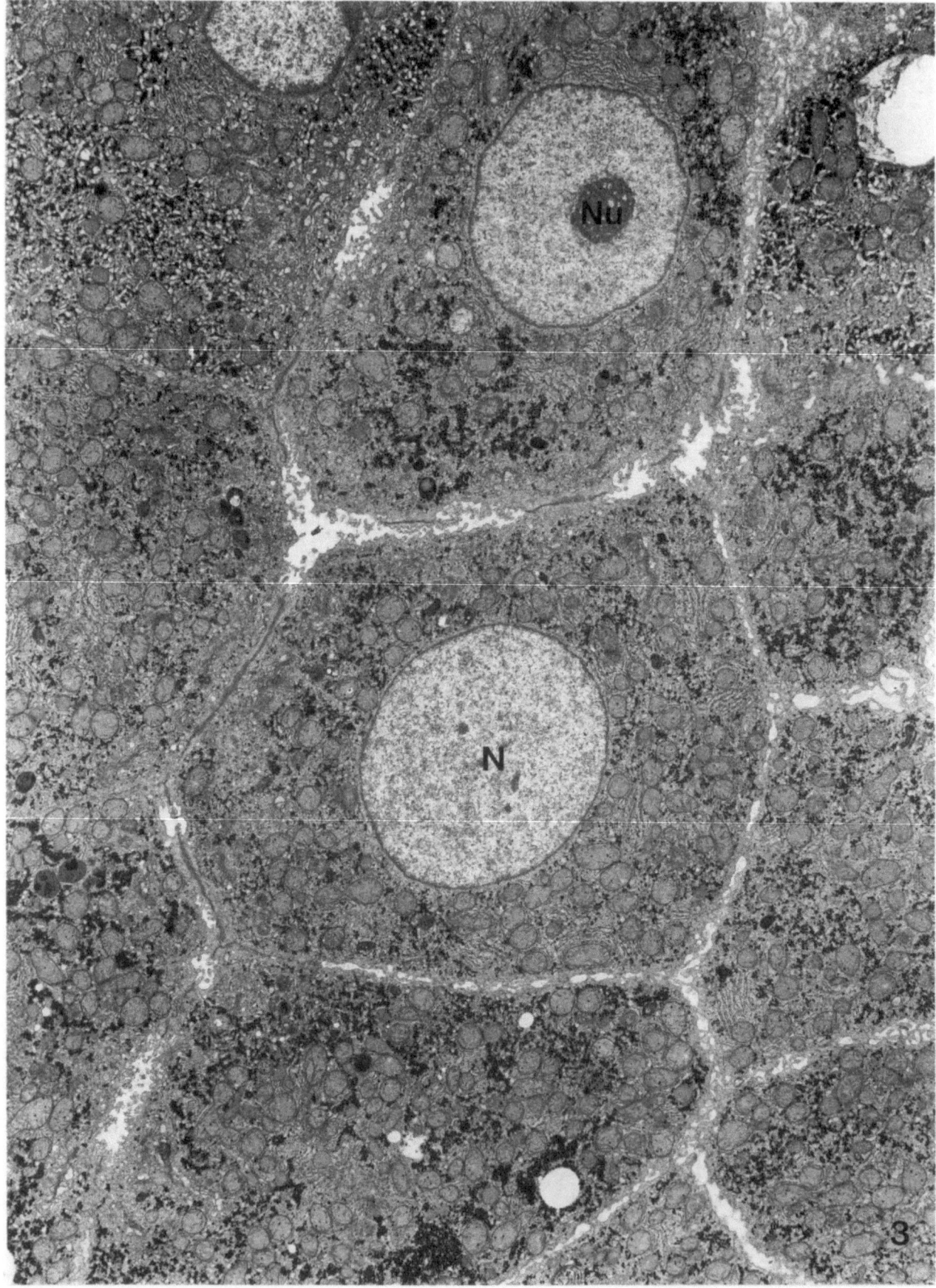

Figure 3   Human liver, at relatively low magnification, showing the topographical relationship of the hepatocytes and bile canaliculi. The nucleus (N) is typically round with scattered chromatin clumps and a prominent nucleolus (Nu). × 5000

(3) A dense, fibrillar component composed of many fine, 5 nm ribonucleoprotein fibres, representing RNA transcripts.

Cytoplasmic inclusions

Liver cells may show many cytoplasmic inclusions, such as glycogen, iron-containing granules and lipid droplets, which are not constant components of the cell. Glycogen inclusions are the most evident and can be readily identified on the basis of their characteristic structure (Figures 3 and 4). In ultrathin sections, stained with lead hydroxide or citrate, glycogen appears as roundish, electron-dense granules, measuring approximately 30 nm in diameter (β particles), or as a collection of granules forming clusters or rosettes (α particles) which can measure up to 200 nm in diameter. Glycogen is more abundant in the SER region of the cell where it tends to be concentrated in masses of variable size from which other cytoplasmic organelles are largely excluded. There are significant species-specific differences in the dimension and ultrastructural appearance of glycogen inclusions. In the human liver, the alpha rosettes are quite uniform in size and are clearly evident in the interstices of the reticulum (Figure 4).

Recent studies on glycogen biosynthesis provide evidence for the existence of two distinct forms of glycogen, i.e. a low- and high-molecular weight glycogen. The low-molecular weight glycogen is prevalently associated with the SER[7], whereas the high-molecular weight form has a high protein/polysaccharide ratio[8] and appears to be associated with the RER. It has been suggested that these two molecular forms of glycogen are related to the differential biosynthesis at the liver of either the smooth or the rough endoplasmic reticulum (Figures 4 and 7).

Plasma membranes

Hepatocytes represent a typical example of epithelial cells, which predominantly function by separating different compartments as well as by transporting, absorbing and secreting materials (Figures 4 and 5). To exert these various functions, the epithelial cells are organized according to a certain polarity, and the plasma membrane presents two domains: the apical domain and the basolateral domain, separated from each other by intercellular tight junctions. On the surface of the hepatocyte, three major domains are evident:

(1) The bile canalicular membrane which corresponds to the apical portion of the membrane of a simple epithelial cell, is very small, covered by microvilli and separated from the lateral membranes by tight junctions;

(2) The lateral region which is flat and rich in intermediate junctions, desmosomes and gap junctions;

(3) The sinusoidal region, which corresponds to the basal portion of the membrane in a simple epithelial cell, is large and covered by microvilli.

This different morphology reflects the distinct functions of the three domains: the bile canalicular membrane is specialized for bile secretion, the lateral region for cell–cell attachment and communication, and the sinusoidal region for the exchange of metabolites with blood[9–11] (Figures 2, 4 and 5).

Using monoclonal antibodies directed against surface antigens of rat hepatocytes, at least two integral membrane proteins have been identified and localized in specific domains: HA4 on the bile canalicular membrane, and CE9 on the lateral and sinusoidal membranes. Due to this specificity, the two proteins can be used as markers of the two domains[12].

Several mechanisms are probably responsible for the generation and maintenance of the cell surface polarity: a selective sorting by the Golgi apparatus of both newly synthesized and recycled plasma membrane proteins, and a directional transport over the cell surfaces by shuttling vesicles, followed by delivery at the final destination, seem to be involved.

In rat hepatocytes, the rate of incorporation of fucose-glycoproteins into the plasma membrane regions is different, being delayed within the bile canalicular portion of the cell surface. Recent results, however, have demonstrated that all integral plasma membrane proteins rapidly reach the basolateral domain first and through similar kinetics; apical proteins are then transported from the basolateral to the apical domain at various rates[13].

Peroxisomes

Peroxisomes were first described by Rhodin[14,15] in the proximal tubular cells of the mouse kidney and subsequently in rat hepatocytes[16,17]. Later studies have shown that these organelles are present in many other vertebrate cells, as well as in protozoa, plants, algae and yeast. Peroxisomes are morphologically defined as small round or oval cytoplasmic organelles measuring about 0.5 μm in diameter. They are bound by a single membrane and contain a finely granular matrix, in which, in some species, dense crystalloid inclusions may be found (Figure 7a). The peroxisomes of normal human, as well as avian, hepatocytes lack a distinct nucleoid, but crystalline nucleoids have been found in human hepatic peroxisomes by Biempica[18] in a liver affected by a complex pathology. Peroxisomes are commonly found at one side of the RER or in the area occupied by SER and glycogen particles. They are smaller than mitochondria and less numerous, the ratio being 1:4. Many pathological conditions and several chemical agents may alter the number and the morphology of peroxisomes. An increase in hepatic peroxisomes has been observed in some species after treatment with hypolipidaemic agents, such as clofibrate and its analogues, and with a new piperazine derivate (BM 15760) which inhibits the biosynthesis of cholesterol[19]. Other drugs which may affect peroxisomes but do not have a hypolipidaemic activity include ethionine, salycilate, thioacetamide[20,21] and ammonium perfluoro-octanate (APED). Peroxisomes of peculiar size have been found in hepatocytes of patients with primary hyperlipoproteinaemia type II and IV[22]. A reduction in the number of peroxisomes associated with a decrease in catalase activity occurs in the liver of tumour-bearing animals and in the liver of patients with glial tumours[23]. Lack of peroxisomes in the liver and kidney has been reported in the cerebro-hepato-renal (Zellweger) syndrome[24] and in the liver of patients with the infantile form of Retsum disease[25].

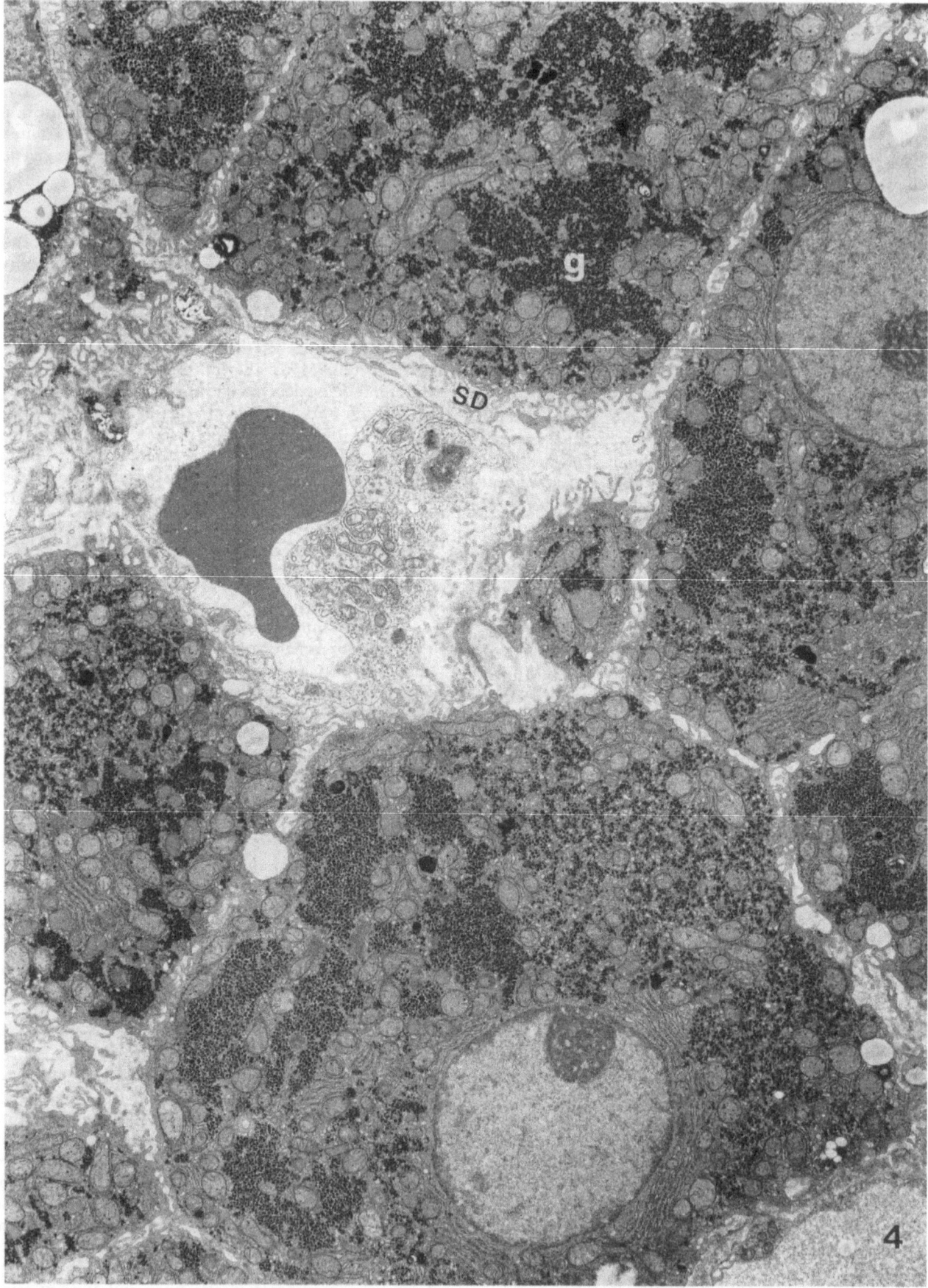

Figure 4   Electron micrograph of part of human liver cells bordering on a sinusoid. Numerous microvilli project into the perivascular space of Disse (SD). Large collections of intensely stained glycogen (g) particles are evident in the cytoplasm. × 6000

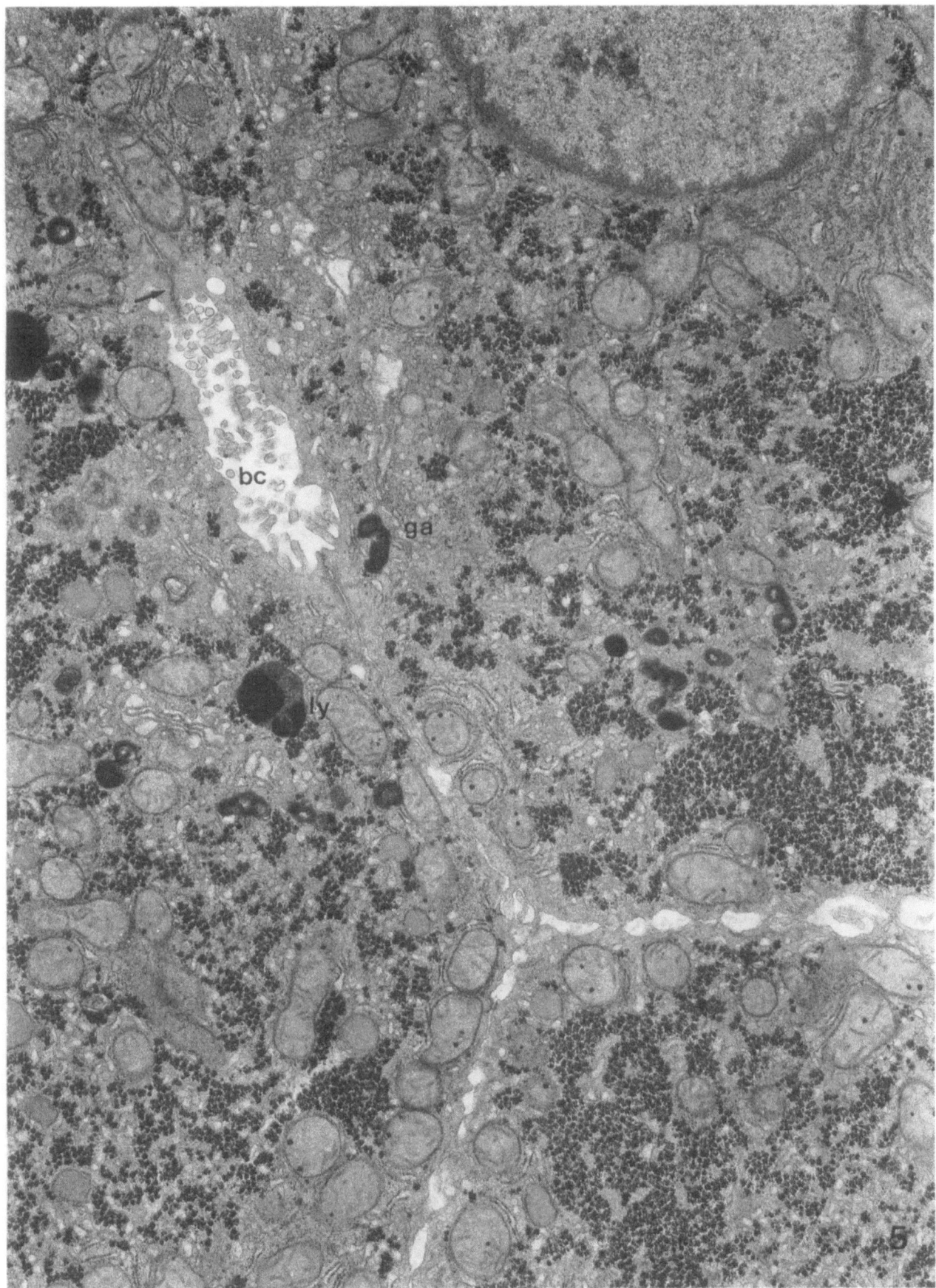

Figure 5 The micrograph shows a typical bile canaliculus (bc) with microvilli that project into its lumen. Along the margins, the membranes are in close contact (arrows) to prevent the escape of its contents into the intracellular space. In the neighbouring cytoplasm, several curving cisternae of a Golgi complex (ga) and lysosomes (ly) can be seen. × 18 000

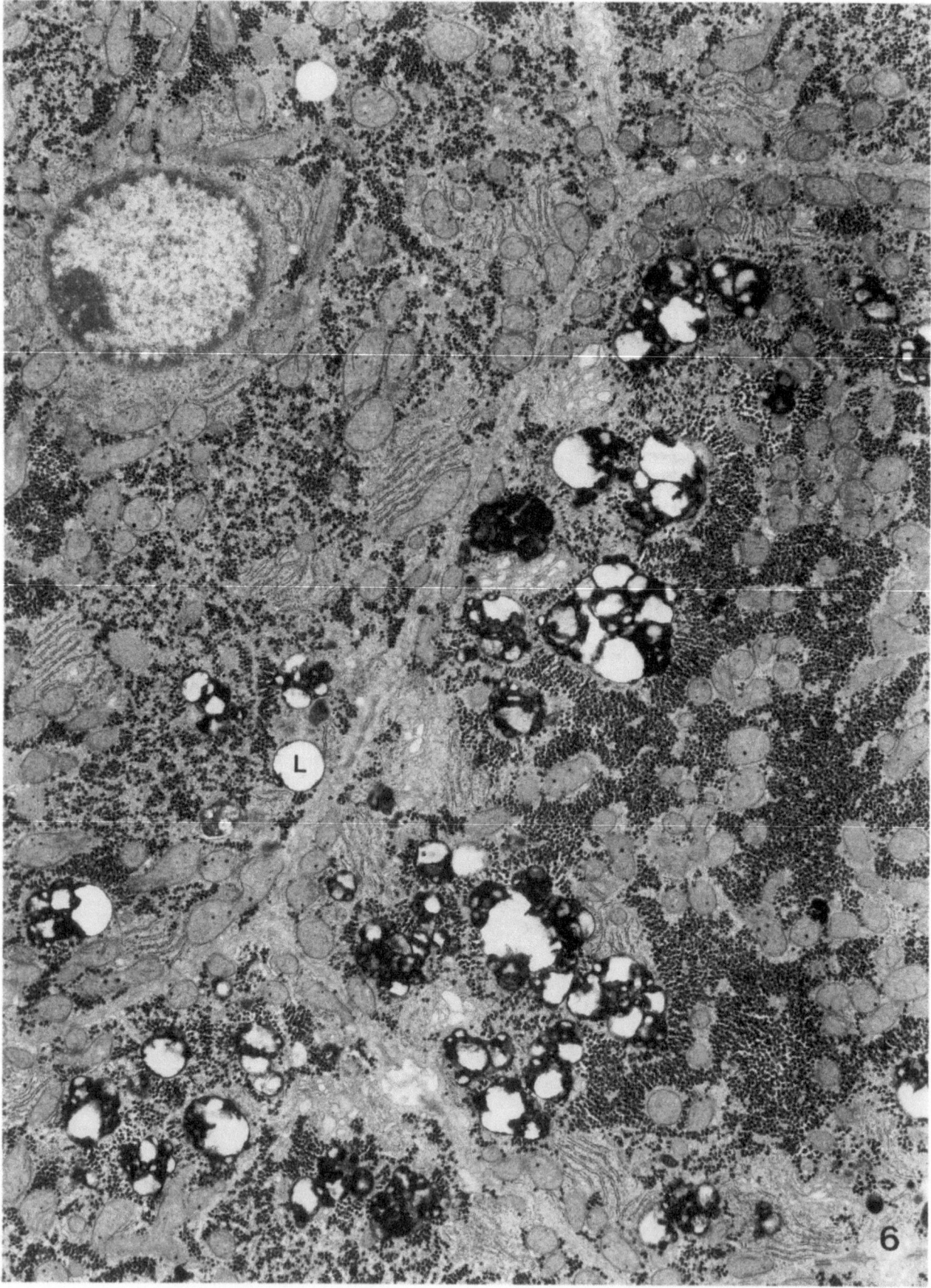

Figure 6 This illustration demonstrates the occurrence of lipofuscin granules (residual bodies) in human liver cells. These granules are composed of electron-dense material. Lipid droplets (L) are found near each bile canaliculus or adjacent to the plasma membranes. × 8000

Mitochondria

The hepatocyte contains numerous well-developed mitochondria (Figures 5 and 7). Electron microscopy studies have shown that mitochondria are bounded by two membranes, the inner of which is folded to form cristae. They are usually spherical or oblong and appear to be randomly distributed in the cytoplasm. Liver mitochondria are membranous organelles of great importance in energy metabolism and in many metabolic reactions, in particular the Krebs tricarboxylic acid cycle coupled to the electron-transport processes, and in the oxidation of fatty acids. Fractions of disrupted mitochondria show that most of the Krebs-cycle enzymes are located in the matrix, and the electron transport and oxidative phosphorylation enzymes form molecular assemblies in or on the inner mitochondrial membrane covering the wall and cristae. Extranuclear circular DNA and prokaryotic-type ribosomes (70S) have been recently found in the mitochondrial matrix, thus suggesting an autosomal genetic control of protein synthesis.

Endoplasmic reticulum

In liver cells, both rough and smooth endoplasmic reticulum are well represented. The rough endoplasmic reticulum comprises numerous cisternae surrounded by ribosomes. The cisternae are often parallel and located in proximity to the mitochondria. The smooth endoplasmic reticulum instead consists of a network of tubules lacking associated ribosomes.

Synthesis of new polypeptides involves the binding of ribosomes to specific sites on membranes of the rough endoplasmic reticulum (ER). Among the newly synthesized proteins released into the lumen of the ER, some are destined for secretion, whereas others remain attached to the ER membranes. In hepatocytes, the major secretory proteins are components of the plasma as albumin and lipoproteins. With the exception of albumin, all secretory proteins contain covalently bound sugar residues which were added in the ER[26]. After synthesis, they are transported and processed through the Golgi complex and then packaged into secretory vacuoles. A specialized area

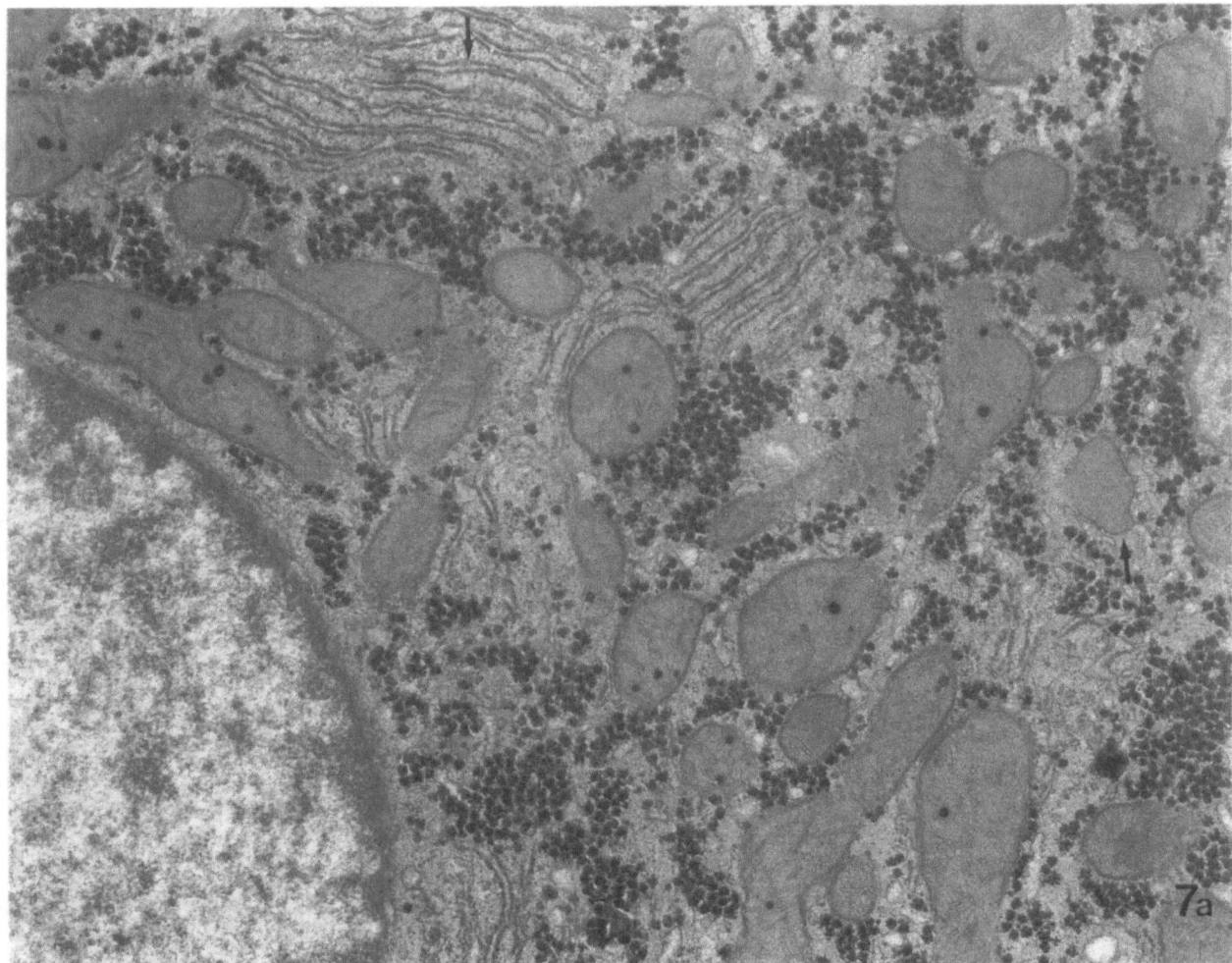

Figure 7   (a) Part of cytoplasm of human hepatocytes, showing the characteristic appearance of the peroxisomes (P). Somewhat smaller and less numerous than the mitochondria (m), these organelles display a uniform matrix of medium density. Glycogen (G). × 16 000.

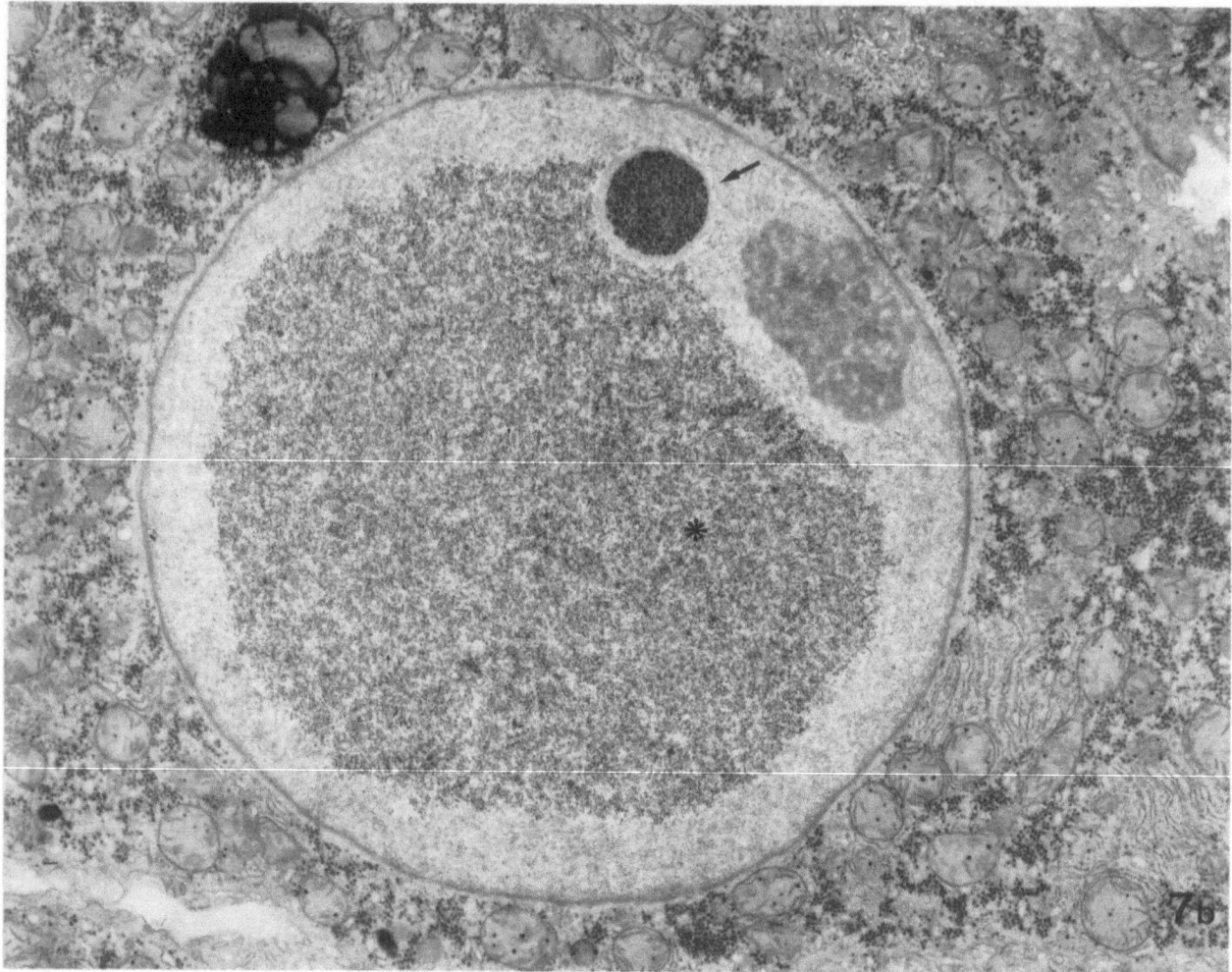

Figure 7 (b) Human adult liver. This electron micrograph shows a nucleus with a large central deposit of glycogen (asterisk) completely surrounded by nucleoplasm. Near the nucleolus a round dense body (arrow) is present separated from the major deposit by a less-dense-material glycogen deposit. No changes are observed in the cytoplasm where mitochondria and other organelles appear normal. × 18 000

of the endoplasmic reticulum has been described and cytochemically identified in hepatocytes. This area has been called GERL (Golgi–endoplasmic reticulum–lysosome) because of its association with the ER and the Golgi complex and because of its high content of hydrolytic enzymes, as in lysosomes[27]. It has been proposed that, in hepatocytes, GERL represents a second population of lipoprotein-containing cisternae and vacuoles which do not derive from the Golgi apparatus (Figure 7a).

At least two hepatic enzymes are considered as markers of the microsomal fraction (corresponding to the endoplasmic reticulum) of liver membranes: the NADPH-cytochrome c reductase and cytochrome P450. These enzymes are also present in the outer nuclear envelope which is continuous with the endoplasmic reticulum and practically identical in composition[28].

Recently, however, some purified antibodies to rough endoplasmic reticulum have been obtained. These antisera recognize four polypeptides present on the luminal side of the ER membranes and represent a useful tool for identifying this organelle[29].

Lysosomes

Lysosomes were originally described as membrane-bound dense bodies which are distinct from mitochondria and contain carbohydrate enzymes. They may vary in size and density, so that no two are exactly alike. They may be irregular in outline, with a homogeneous dense content, or nearly spherical, with very dense granular material dispersed in a fine matrix of lower density. Some may contain one or more lipid-like droplets of medium density in association with electron-dense material of a granular nature. In liver cells, lysosomes may be found in close association with bile canaliculi or along the plasma membranes. Lysosomes can be distinguished, on the basis of size and fine structure, as:

(1) Primary lysosomes which measure about 100 nm and are not yet involved in a digestive event.

(2) Secondary lysosomes that have been functionally active and contain enzymes with a variable and heterogeneous ultrastructural appearance.

(3) Residual bodies containing enzymes and a conglomerate of undigested residue derived from lysosomal activity. These are larger than primary and secondary lysosomes, may be detected by light microscopy and are more readily evident in the elderly or in patients treated with a variety of pharmaceuticals (i.e. antalgics, antibiotics and hormones). Residual bodies are also known as lipofuscins or age pigments.

(4) Autophagic vacuoles, which contain portions of sequestered cytoplasmic organelles destined for degradation by fusion with primary or secondary lysosomes[30] (Figures 5 and 6).

Lysosomes contain several proteolytic enzymes having an acidic pH optimum in the range of 4.5–5.5, lipids and carbohydrates (10% of liver glycogen is contained in lysosomes). Lysosomal activity requires energy (ATP) which is probably utilized in sustaining a low pH and for the internalization of cytoplasm into lysosomes[31,32]. Inhibitors of protein synthesis tend to decrease lysosomal activity relatively rapidly. Lysosomes play a key role in a variety of cellular metabolic pathways in both physiological and pathological conditions, including the digestion of micro-organisms, the migration of inflammatory cells and neoplastic spread and metastasis[33,34]. The genetically determined lack or malfunction of specific lysosomal enzymes may cause a substrate accumulation resulting in storage diseases[35]. Alterations may also involve the transport of degradation products, as is the case in one lethal disease, nephropathic cystinosis[36].

The Golgi apparatus

In the last few years, because of its central role in intracellular traffic control, the Golgi apparatus has become one of the most studied cellular organelles[37]. Many cellular functions are elicited by the Golgi complex: the transport, processing and sorting of newly synthesized components, i.e. membrane glycoproteins and glycolipids, secretory products and lysosomal enzymes, and traffic control in endocytosis and recycling.

The Golgi complex is composed of a group of flat parallel cisternae with dilated rims; it shows a clear heterogeneity in composition, which has been evidenced by cytochemical methods, and a polarity that is morphologically distinguishable in some tissues, such as the liver. In fact, the Golgi apparatus shows two distinct sides: the *cis* part, in proximity to the endoplasmic reticulum, and the *trans* part, which is close to the secretory granules; the transport of newly synthesized components is vectorial from the *cis* to the *trans* sides (Figure 5).

The compositional heterogeneity due to processing enzymes, such as glycosyltransferases and mannosidases, led investigators to propose the existence of at least three different subcompartments: the *cis,* the middle, and the *trans* subcompartments. Very recently, a new model for the exit site of the Golgi complex has been suggested[38]; in this model, the last Golgi compartment on the *trans* side is said to be a specialized organelle, the *trans* Golgi network (TGN), responsible for the sorting of proteins to lysosomes, plasma membranes or secretory vesicles. This tubular reticulum probably corresponds to the structures described by Novikoff[39] and which have been called GERL (Golgi–endoplasmic reticulum–lysosome).

Extracellular matrix

The extracellular matrix is a collection of macromolecules that surrounds the plasma membrane of a cell and comprises the substratum on which the cell may be attached. However, the extracellular matrix should not be considered just as an amorphous support for the cell. Because of its strategic location, it plays an important role in determining certain fundamental cell features, such as shape, adherence to other cells and tissue components, and perception of the external milieu. All of these aspects are related to the regulation of cell growth and differentiation[40–42].

The major representative components of the extracellular matrix are the collagen types I–V, the procollagens, elastin, the glycoproteins (for example, fibronectin and laminin) and the proteoglycans. Newly discovered types of collagen (types VI–IX) and glycoproteins have been described recently.

In normal human liver, 4% of the total protein is collagenous, 53% of the total interstitial collagen is type I, and 47% is type III. In contrast, in cirrhotic human livers, 10% of the total protein is collagenous, 75% of the interstitial collagen is type I, and 25% is type III[43].

Electron immunohistochemical studies have shown the specific localization of each extracellular matrix component in normal liver. Interstitial type I collagen is distributed in the liver capsule, portal stroma and in Disse's space, often in direct contact with the hepatocyte plasmalemma, but along the sinusoidal wall at points of branching or inflection. All basement membranes (ductal, neural and vascular) are composed of type IV collagen, whereas only deposits of type IV can be found along the sinusoidal wall. Laminin, in contrast, codistributes with type IV collagen in all basement membranes, but not in the sinusoidal wall. Fibronectin is visible in the liver capsule and portal stroma, but not in basement membranes; it is shown to form an almost continuous structure in direct contact with the hepatocyte microvilli; also, this glycoprotein is the major extracellular matrix constituent of Disse's space[44].

These data provide a new image of Disse's space: rather than being an empty space, it contains a complex extracellular matrix, where type I collagen forms the scaffold of the hepatic lobule, being in direct contact with hepatocytes and endothelial cells. In addition, type IV collagen is not associated with laminin forming a basement membrane, but is found free in deposits. Hepatocytes and endothelial cells lack a basement membrane, being separated by an extracellular matrix containing mainly fibronectin, type I collagen and occasional deposits of type IV collagen.

References

1. Peschle, C., Migliaccio, G., Lazzaro, D., Petti, S., Mancini, G., Carè, A., Russo, G., Mastroberardino, G., Migliaccio, A. R. and Testa, U. (1984). *Blood Cells,* 10, 427–432
2. Moore, K. L. (1982). *The Developing Human,* 3rd Edn. (Philadelphia: W. B. Saunders)
3. Kelemen, E., Calvo, W. and Fliedner, T. M. (1979). *Atlas of*

Human Hemopoietic Development. (New York: Springer-Verlag)

4. Lovol, A. V. (1968). Quantitative stereological description of the ultrastructure of normal rat liver parenchymal cells. *J. Cell Biol.*, **37**, 27–31

5. Alberts, B., Dennis, B., Lewis, J., Raff, M., Roberts, K. and Watson, J. (1983). *Molecular Biology of the Cell.* (New York: Garland Publ. Inc.)

6. Caramia, F. G., Chergo, G. F. and Menghini, G. (1967). A glycogen body in liver nuclei. *J. Ultrastruct. Res.*, **19**, 573–585

7. De Man, J. C. H. and Blok, A. P. R. (1966). Glycogen biosynthesis in liver. *J. Histochem. Cytochem.* **14**, 135–139

8. Calder, P. C. and Geddes, R. (1983). Ordered synthesis and degradation of liver glycogen involving 2-amino-2-deoxy-D-glucose. *Carbohydrate Res.*, **118**, 233–238

9. Simons, K. and Fuller, S. D. (1985). Cell surface polarity in epithelia. *Ann. Rev. Cell Biol.*, **1**, 243–88

10. Evans, W. H., Flint, N. A. and Vischer, P. (1980). Biogenesis of hepatocyte plasma membrane domains. *Biochem. J.*, **192**, 903–910

11. Hubbard, A. L., Wall, D. A. and Ma, A. (1983). Isolation of rat hepatocyte plasma membrane. I. Presence of the three major domains. *J. Cell Biol.*, **96**, 217–229

12. Hubbard, A. L., Bartles, J. R. and Braiterman, L. T. (1985). Identification of rat hepatocyte plasma membrane proteins using monoclonal antibodies. *J. Cell Biol.*, **100**, 1115–1125

13. Bartles, J. R., Feracci, H. M., Stieger, B. and Hubbard, A. L. (1987). Biogenesis of the rat hepatocyte plasma membrane in vivo: comparison of the pathways taken by apical and basolateral proteins using subcellular fractionation. *J. Cell Biol.*, **105**, 1241–1251

14. Rhodin, J. (1954). Correlation of ultrastructural organization and function in normal and experimentally changed proximal convoluted tubule cells of mouse kidney. Thesis, Karolinska Institute, Stockholm, Aktiebolaget Godvil

15. Rhodin, J. (1956). Further studies on the nephron ultrastructure in mouse terminal part of proximal convolution. In *Proceedings of the Stockholm Conference of Electron Microscopy*, pp. 1–76. (Stockholm: Almqvist and Wiksell)

16. Gansler, H. and Rouiller, C. (1956). Modifications physiologiques et pathologiques du chondriome. Etude au microscope electronique. *Schweiz. Z. Path. bakt.*, **19**, 217–221

17. Rouiller, C. and Bernard, W. (1956). Microbodies and the problem of mitochondrial regeneration in liver cells. *J. Biophys. Biochem. Cytol.*, **2**, 355–361

18. Biempica, L. (1966). Human hepatic microbodies with crystalloid cores. *J. Cell Biol.*, **29**, 383–387

19. Baumgart, E., Stagmeier, K., Schmidt, F. H. and Fahimi, H. D. (1987). Proliferation of peroxisomes in pericentral hepatocytes of rat liver after administration of a new hypocholesterolemic agent (BM 15766). Sex-dependent ultrastructural differences. *Lab. Invest.*, **56**, 554–64

20. Svoboda, D. J., Grady, H. and Azarnoff, D. (1977). Microbodies in experimentally altered cells. *J. Cell Biol.*, **35**, 127–131

21. Pastoor, T. P., Lee, K. P., Perri, M. A. and Gillies, P. J. (1987). Biochemical and morphological studies of ammonium perfluorooctanoate-induced hepatomegaly and peroxisome proliferation. *Exp. Mol. Pathol.*, **47**, 98–102

22. Gariot, P., Foliguet, B., Drouin, P., Barrat, E., Genton, P. and Debry, G. (1986). Hypertrophy of liver peroxisomes in type II and type IV hyperproteinemia. *Atherosclerosis*, **59**, 257–262

23. Sima, A. A. F. (1980). Peroxisomes (microbodies) in human glial tumours. A cytochemical ultrastructural study. *Acta Neuropathol.*, **51**, 113–117

24. Goldfischer, S. (1979). Peroxisomes in disease. *J. Histochem. Cytochem*, **27**, 1371–1376

25. Roels, F., Cornelis, A., Poll-The, B. Y., Aubourg, P., Ogier, H., Scotto, J. and Saudubray, J. M. (1986). Hepatic peroxisomes are deficient in infantile Refsum disease: a cytochemical study of 4 cases. *Am. J. Med. Genet.*, **25**, 257–262

26. Bergeron, J. J. M., Borts, D. and Cruz, J. (1978). Passage of serum-destined proteins through the Golgi apparatus of the rat liver. An examination of heavy and light Golgi apparatus. *J. Cell Biol.*, **76**, 87–97

27. Novikoff, A. B. and Novikoff, P. M. (1977). Cytochemical contributions to differentiating GERL from the Golgi apparatus. *Histochem. J.*, **9**, 525–551

28. Masuura, S., Masuda, R., Omori, K., Negishi, M. and Tashiro, Y. (1981). Distribution and induction of cytochrome P450 in rat liver nuclear envelope. *J. Cell Biol.*, **91**, 212–220

29. Louvard, D., Reggio, H. and Warren, G. (1982). Antibodies to the Golgi complex and the rough endoplasmic reticulum. *J. Cell Biol.*, **92**, 92–107

30. Glaumann, H. and Marzella, L. (1981). Degradation of membrane components by Kupffer cell lysosomes. *Lab. Invest.*, **45**, 479–481

31. Kovacs, A. L., and Seglen, P. O. (1981). Inhibition of hepatocytes protein degradation by methylamminopurines and inhibitors of protein synthesis. *Biochem. Biophys. Acta*, **676**, 213–218

32. Grinde, B. (1985). Autophagy and lysosomal proteolysis in the liver. *Experientia*, **41**, 1089–1094

33. Sloane, B. F., Dunn, J. R. and Honn, K. V. (1981). Lysosomal cathepsin B: correlation with metastatic potential. *Science*, **212**, 1151–1156

34. Liotta, L. A. (1982). Tumor extracellular matrix. *Lab. Invest.*, **47**, 112–118

35. Hers, H. G. and Van Hoof, F. (1973). *Lysosomes and Storage Disease.* (New York: Academic Press)

36. Gahl, W. A., Bashann, N., Tietze, F., Bernardini, I. and Schulman, J. D. (1982). Cystine transport is defective in isolated leukocyte lysosomes from patients with cystinosis. *Science*, **217**, 1263–1264

37. Farquhar, M. G. (1985). Progress in unrevealing pathways of Golgi traffic. *Annu. Rev. Cell Biol.*, **1**, 447–488

38. Griffith, G. and Simmons, K. (1986). The *trans* Golgi network: sorting of the exit site of the Golgi complex. *Science*, **234**, 438–443

39. Novikoff, A. B. (1976). The endoplasmic reticulum: a cytochemic view. *Proc. Natl. Acad. Sci. USA*, **73**, 2781–2787

40. Hay, E. D. (1981). Extracellular matrix. *J. Cell Biol.*, **91**, 205s

41. Piez, K. A. and Reddi, A. H. (eds.) (1984). *Extracellular Matrix Biochemistry* (New York: Elsevier)

42. Miller, E. J. and Gay, S. (1982) Collagen: An overview. *Meth. Enzymol.*, **82**, 3–7

43. Seyer, J. M., Hucheson, E. T. and Kang, A. H. (1977). Collagen polymorphism in normal and cirrhotic human liver. *J. Clin. Invest.*, **59**, 241–245

44. Martinez-Hernandez, A. (1984). Electron immunohistochemical studies in normal rat liver. *Lab. Invest.*, **51**, 57–61

2

Structure and function of the hepatic sinusoidal wall

L. BOUWENS, A. GEERTS and E. WISSE

The hepatic blood capillaries, called sinusoids because they have a tortuous course, are lined by a wall of cells which, at the same time, form a barrier and a pathway for exchange between the blood and the hepatic parenchyma. This wall is composed of three different cell types: the endothelial cell, the Kupffer cell and the pit cell. Behind the sinusoidal lining, a fourth sinusoidal cell type occurs, the fat-storing or Ito cell, which will be discussed in another chapter. It has become clear that these cells serve a number of different functions important during both homoeostasis and pathological conditions[1].

ENDOTHELIAL CELLS (Figures 1–4)

Sinusoidal endothelial cells form a continuous but fenestrated lining of the hepatic sinusoids[2]. In the rat, the fenestrae or pores have an average diameter of 105 nm in the centrolobular areas of the liver and of 111 nm in periportal areas when measured on scanning electron micrographs after critical point drying of the tissue. In plastic embedded tissue, the diameter of the fenestrae[3] was found to be 150–175 nm. The endothelial fenestrae lack a diaphragm and are organized in groups called sieve

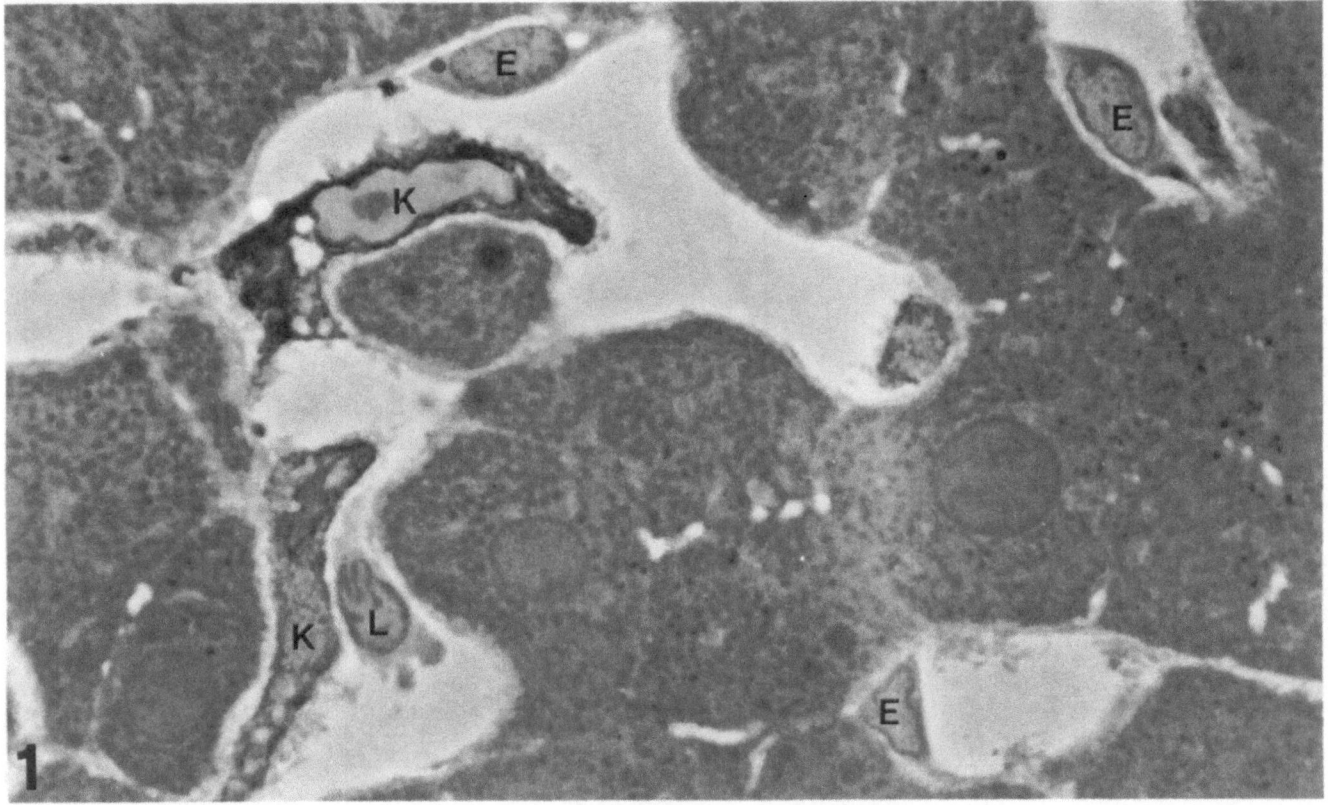

Figure 1 Light micrograph of a semithin liver section. Several endothelial cells (E), Kupffer cells (K) and a leukocyte (L) are seen in or along the sinusoids. The Kupffer cells are stained for endogenous peroxidase activity in the cytoplasm (rough endoplasmic reticulum) and the nuclear envelope. × 1800

13

plates. These sieve plates represent the major characteristic used to recognize the endothelial cell in electron
microscopy. In low pressure perfusion-fixed liver, only
fenestrae occur. Gaps, defined as endothelial openings,
with diameter of at least twice the average diameter of
the fenestrae have been described inter- and intra-
cellularly[3] but are most probably artefacts due to the
fixation procedure. The fenestrated endothelium filters
particulate material, including chylomicrons, during
passage through the sinusoids[4,5]. In these studies, it was
shown that chylomicrons with a diameter exceeding
300 nm are excluded from the space of Disse. Smaller
chylomicrons and their remnants, which are rich in cholesterol, are seen in the space of Disse. Thus, through the
filtration effect of the fenestrated endothelium, parenchymal cells preferentially take up cholesterol-rich remnants, whereas the large triglyceride-rich chylomicrons

remain in circulation. This selective uptake mechanism
may be important in preventing atheroma formation[6,7].

Several substances have been demonstrated to induce
changes in the diameter of liver fenestrae. Alcohol
enlarges fenestrae[8,9] but decreases their number per unit
area[9]. The enlargement of the fenestrae may allow larger
chylomicrons to penetrate the space of Disse and therefore contribute to the development of fatty liver, a well-
known condition after alcohol abuse. Other conditions
which cause enlargement of the fenestrae include high
portal pressure[10-12], CCl_4 (carbon tetrachloride) intoxication[13], hypoxia, irradiation and endotoxin[14].

Sinusoidal endothelial cells also take part in the hepatic
clearance of various test substances[15]. Materials such as
latex beads[16,17], colloidal sulphur, silver iodide and
carbon[16], Thorotrast[18], Frog-virus[19], heat aggregated
albumin[20], immune complexes[21], ferritins[22] and lipo-

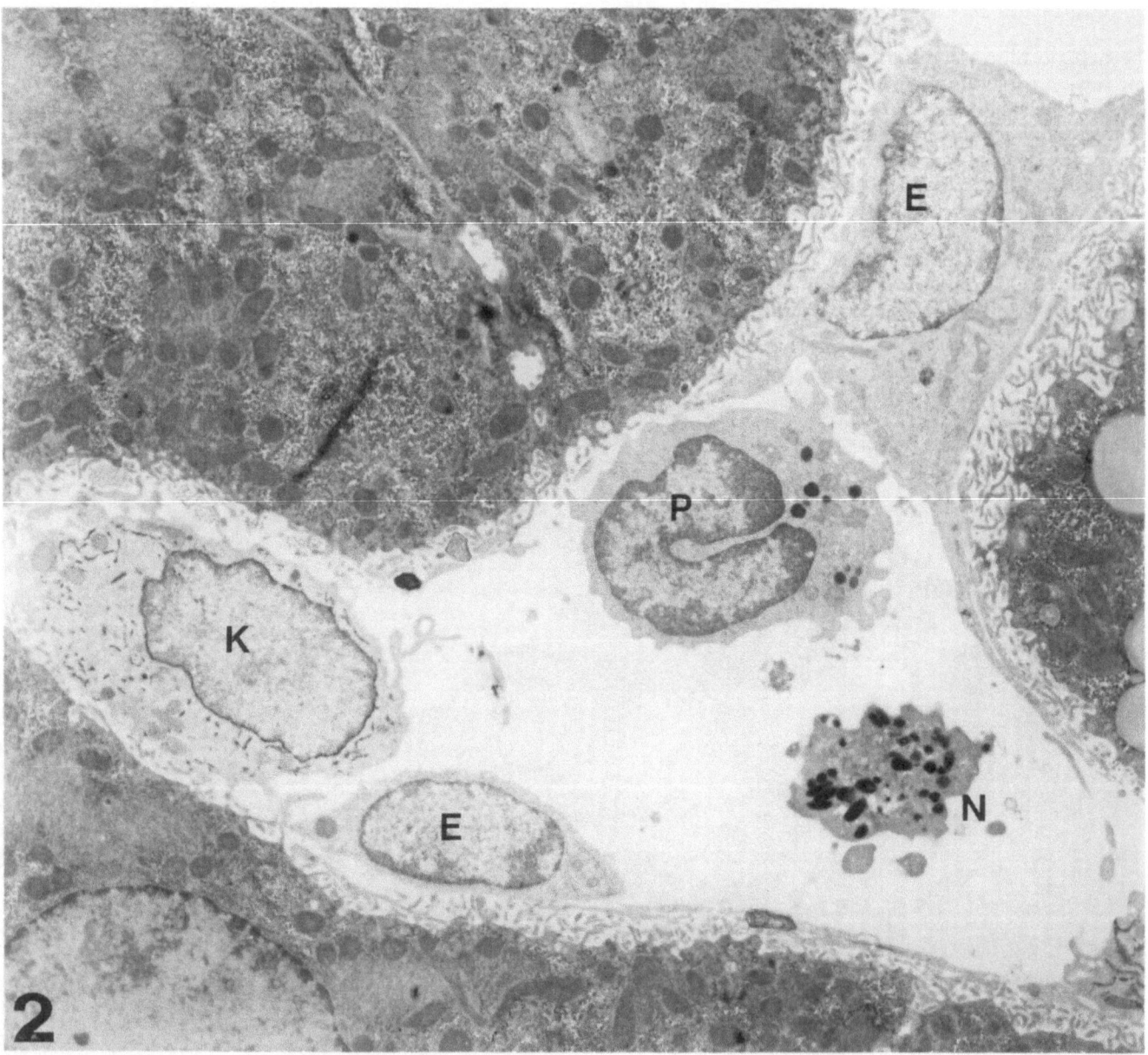

Figure 2 Transmission electron micrograph (TEM) of a sinusoid with two endothelial cells (E), a Kupffer cell (K) with peroxidase
activity in the nuclear envelope and rough endoplasmic reticulum, a pit cell (P) with an indented nucleus and characteristic dense
cytoplasmic granules. A portion of a neutrophilic granulocyte (N) is also seen in the sinusoidal lumen. × 7000

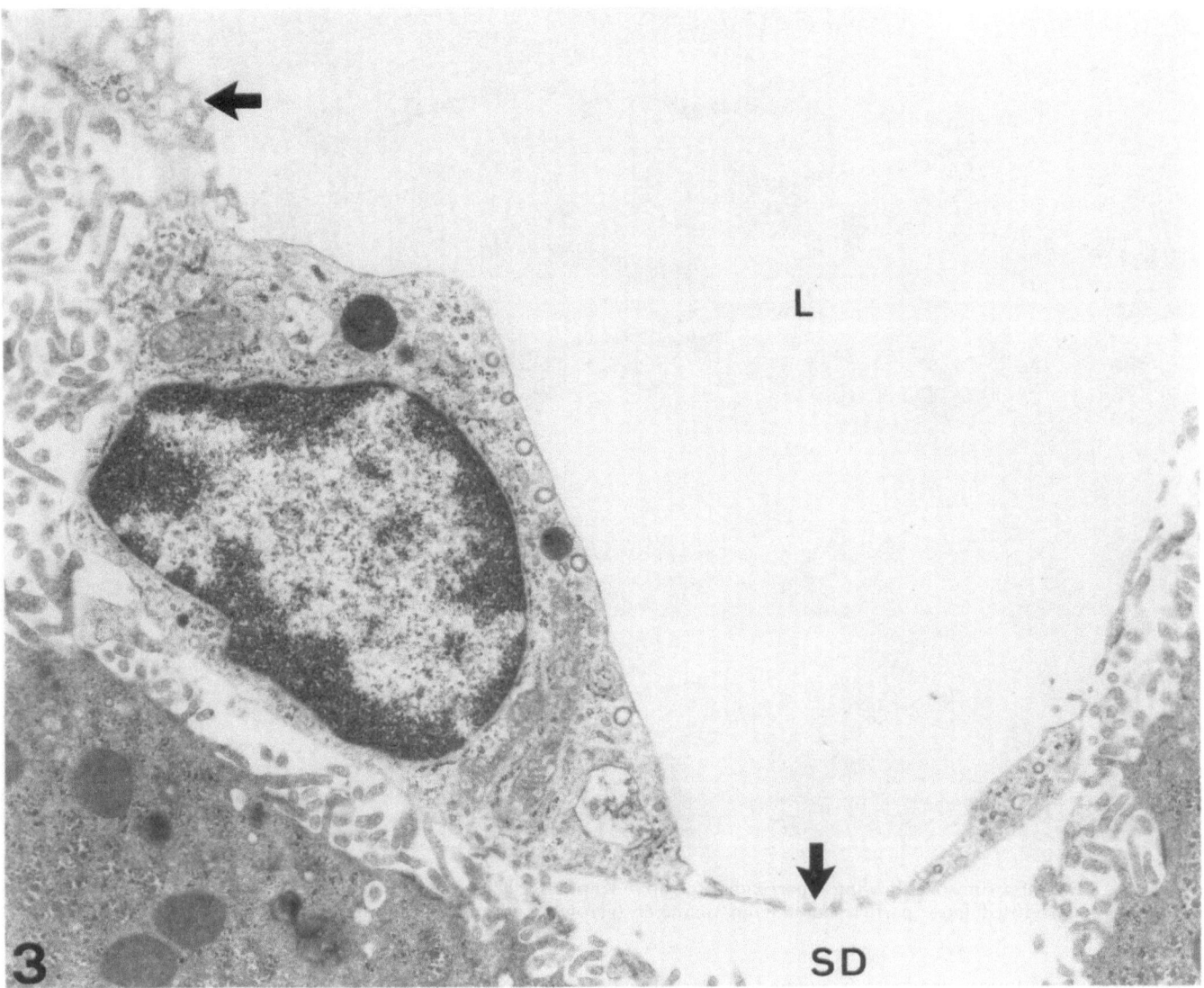

Figure 3 TEM of a sinusoidal endothelial cell. Note the fenestrations arranged in sieve plates (arrows) and the pinocytotic vesicles pinching off from the cell membrane at the luminal side. L = sinusoidal lumen. SD = space of Disse. × 15 600

proteins[23], as well as monodispersed molecules, such as horseradish peroxidase[16], are taken up by these cells. Endothelial cells endocytose material by pinocytosis either with or without prior adsorption of the compound on receptors on the cell membrane[15,16,23]. It has recently been demonstrated that endothelial cells can also ingest larger particles by phagocytosis, but this occurs only when the Kupffer cells have been eliminated using compounds toxic for macrophages[24]. Sinusoidal endothelial cells often contain many lysosomes of variable size and shape, and numerous pinocytotic structures can be seen in transmission electron microscopy[2,18].

KUPFFER CELLS (Figures 1, 2, 4–7)

Kupffer cells represent the largest population of macrophages in the mammalian body and they are strategically positioned within the hepatic sinusoidal vasculature[25]. Together with the endothelial cells, they constitute the most active part of the reticuloendothelial system (RES); this is shown by the fact that 75–90% of i.v. injected test substances, such as colloidal gold and latex particles, are cleared by the liver[26,27]. Kupffer cells are well char-

acterized by electron microscopy[25]. They are found on or between endothelial cells and sometimes also in the space of Disse. They have a variable shape with many cytoplasmic extensions and contain a large number of lysosomes and phagosomes of varying size, density and shape. Furthermore, these macrophages are characterized by some peculiar ultrastructural features, such as worm-like surface invaginations, annulate lamellae and a surface 'fuzzy coat'[25]. In light microscopy, the best characteristic by which to recognize Kupffer cells, at least in the rat, is the cytochemical localization of the peroxidase enzyme. Electron microscopic studies have shown that all rat Kupffer cells contain peroxidase activity in their nuclear envelope and endoplasmic reticulum whereas other liver cells are devoid of peroxidase activity[25].

Kupffer cells are able to clear a large variety of substances from the blood. Endogenous and exogenous substances which can be endocytosed include viruses[28], bacteria and yeast particles, material leaked from the gastrointestinal tract, such as enzymes and bacterial toxins, latex beads, colloidal gold, Thorotrast, cells like erythrocytes, thrombocytes and leukocytes, hormones like insulin, antigens and immune complexes, fibrin and

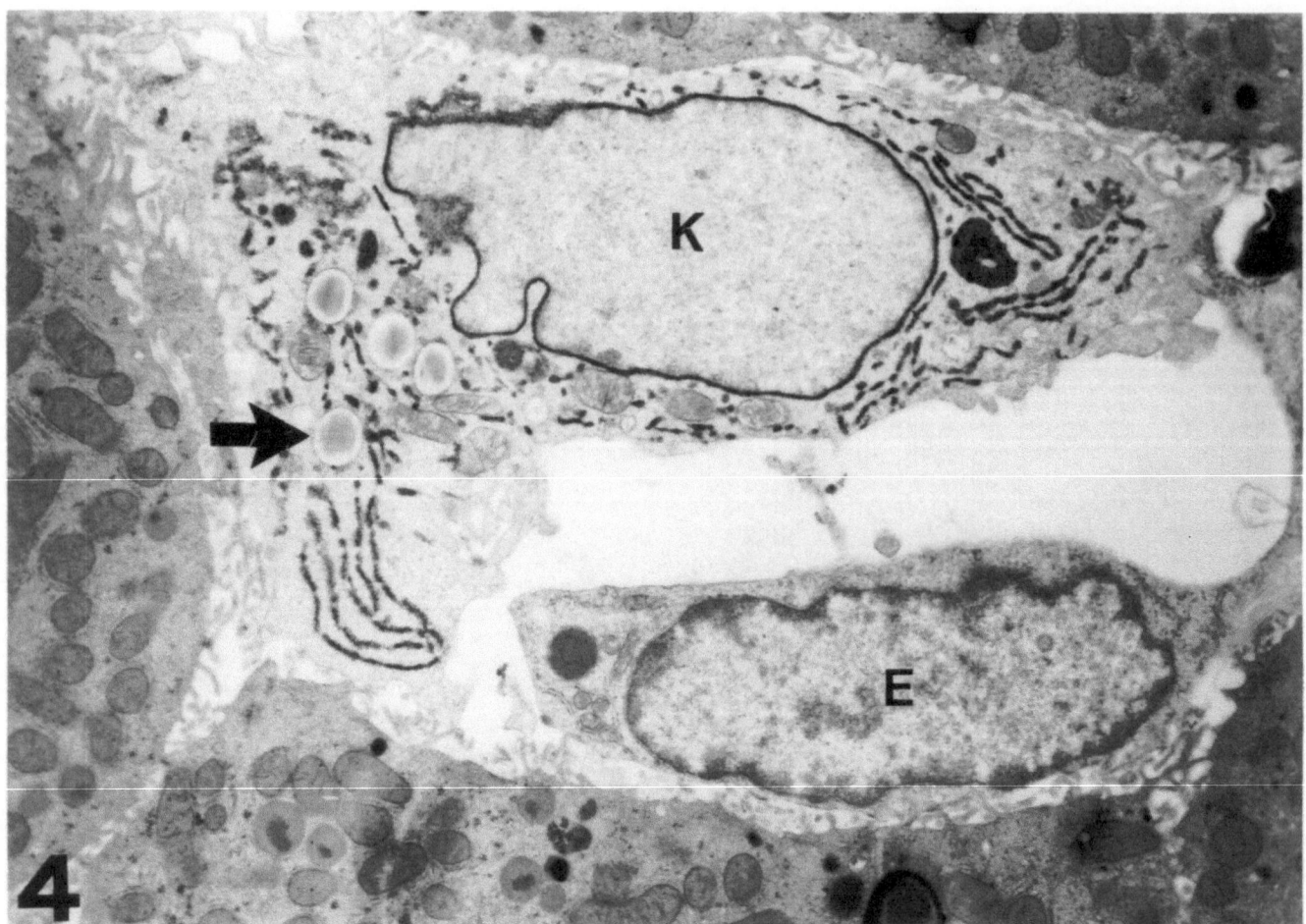

Figure 4   TEM of a sinusoid showing a peroxidase positive Kupffer cell (K) and a negative endothelial cell (E). The Kupffer cell contains phagocytosed latex particles of 0.8 μm diameter (arrow). Endothelial cells do not normally phagocytose these particles. × 11 400

fibrinogen degradation products (reviewed in references 23 and 29), parasites[30], tumour cells[31] and liposomes[32]. Kupffer cells degrade haemoglobin from cleared erythrocytes and play an important role in the storage and release of iron[33].

The process of endocytosis, i.e. phagocytosis and pinocytosis, is mainly receptor mediated, and several receptors have been demonstrated on Kupffer cells, e.g. Fc and C3 receptors, N-acetyl-D-galactosamine receptors, N-acetylglucosamine/mannose receptors and others (reviewed in references 16, 23 and 29). Exogenous particulate material, such as latex, can be taken up by non-receptor-mediated phagocytosis. Impaired function of complement and/or Fc receptors on Kupffer cells has been proposed to play an important role in the pathogenesis of tissue injury in several liver diseases[29,34].

Kupffer cells are the principal site for the removal of circulating endotoxin as it was observed, amongst other methods, after injection of radioactively labelled endotoxin[35–40]. There is evidence that endotoxin plays a key role in liver injury in many pathological conditions (for a review, see reference 41). There is no doubt that Kupffer cells play a major role in protecting the liver and the host from endotoxins.

After stimulation by phagocytosable material or inflammatory/immunomodulating agents, including endotoxin, Kupffer cells release prostaglandins and leukotrienes[42,43], interleukin-1[44,45], parenchymal cell-stimulating factor[46], interferon[47,48] and tumour necrosis factor[49]. These substances participate in the resistance of the host to infection and disease. Interleukin-1 and parenchymal cell-stimulating factor induce the acute-phase response during inflammation and stimulate hepatocytes to produce acute-phase proteins (proteinase inhibitors)[44]. Interferons are known for their antiviral and antitumour effects. The latter property is shared by tumour necrosis factor.

Kupffer cells are among the first members of the macrophage system to encounter immunogens absorbed from the lumen of the intestine and it has been shown that Kupffer cells have the potential to participate in the induction of antigen-specific immune responses. It has been proposed that, under normal circumstances and as a result of local environmental influences, the Kupffer cell functions primarily as an antigen-sequestering cell, whereas, in pathological conditions (acute or chronic inflammation), the normal constraint of its immunological function is disrupted[50,51]. Under experimental conditions of liver inflammation, caused by the intravenous injection of particulate material derived from yeast cells[52–54] or bacteria (L.B., unpublished observation), accumulation and proliferation of lymphocytes, with maturation to plasma cells, is observed in rat liver sinusoids. In many pathological conditions, lymphocyte infil-

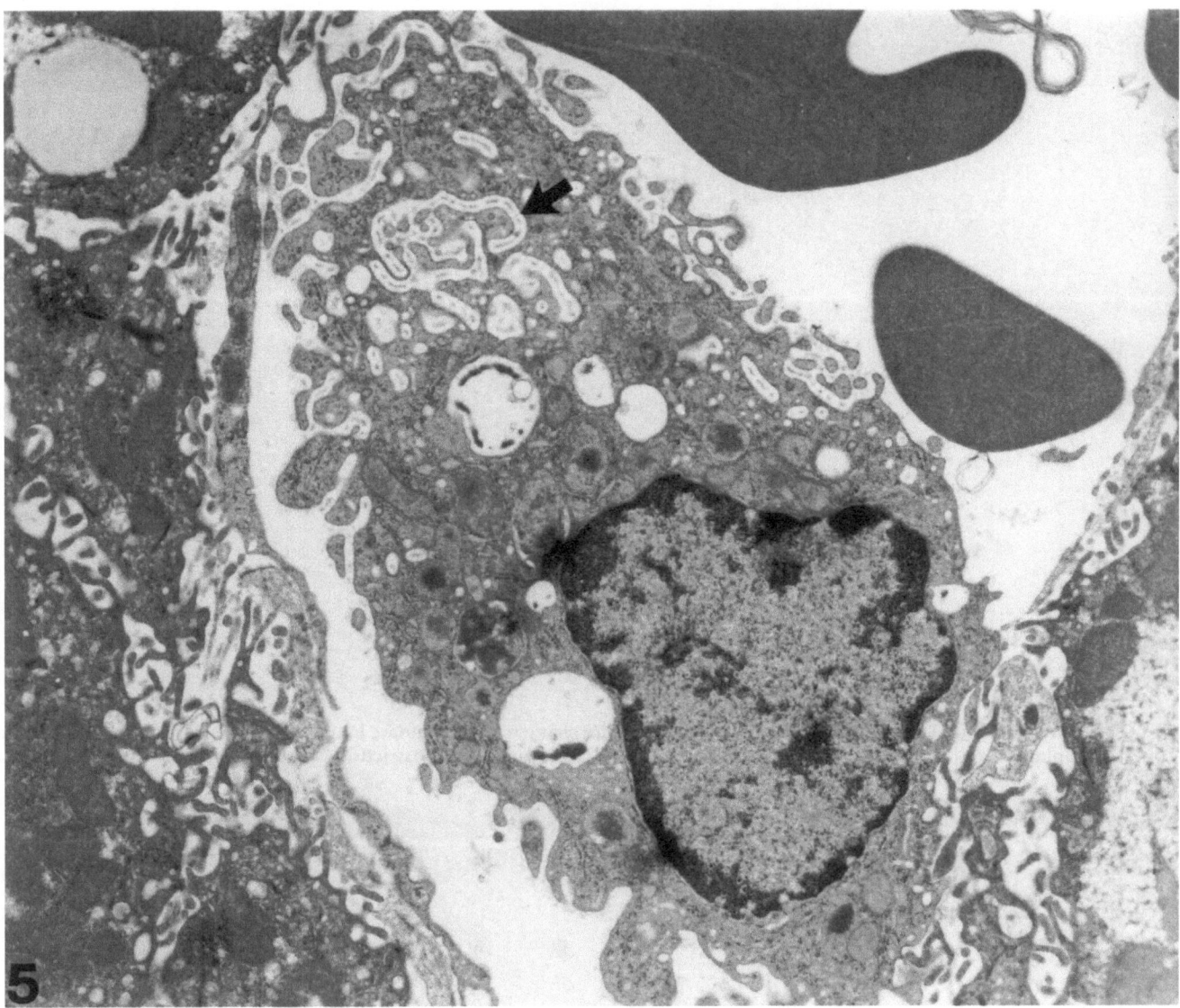

Figure 5   TEM of a Kupffer cell within the sinusoidal lumen. The cell contains numerous 'worm-like structures' (arrow) which are characteristic for Kupffer cells. These surface invaginations contain the same 'fuzzy' material present on the cell surface (the 'fuzzy coat'). A few erythrocytes are seen in the upper right-hand corner. × 11 700

tration is observed in the liver. In such circumstances, Kupffer cells may initiate immune responses which participate in the tissue damage and they might then become a major determinant of clinical outcome.

In vitro studies have shown that Kupffer cells are cytotoxic against intracellular parasites and against tumour cells, at least when they are activated by lymphokines and/or endotoxin[55-59]. These studies indicate that Kupffer cells may play a role in the destruction of tumour cells and thus be important in host defence against neoplasia and metastasis. In a rat model of liver metastasis, depression of the Kupffer cell activity by the injection of silica, gadolinium chloride or human red cells, increased the number of metastases whereas stimulation with zymosan or *Corynebacterium parvum* reduced the number of liver metastases in the animals[60].

Certain Kupffer cell functions, such as intracellular (parasite) and extracellular (tumour) cytotoxicity, are expressed only after activation of the cells, for instance by lymphokines (see above). The activating conditions which were used *in vitro* may occur also *in vivo*, for

example during acute or chronic inflammation. In experimental models of inflammation, however, it has been shown that, in addition to the resident Kupffer cell population, immigrant macrophages (monocytes) are recruited to the liver. Furthermore, the resident mature Kupffer cells were shown to differ functionally from the newly recruited monocyte-derived macrophages. Reported differences include fungicidal activity in *Corynebacterium parvum*-treated rats[61], secretion of hydrogen peroxide in *Listeria monocytogenes*-treated mice[62], and lysosomal enzyme release in *Corynebacterium parvum*-treated rats[63]. In these studies, the resident macrophages were deficient in the investigated function compared with the recently recruited cells. Thus, in the light of these functional differences, it is important to distinguish the two hepatic macrophage subpopulations during inflammatory conditions *in vivo*. The relative significance of both populations, the resident and the recently immigrated macrophages, in terms of cell numbers and functional activity, depends on the experimental or pathological conditions. It has been shown that in certain experimental situations,

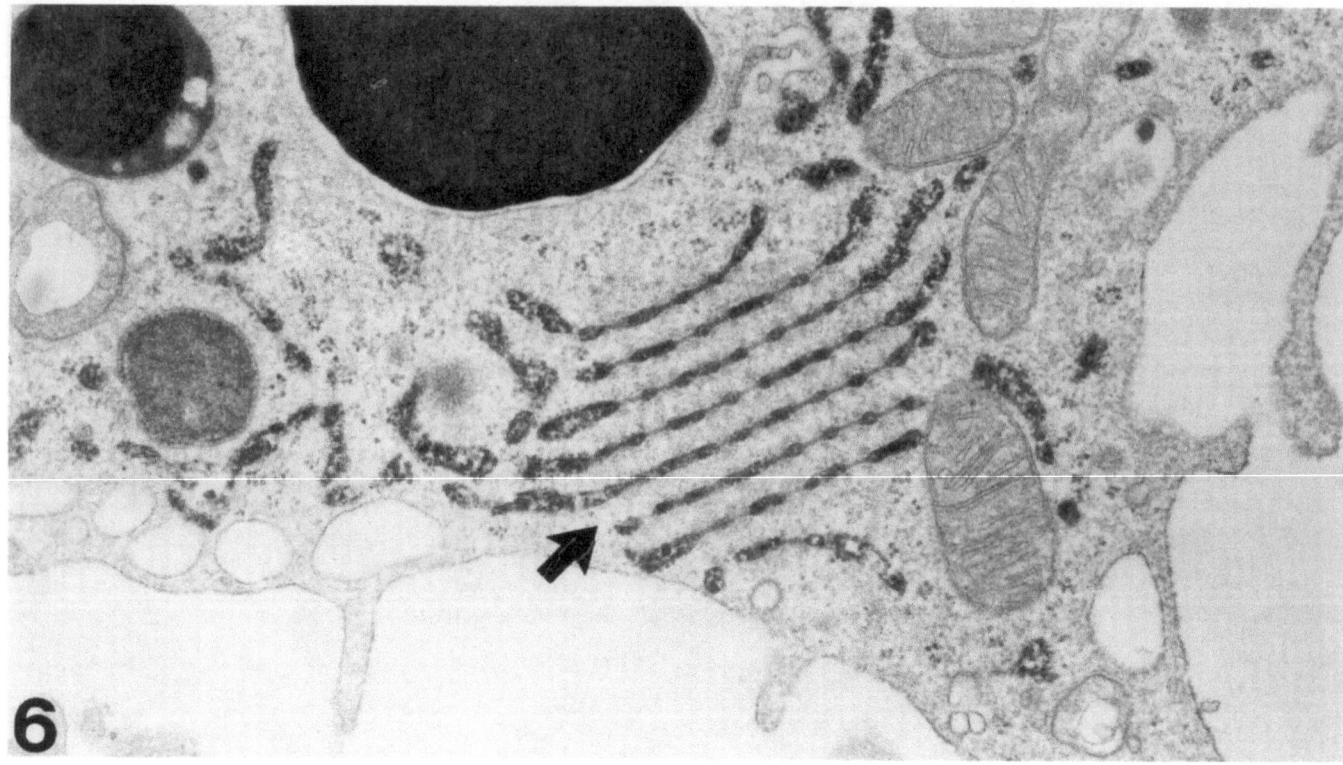

Figure 6 Detail (TEM) of a Kupffer cell's cytoplasm showing the characteristic annulate lamellae (arrow). These are parallel stacks of rough endoplasmic reticulum (containing peroxidase activity) with pore-like constrictions. The function of this structure is not clear. × 34 700

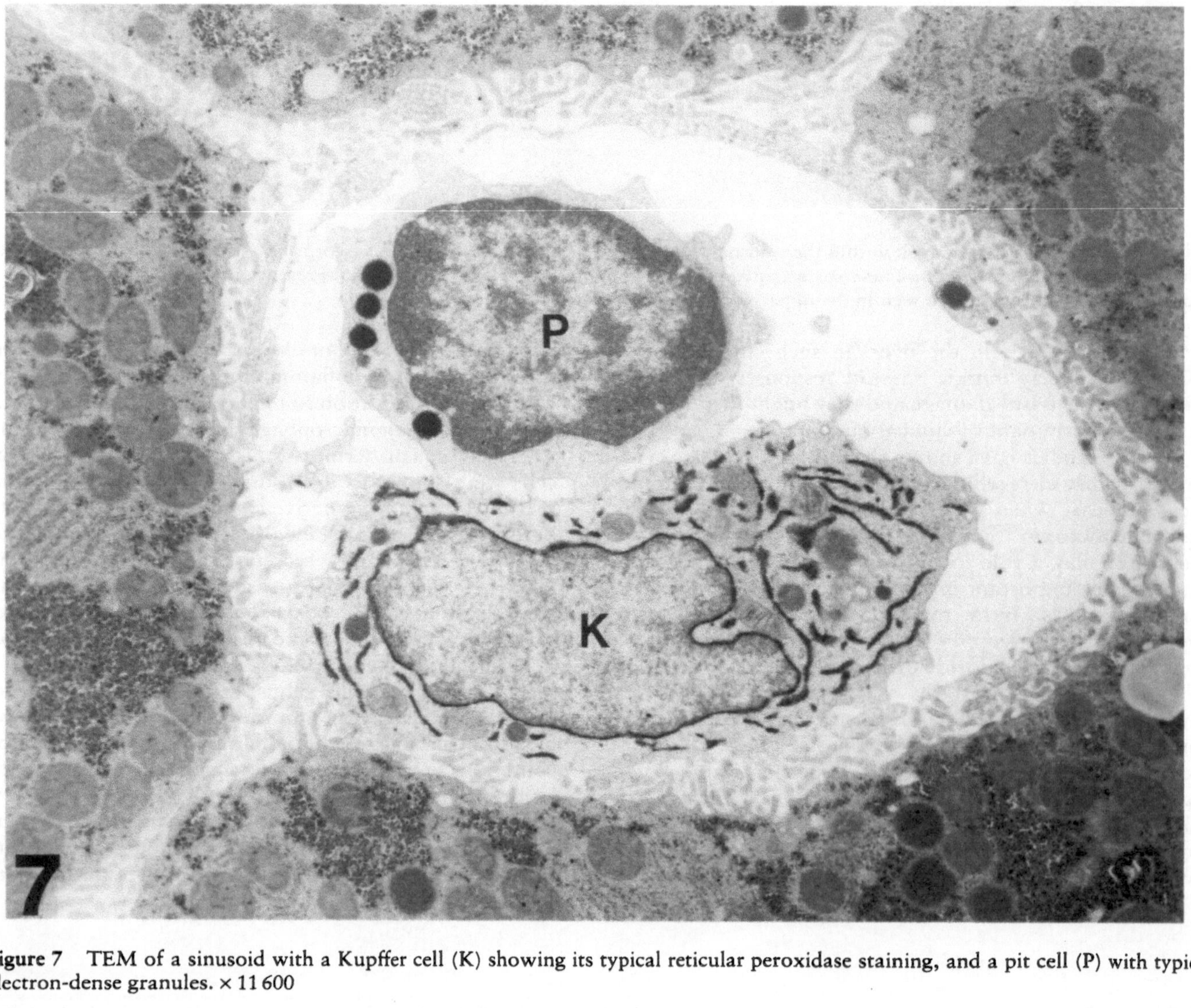

Figure 7 TEM of a sinusoid with a Kupffer cell (K) showing its typical reticular peroxidase staining, and a pit cell (P) with typical electron-dense granules. × 11 600

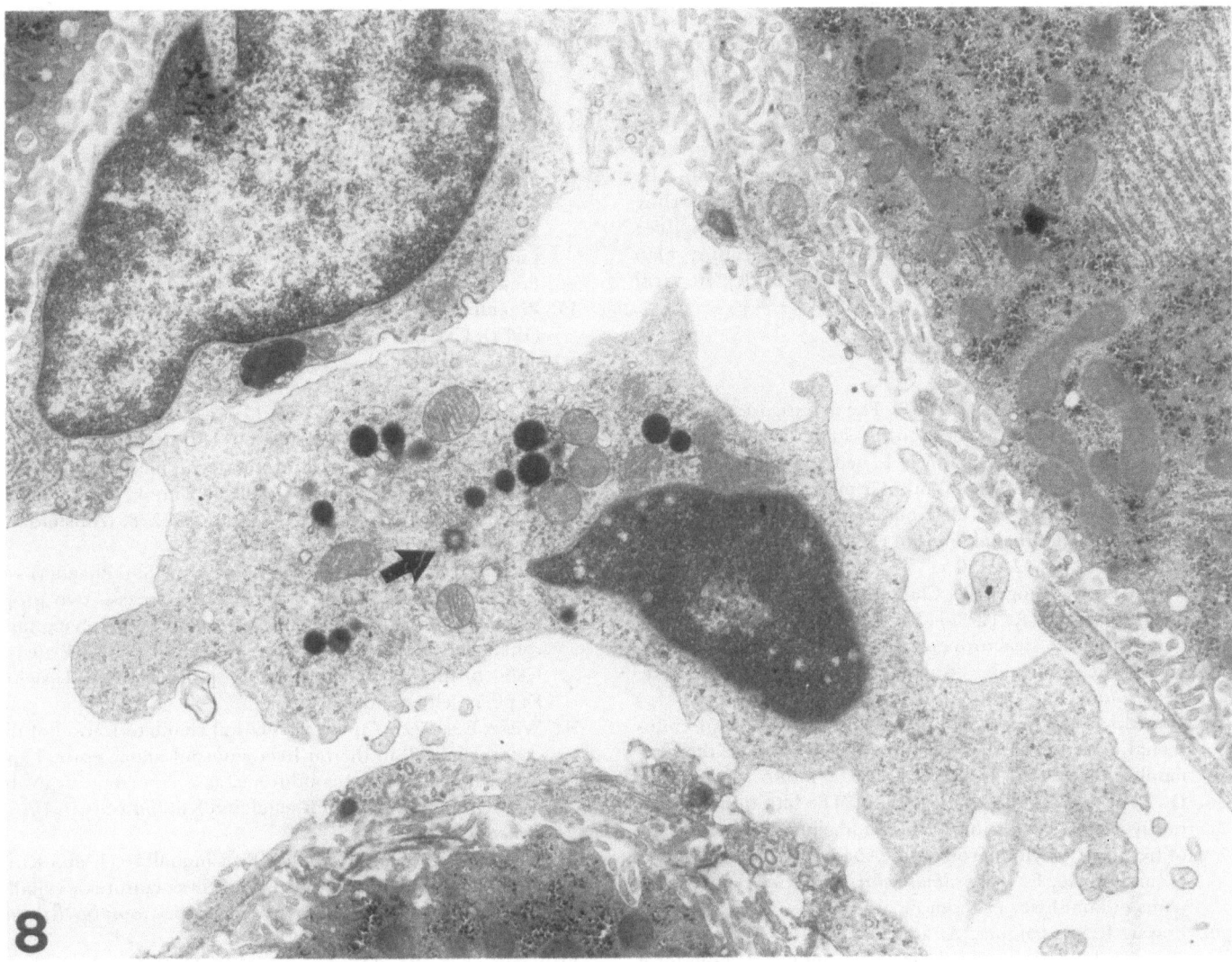

Figure 8   TEM of a pit cell present in the sinusoidal lumen. Pit cells have a characteristic polar organization of the cytoplasm with all organelles at one end of the nucleus. Most dense granules are found close to the cytocentre. The arrow points to a centriole in the cytocentre. × 13 500

such as liver regeneration after partial hepatectomy and during a zymosan-induced inflammatory reaction, Kupffer cells multiply locally by mitotic division[52–54]. In addition, monocytes have been shown to immigrate and marginate temporarily in the liver sinusoids during a zymosan-induced inflammation[64], and it has been suggested that these cells can differentiate into Kupffer cells under certain conditions[64,65]. In the normal physiological state, however, Kupffer cells are long-living cells which replicate independently from the monocytes[66].

PIT CELLS (Figures 2, 7 and 8)

Pit cells were described for the first time in 1970 by Wisse and Daems[67] but received their name in a second paper in 1976[68]. These cells are well characterized morphologically by electron microscopy but their function remains uncertain. They are found adherent to the sinusoidal endothelium or to Kupffer cells; thus in the sinusoidal lumen, and have a characteristic polar organization of the cytoplasm. Most organelles are found at one end of the nucleus, often concentrated near the cytocentrum. The latter is composed of a well-developed Golgi complex

and centrioles. The most characteristic organelles are electron-dense granules with specific ultrastructure, multivesicular bodies and rod-cored vesicles[67–69]. Pit cells contain many free ribosomes or polyribosomes but only sparse single strands of endoplasmic reticulum.

Originally, it was suggested that pit cells might represent endocrine cells but evidence for this was never obtained[68]. More recently, Kaneda et al.[70] proposed that pit cells, which also occur in various other organs as well as in the peripheral blood, would represent large granular lymphocytes (LGL). LGL are known as the morphological (light microscopic) equivalent of natural killer (NK) cells in the human, mouse and rat[71–73]. Conclusive evidence for the NK nature of pit cells has now been given by Bouwens et al.[74] who established a method for the isolation and purification of pit cells from rat liver. They found that cell suspensions enriched in pit cells (up to 90%) and containing virtually no monocytes or macrophages, had a strong lytic activity against YAC-1 lymphoma cells, the most commonly used targets for NK cells in rodents in vitro. Furthermore, this lytic activity was completely suppressed by treatment of the pit cells with anti-asialo GM1 (and complement), an antibody that reacts strongly with NK cells[74]. Also, the isolated pit cells have the morphology of LGL when observed by light microscopy in cytosmear preparations stained with Giemsa, i.e. they have prominent azurophilic granules near the nuclear notch[74]. These granules are probably the ones which constitute the most specific characteristic of the pit cells at the electron microscopic level. Since pit cells must be regarded as the tissue equivalent of LGL/NK cells, they may represent an important function of the healthy liver in controlling neoplasia and metastasis. They may also play a role in the pathogenesis of tissue injury in viral hepatitis.

References

1. Wisse, E. and Knook, D. (1979) The investigation of sinusoidal cells: A new approach to the study of liver function. In Popper, H. and Schaffner, F. (eds.) *Progress in Liver Diseases*, 153–171. (New York: Grune and Stratton)

2. Wisse, E. (1970). An electron microscopic study of the fenestrated endothelial lining of rat liver sinusoids. *J. Ultrastruct. Res.*, 31, 125–150

3. Wisse, E., De Zanger, R., Charels, K., Van Der Smissen, P. and McCuskey, R. (1985). The liver sieve: considerations concerning the structure and function of endothelial fenestrae, the sinusoidal wall and the space of Disse. *Hepatology*, 5, 683–692

4. Naito, M. and Wisse, E. (1978). Filtrating effect of endothelial fenestrations on chylomicron transport in the neonatal rat liver. *Cell Tissue Res.*, 190, 371–382

5. De Zanger, R. and Wisse, E. (1982). The filtration effect of rat liver fenestrated sinusoidal endothelium on the passage of (remnant) chylomicrons to the space of Disse. In Knook, D. and Wisse, E. (eds.) *Sinusoidal Liver Cells*, pp. 69–76. (Amsterdam: Elsevier Biomedical Press)

6. Fraser, R., Bosanquet, A. and Day, N. (1978). Filtration effect of chylomicrons by the liver may influence cholesterol metabolism and atherosclerosis. *Atherosclerosis*, 29, 113–123

7. Wright, P., Smith, K., Day, W. *et al.* (1983). Small liver fenestrae may explain the susceptibility of rabbits to atherosclerosis. *Atherosclerosis*, 3, 344–348

8. Fraser, R., Bowler, L. and Day, W. (1980). Damage of rat liver sinusoidal endothelium by ethanol. *Pathology*, 12, 371–376

9. Mak, K. and Lieber, C. (1984). Alterations in the endothelial fenestration in liver sinusoids of baboons fed alcohol: a scanning electron microscopical study. *Hepatology*, 4, 386–391

10. Nopanitaya, W., Lamb, J., Grisham, J. and Carson, J. (1976). Effect of hepatic venous outflow obstruction on pores and fenestrations in sinusoidal endothelium. *Br. J. Exp. Pathol.*, 57, 604–609

11. Frenzel, H., Kremer, B., Richter, I. and Hucker, H. (1976). Der Einfluss des Perfusiondruckes bei der Perusionsfixation auf die Feinstruktur der Lebersinusoide. Transmissions- und Rasterelectronenmikroskopische Untersuchung, *Res. Exp. Med.*, 168, 229–241

12. Fraser, R., Bowler, L., Day, W., Dobbs, B., Johnson, H. and Lee, D. (1980). High perfusion pressure damages the sieving ability of sinusoidal endothelium in rat livers, *Br. J. Exp. Pathol.*, 61, 222–228

13. Fraser, R., Bowler, L., De Zanger, R. and Wisse, E. (1982). Agents related to fibrosis, such as alcohol and CCl4 acutely affect endothelial fenestrae which may cause fatty liver. In Gerlach, U., Pott, G., Rauterberg, J. and Voss, B. (eds.) *Connective Tissue of the Normal and Fibrotic Human Liver*, pp. 159–160. (Stuttgart: Georg Thieme Verlag)

14. Frenzel, H., Kremer, B. and Hucker, H. (1977). The liver sinusoids under various pathological conditions. A TEM and SEM study of rat liver after respiratory hypoxy, telecobalt-irradiation and endotoxin application. In Wisse, E. and Knook, D. (eds.) *Kupffer Cells and other Sinusoidal Liver Cells*, pp. 213–222. (Amsterdam: Elsevier Biomedical Press)

15. Praaning-Van Dalen, D., Brouwer, A. and Knook, D. (1981). Clearance capacity of rat liver Kupffer, endothelial and parenchymal cells. *Gastroenterology*, 81, 1036–1044

16. Praaning-Van Dalen, D., De Leeuw, A., Brouwer, A., De Ruiter, G. and Knook, D. (1982). Ultrastructural and biochemical characterization of endocytic mechanisms in rat liver Kupffer and endothelial cells. In Knook, D. and Wisse, E. (eds.) *Sinusoidal Liver Cells*, pp. 271–278, (Amsterdam: Elsevier Biomedical Press)

17. Steffan, A., Gendrault, J. and Kirn, A. (1986). Phagocytosis and surface modulation of fenestrated areas – two properties of murine endothelial liver cells (EC) involving microfilaments. In Kirn, A., Knook, D. and Wisse, E. (eds.) *Cells of the Hepatic Sinusoid*, pp. 483–488. (Rijswijk: Kupffer Cell Foundation)

18. Wisse, E. (1972). An ultrastructural characterization of the endothelial cell in the rat liver sinusoid under normal and various experimental conditions, as a contribution to the distinction between endothelial and Kupffer cells. *J. Ultrastruct. Res.*, 38, 528–562

19. Steffan, A., Lecerf, F., Keller, F., Cinqualbre, J. and Kirn, A. (1981). Biologie generale: isolement et culture de cellules endotheliales de foie humain et murin. *Comptes Rendus Acad. Sci. Paris*, 292, 809–815

20. Brouwer, A., Barelds, R. and Knook, D. (1985). Age-related changes in the endocytic capacity of rat liver Kupffer and endothelial cells. *Hepatology*, 3, 362–366

21. Van Der Laan-Klamer, S., Brouwer, A., Atmosoerodjo-Briggs, J., Harms, G. and Hardonk, M. (1986). Binding of heterologous immune complexes to cultured rat liver endothelial cells. In Kirn, A., Knook, D. and Wisse, E. (eds.) *Cells of the Hepatic Sinusoid*, pp. 119–124. (Rijswijk: Kupffer Cell Foundation)

22. Ghitescu, L. and Fixman, A. (1984). Surface charge distribution on the endothelial cell of liver sinusoids. *J. Cell. Biol.*, 99, 639–647

23. Praaning-Van Dalen, D., De Leeuw, A., Brouwer, A. and Knook, D. (1982). Endocytosis by sinusoidal liver cells: summary of a round table discussion. In Knook, D. and Wisse, E. (eds.) *Sinusoidal Liver Cells*, pp. 517–524. (Amsterdam: Elsevier Biomedical Press)

24. Steffan, A., Gendrault, J., McCuskey, R., McCuskey, P. and Kirn, A. (1986). Phagocytosis, an unrecognized property of murine endothelial liver cells. *Hepatology*, 6, 830–836

25. Wisse, E. (1974). Observations on the fine structure and peroxidase cytochemistry of normal rat liver Kupffer cells. *J. Ultrastruct. Res.*, 46, 393–426

26. Singer, J., Adlersberg, L., Hoenig, E., Ende, E. and Tchorsch, Y. (1969). Radiolabeled latex particles in the investigation of phagocytosis in vivo: clearance curves and histological observations. *J. Reticuloend. Soc.*, 6, 561–589

27. Singer, J., Adlersberg, L. and Sadek, M. (1972). Long-term

observation of intravenously injected colloidal gold in mice. *J. Reticuloend. Soc.*, 12, 658–671

28. Gendrault, J., Steffan, A., Bingen, A. and Kirn, A. (1980). Uptake of frog virus 3 by Kupffer cells in vivo and in vitro. In Leihr, H. and Grun, M. (eds). *The Reticuloendothelial System and the Pathogenesis of Liver Disease*, pp. 221–228. (Amsterdam: Elsevier)

29. Jones, E. and Summerfield, J. (1982). Kupffer cells. In Arias, I., Popper, H., Schachter, D. and Shafritz, D. (eds). *The Liver: Biology and Pathology*, pp. 507–523. (New York: Raven Press)

30. Meis, J., Verhave, J., Jap, P. and Meuwissen, J. (1982). The role of Kupffer cells in the trapping of malarial sporozoites in the liver and the subsequent infection of hepatocytes. In Knook, D. and Wisse, E. (eds). *Sinusoidal Liver Cells*, pp. 429–436. (Amsterdam: Elsevier Biomedical Press)

31. Roos, E. and Dingemans, K. (1977). Phagocytosis of tumor cells by Kupffer cells in vivo and in the perfused mouse liver. In Wisse, E. and Knook, D. (eds). *Kupffer Cells and Other Liver Sinusoidal Cells*, pp. 183–190. (Amsterdam: Elsevier Biomedical Press)

32. Dijkstra, J., Van Galen, W., Roerdink, F., Regts, D. and Scherphof, G. (1982). Uptake of liposomes by Kupffer cells in vitro. In Knook, D. and Wisse, E. (eds). *Sinusoidal Liver Cells*, pp. 297–304. (Amsterdam: Elsevier Biomedical Press)

33. Fillet, G., Cook, J. and Finch, C. (1974). Storage iron kinetics. VII. A biological model for reticuloendothelial iron transport. *J. Clin. Invest.*, 53, 1527–1533

34. Loegering, D. (1986). Review article: Kupffer cell complement receptor clearance function and host defense. *Circ. Shock*, 20, 321–333

35. Mathison, J. and Ulevitch, R. (1979). The clearance, tissue distribution and cellular localization of intravenously injected lipopolysaccharide in rabbits. *J. Immunol.*, 123, 2133–2143

36. Ramadori, G., Hopf, U., Galanos, C., Freudenberg, M. and Meyer zum Buschenfelde, K. (1980). In vitro and in vivo reactivity of lipopolysaccharides and lipid A with parenchymal and non-parenchymal liver cells in mice. In Liehr, H. and Grun, M. (eds). *The Reticuloendothelial System and the Pathogenesis of Liver Disease*, pp. 285–294. (Amsterdam: Elsevier)

37. Maier, R. and Ulevitch, R. (1981). The response of isolated rabbit hepatic macrophages (H-M macrophage) to lipopolysaccharide (LPS). *Circ. Shock*, 8, 165–181

38. Praaning-Van Dalen, D., Brouwer, A. and Knook, D. (1976). Clearance capacity of rat liver Kupffer, endothelial and parenchymal cells. *Gastroenterology*, 70, 82–84

39. Ruiter, D., van Der Meulen, J., Brouwer, A. *et al.* (1981). Uptake by liver cells of endotoxin following its intravenous injection. *Lab. Invest.*, 45, 38–45

40. Freudenberg, M., Freudenberg, N. and Galanos, C. (1982). Time course of cellular distribution of endotoxin in liver, lungs and kidneys of rats. *Br. J. Exp. Pathol.*, 63, 56–65

41. Nolar, J. and Camara, P. (1982). Endotoxin, sinusoidal cells, and liver injury. In Popper, H. and Schaffner, F. (eds). *Progress in Liver Diseases*, Vol. 7, pp. 361–376. (New York: Grune and Stratton)

42. Birmelin, M. and Decker, K. (1984). Synthesis of prostanoids and cyclic nucleotides by phagocytosing rat Kupffer cells. *Eur. J. Biochem.*, 142, 219–225

43. Decker, K., Dieter, P., Henninger, H., Eyhorn, S. and Birmelin, M. (1986). The arachidonoids released by rat Kupffer cells in response to phagocytic stimuli. In Kirn, A.,

Knook, D. and Wisse, E. (eds). *Cells of the Hepatic Sinusoid*, pp. 65–70. (Rijswijk: Kupffer Cell Foundation)

44. Bauer, J., Birmelin, M., Northoff, G. *et al.* (1984). Induction of rat alpha 2-macroglobulin in vivo and in hepatocyte primary cultures: synergistic action of glucocorticoids and a Kupffer cell-derived factor. *FEBS Lett.*, 177, 89–94

45. Bauer, J., Tran-Thi, T., Northoff, H. *et al.* (1986). The acute-phase induction of alpha 2-macroglobulin in rat hepatocyte primary cultures: action of a hepatocyte-stimulating factor, triiodothyronine and dexamethasone. *Eur. J. Cell. Biol.*, 40, 86–93

46. Wolosky, B. and Fuller, G. (1985). Identification and partial characterization of hepatocyte-stimulating factor from leukemia cell lines: comparison with interleukin-1. *Proc. Natl. Acad. Sci. USA*, 82, 1443

47. Neumann, C. and Sorg, C. (1978). Immune interferon. II. Different cellular site for the production of murine macrophage migration inhibitory factor and interferon. *Eur. J. Immunol.*, 8, 582–589

48. Kirn, A., Gut, J. and Gendrault, J. (1982). Interaction of viruses with sinusoidal cells. In Popper, H. and Schaffner, F. (eds). *Progress in Liver Diseases*, Vol. 7, pp. 377–392. (New York: Grune and Stratton)

49. Decker, T., Lohmann-Matthes, M. and Gifford, G. E. (1987). Cell-associated necrosis factor (TNF) as a killing mechanism of activated cytotoxic macrophages. *J. Immunol.*, 138, 957–962

50. Rogoff, T. and Lipsky, P. (1981), Role of the Kupffer cells in local and systemic immune responses. *Gastroenterology*, 80, 854–860

51. Ramadori, G., Dienes, H., Burger, R., Meuer, S., Rieder, H. and Meyer zum Buschenfelde, K. (1986). Expression of Ia-antigens on guinea pig Kupffer cells. Studies with monoclonal antibodies. *J. Hepatol.* 2, 208–217

52. Bouwens, L., Baekeland, M. and Wisse, E. (1984). Importance of local proliferation in the expanding Kupffer cell population of rat liver after zymosan stimulation and partial hepatectomy. *Hepatology*, 4, 213–219

53. Bouwens, L., Baekeland, M. and Wisse, E. (1986). Cytokinetic analysis of the expanding Kupffer-cell population in rat liver. *Cell. Tissue Kinet.*, 19, 217–226

54. Bouwens, L., Knook, D. and Wisse, E. (1986). Local proliferation and extrahepatic recruitment of liver macrophages (Kupffer cells) in partial-body irradiated rats. *J. Leukocyte Biol.*, 39, 687–697

55. Decker, T., Kiderlen, A. and Lohmann-Matthes, M. (1985). Liver macrophages (Kupffer cells) as cytotoxic effector cells in extracellular and intracellular cytotoxicity. *Infect. Immun.*, 50, 358–364

56. Daemen, T., Veninga, A., Roerdink, F. and Scherphof, G. (1986). In vitro activation of rat liver macrophages to tumoricidal activity by free or liposome-encapsulated muramyl dipeptide. *Cancer Res.*, 46, 4330–4335

57. Cohen, S., Salazar, D., Von Muenchhausen, W., Werner-Wasik, M. and Nolan, J. (1985). Natural antitumor defense system of the murine liver. *J. Leukocyte Biol.*, 37, 559–569

58. Malter, M., Friedrich, E. and Suss, R. (1986). Liver as a tumor cell killing organ: Kupffer cells and natural killers. *Cancer Res.*, 46, 3055–3060

59. Xu, Z., Bucana, C. and Fidler, I. (1984). In vitro activation of murine Kupffer cells by lymphokines or endotoxins to lyse syngeneic tumour cells. *Am. J. Pathol.*, 117, 372–379

60. Pearson, H., Anderson, J., Chamberlain, J. and Bell, P. (1986). The effect of Kupffer cell stimulation or depression

on the development of liver metastases in the rat. *Cancer Immunol. Immunother.*, **23**, 214–216

61. Sawyer, R., Moon, R. and Beneke, E. (1981). Trapping and killing of Candida albicans by Corynebacterium parvum-activated livers. *Infect. Immun.*, **32**, 945–950

62. Lepay, D., Steinman, R., Nathan, C., Murray, H. and Cohn, Z. (1985). Liver macrophages in murine Listeriosis. Cell-mediated immunity is correlated with an influx of macrophages capable of generating reactive oxygen intermediates. *J. Exp. Med.*, **161**, 1503–1512

63. Tanner, A., Keyhani, A. and Wright, R. (1983). The influence of endotoxin in vitro on hepatic macrophage lysosomal enzyme release in different rat models of hepatic injury. *Liver*, **3**, 151–160

64. Bouwens, L. and Wisse, E. (1985). Proliferation, kinetics, and fate of monocytes in rat liver during a zymosan-induced inflammation. *J. Leukocyte Biol.*, **37**, 531–543

65. Deimann, W. and Fahimi, H. (1979). The appearance of transition forms between monocytes and Kupffer cells in the liver of rats treated with glucan. *J. Exp. Med.*, **149**, 883–897

66. Bouwens, L., Baekeland, M., De Zanger, R. and Wisse, E. (1986). Quantitation, tissue distribution and proliferation kinetics of Kupffer cells in normal rat liver. *Hepatology*, **6**, 718–722

67. Wisse, E. and Daems, W. (1970). Fine structural study on the sinusoidal lining cells of rat liver. In Van Furth, R. (ed.) *Mononuclear Phagocytes*, pp. 200–215. (Oxford: Blackwell)

68. Wisse, E., Van't Noordende, J., Van der Meulen, J. and Daems, W. (1976). The pit cell: description of a new type of cell occurring in rat liver sinusoids and peripheral blood. *Cell. Tissue Res.*, **173**, 423–435

69. Kaneda, K. and Wake, K. (1983). Distribution and morphological characteristics of the pit cells in the liver of the rat. *Cell. Tissue Res.*, **233**, 485–505

70. Kaneda, K., Dan, C. and Kaneda, K. (1983). Pit cells as natural killer cells. *Biomed. Res.*, **4**, 567–576

71. Timonen, T., Ortaldo, J. and Herberman, R. (1981). Characteristics of human large granular lymphocytes and relationship to natural killer and K cells. *J. Exp. Med.*, **153**, 569–582

72. Luini, W., Boraschi, D., Alberti, S., Aleotti, A. and Tagliabue, A. (1981). Morphological characterization of a cell population responsible for natural killer activity. *Immunology*, **43**, 663–668

73. Reynolds, C., Timonen, T. and Herberman, R. (1981). Natural killer (NK) cell activity in the rat. I. Isolation and characterization of the effector cells. *J. Immunol.*, **127**, 282–287

74. Bouwens, L., Remels, L., Baekeland, M., Van Bossuyt, H. and Wisse, E. (1987). Large granular lymphocytes or 'Pit cells' from rat liver: isolation, ultrastructural characterization and natural killer activity. *Eur. J. Immunol.*, **17**, 37–42

3

Liver perivascular cells revealed by gold- and silver-impregnation methods and electron microscopy

K. WAKE

INTRODUCTION

Scientific interest in the perivascular cells of the liver began over one hundred years ago, in 1876, with the discovery of 'Sternzellen' (stellate cells) by von Kupffer[1]. After much controversy through several decades, however, the theory that the perisinusoidal stellate cells play metabolic roles in retinol (vitamin A) storage and collagen synthesis in the liver, has rather recently been established (see Wake, 1980)[2].

This chapter deals with our current progress in research on the liver's perivascular cells, reviewed along with other relevant information. Studies based on both classical and modern techniques have been undertaken in our laboratory, and they appear to verify observations made by earlier investigators. Further, these studies add many essential aspects, previously overlooked and neglected, concerning the above cells, i.e. the distribution, general and fine structures, and differentiation as related to function of the cells. To aid the reader's understanding, this chapter begins with a brief historical outline.

HISTORICAL PERSPECTIVE OF PERIVASCULAR CELLS OF THE LIVER

In 1876, Kupffer[1] wrote his memorable work in which he described star-shaped cells scattered in the hepatic lobule, which he examined using a modification of Gerlach's gold chloride method. These cells were named 'Sternzellen' (stellate cells). In his treatise, we find a clear reference to the discovery that stellate cells were located peri-sinusoidally and that they were different from phagocytic cells. Rothe (1882)[3] confirmed the existence of stellate cells in livers of several species of mammals and a bird. Another important description in relation to these cells was that of **inclusion bodies** in the cytoplasm[3]. These globular structures appear as clear spots in the gold-precipitated cytoplasm. At that time, these bodies were thought to be **small nuclei**. Not until more than eight decades had elapsed were the unidentified inclusions proved to be lipid droplets containing retinol in the form of retinyl ester[4,5].

Twenty-two years after Kupffer's first paper, however,

a mistaken alternative view, based on phagocytosis of India ink particles, was proposed by Kupffer himself[6,7]. According to Kupffer[7], the inclusion bodies in stellate cells were 'fragments of erythrocytes' which were taken up from the circulation. He concluded that stellate cells were the special endothelial cells of the sinusoids. This misinterpretation led to deep-rooted confusion in liver histology. The revised concepts were not challenged for several decades, since many researchers continued to believe that perisinusoidal cells did not exist in the liver, or that if ever they did exist, they must be of a special type of reticuloendothelial phagocytic cell. For example, it was repeatedly claimed, in over forty papers published during the period from about 1930 to 1970, that retinol is stored in the reticuloendothelial Kupffer cells of the liver[2].

Meanwhile, after Rothe, several perivascular cells in the hepatic lobule were discovered by the use of silver-impregnation methods. The pioneer investigation, using Golgi's silver method, was carried out in 1893 by Berkley[8] who described the scattered yellowish granular bodies, lying between the hepatocytes and the adjacent vascular walls, that were not visible by the usual staining methods, suggesting that the majority of these cells were the stellate cells originally cited by Kupffer[1]. He called these cells 'granular cells'. Shortly afterwards, Dogiel[9] reported special star-shaped cells whose cytoplasmic processes surrounded the walls of capillaries in dog liver. In 1923, Zimmermann[10] developed the idea of the existence of perivascular cells, not only in the liver, but also generally in the other organ system. With the improvement of Golgi's silver technique by Zimmermann, the dendritic processes of these cells, designated 'pericytes', could be discerned as longer with striking branchings surrounding the sinusoidal walls. Unfortunately, however, this key paper describing the perivascular cells of the liver attracted virtually no attention from investigators. Thus, there was no reinvestigation after Zimmermann's studies using the unbelievably fruitful method of Golgi. Suzuki[11,12] reported the 'interstitial cells' by the use of his own modification of Bielschowsky's silver-impregnation technique. This silver method revealed characteristically the innervation of autonomic nerve fibres for the peri-vascular cells. Suzuki contributed his valuable suggestion that the silver-impregnated 'interstitial cells' might be the original stellate cells of Kupffer (1876)[1].

In another study on perivascular cells of the hepatic lobule, the cells were documented as 'fat-storing cells' of Ito[13]. Ito found the cells containing lipid droplets in the human liver, putting forward the misleading idea that 'the fat droplets' in the cytoplasm were not derived from the blood stream but from glycogen[14]. However, the advent of electron microscopy made it possible for his group[15] to be the first to establish correctly the perisinusoidal location of these cells.

A new development in this confusing history reinstated the perisinusoidal stellate cells as the retinol-storage cells. Nakane[16] reported that retinol was stored in the fat-storing cells and Wake[4] demonstrated it in the interstitial cells. Afterwards, both cells were proved[5] to be a single one, identical to the gold-reactive cells of Kupffer. Gold precipitates occur primarily on the surface of retinol-containing lipid droplets[5,17]. Hirosawa and Yamada[18] showed storage of retinol in these lipid droplets by the use of autoradiography of [14C]retinol. The pericytes of Zimmermann were similarly demonstrated to be stellate cells, since, following administration of excess retinol to the animal, the Golgi-stained pericytes increased the volume of their cell bodies, which contained numerous lipid droplets[19]. Therefore, the various perivascular cells in the hepatic lobule advocated by numbers of research workers in the past using different methodological approaches finally proved to be identical. Investigators and their followers had put forward their belief that they had 'discovered a new type of cell' in the liver, without comparing and confirming the results obtainable by other staining methods, since the cells demonstrated by one technique could appear to be different from exactly the same cells but demonstrated by other techniques.

In the present chapter, the nomination, 'stellate cells (Sternzellen)', as first designated by the discoverer of this cell type, *Carl von Kupffer*, will be given to the perisinusoidal cells in the liver, and also to the retinol-storing cells located in the interstitium of the liver and extrahepatic organs, all of which are gold-reactive in nature. Aterman[20] proposed the nomenclature of these cells as 'parasinusoidal cells' in his recent review paper.

According to the current state of hepatology, in its anatomical aspect, we know that there exist five different kinds of cells in the liver parenchyma: (1) parenchymal cells (hepatocytes), (2) endothelial cells of the sinusoid, (3) Kupffer cells (liver macrophages), (4) stellate cells (fat-storing cells, vitamin A-storing cells, interstitial cells, or lipocytes), and (5) pit cells (liver-associated large granular lymphocytes, or NK cells)[21-24]. The latter four kinds of cells are comprehensively called 'liver sinusoidal cells'.

DISTRIBUTION OF STELLATE CELLS

Kupffer's gold chloride method offers several advantages for analysis of the distribution of retinol-storing stellate cells in the liver and other extrahepatic organs[25]. Although fluorescence microscopy for retinol is also available for this purpose, as the fluorescence rapidly fades away during the examination, it is difficult to study the relationship between fluorescent sources and the surrounding tissue. In contrast, the gold deposits occur primarily on the surface of the lipid droplets which contain

retinol in the cytoplasm of the stellate cells and then diffuse into the nearby cytoplasm of perikarya and thick cytoplasmic processes[26], thus remaining permanent in the histological preparation.

Liver

In the livers of mammalian species, gold-reactive cells are found only within the hepatic lobule[5] (Figures 1 and 2), while in certain lower vertebrates, such as lampreys, myxinoides and eels, these cells are distributed not only in the hepatic parenchyma, but also in the interstitial connective tissue[27-29]. All fibroblast-like cells in the interstitium store abundant retinol in the liver of the adult lamprey, *Lampetra japonica*, caught during the spawning migration. No distinction, therefore, can be recognized between the perisinusoidal stellate cells and the interstitial fibroblast-like cells of the liver in the lower vertebrates in terms of retinol storage.

Extrahepatic organs

In addition, almost all fibroblast-like cells in the splanchnic organs in the lamprey contain large amounts of retinol[27,29]. Gold-deposited cells are abundant in the lamina propria, submucosa, muscle layers and adventitia of the digestive canal. Retinol-storing cells that occur in renal glomeruli are equivalent to the mesangial cells in mammalian kidneys. Numerous stellate cells are distributed in the interstitium surrounding the convoluted renal tubules and in the dense connective tissue of the renal capsule and Bowman's capsule. Gold-impregnated stellate cells are also seen in the interstitium of the pancreas, gonads and heart of the animal. Pillar cells in gill filaments are found to be retinol-storing cells[19].

In contrast, retinol-storing cells are sparse or absent in somatic tissues, such as dermis, subcutaneous connective tissue, notocord and nervous system, in the lamprey. In the skeletal muscles, small numbers of gold-reactive cells, which differ somewhat from the adipose cells, are scattered among muscle fibres. In an attempt to account for the vast distribution in many splanchnic organs in lower vertebrates on the one hand, and the very limited localization in the liver of mammals on the other hand, an idea describing these peculiar features of gold-sensitive cells is tentatively given in the text (see 'Differentiation of stellate cells').

LOCATION OF STELLATE CELLS IN THE LIVER

In order to examine the location of the stellate cells in the liver, gold-stained sections of the liver are subjected to sonication in 1% aqueous boric acid to remove parenchymal cells, leaving a network of the sinusoids and the surrounding reticular fibres[25]. In these sinusoid-network preparations, stellate cells in the hepatic lobules appear to be adherent to the outer surface of the endothelium at fairly regular intervals. They lie with nucleus-to-nucleus distances of $39.6 \pm 11.2\,\mu m$ in man, $77.0 \pm 16.1\,\mu m$ in Rhesus monkey, $21.0 \pm 7.8\,\mu m$ in chick, and $21.6 \pm 7.6\,\mu m$ in eel, *Anguilla japonica*. The spaces between each pair of nuclei reflect the area occupied by cytoplasmic processes of neighbouring stellate cells (see the next section). From this regularity of distribution, it may be said, in

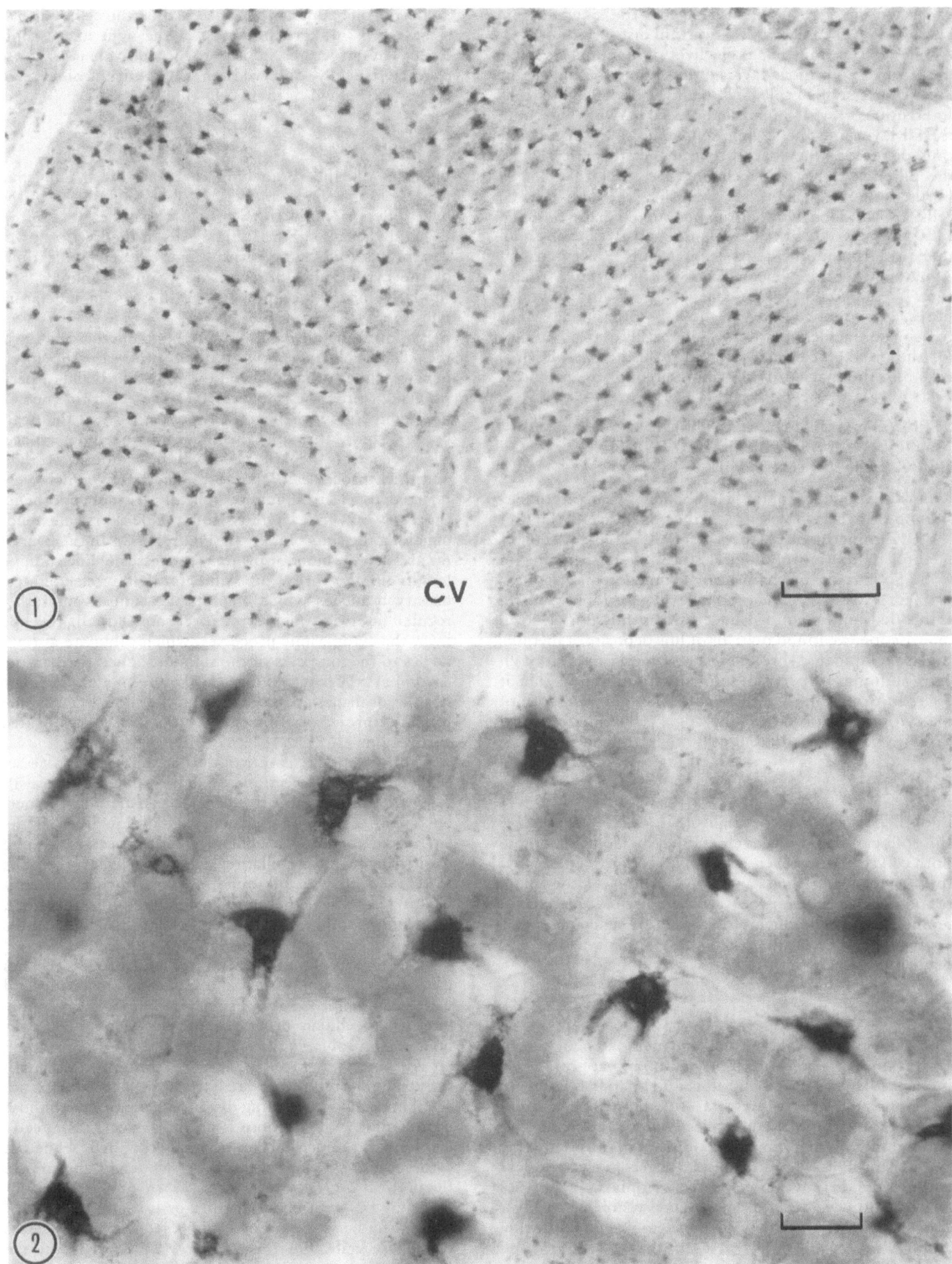

Figure 1 Low magnification view of gold chloride preparation of hog liver. Sternzellen (stellate cells) are distributed regularly in hepatic lobules and no reaction occurs in the interlobular connective tissue. Kupffer's gold chloride method. CV, central vein. Bar, 100 μm (× 190)

Figure 2 Stellate cells in human liver. Gold chloride method. Bar, 20 μm (× 750)

other words, that along their stretch the sinusoids are equipped with stellate cells at certain distances.

The wall of sinusoids in the liver of mammals is made up of three concentric layers – the endothelial layer, the layer of the stellate cells and the layer of collagen fibrils. Interrupted basal lamina is interposed between the endothelial layer and the stellate cells. The space of Disse is thus defined as the space between the stellate cells and the parenchymal cells, including the layer of collagen fibrils. In lamprey liver, however, since the parenchymal cells are studded with an uninterrupted basal lamina, there exist two distinct basal laminae between the endothelial cells and the parenchymal cells[29,30,31,32]. In this Agnatha, therefore, elements of the connective tissue, such as the stellate cells, collagen fibrils and oxytalan fibres, are confined between those basal laminae[29]. The perisinusoidal location of the stellate cells is an advantage for the uptake of retinol released from the parenchymal cells into the space of Disse and the blood stream[33].

STELLATE CELLS (PERICYTES) AND MYOFIBROBLASTS REVEALED BY USING GOLGI'S SILVER METHOD

Golgi's silver impregnation method helps us in our understanding of the whole view of the stellate cells (Figures 3–8). Zimmermann[10], in particular, applied Golgi's method to the morphological study of the pericytes in liver. So far, its mechanism of staining remains unexplained. However, when Golgi's preparations were re-embedded and examined under a transmission electron microscope, we found myriads of fine deposits of metallic silver disseminated throughout the cytoplasm (Figure 9). This staining property is surprisingly unique in that it offers information over the whole length and breadth of the cytoplasmic processes of a single cell, while, in many cases, it leaves the adjacent cells completely unstained.

Stellate cells (pericytes)

Endothelial cells and perisinusoidal stellate cells of the sinusoid can be unselectively stained by Golgi's method. Both cell types, however, are easily distinguished because the former show thick and thin portions of the membranous cytoplasmic processes[34], while the stellate cells, no matter how complicated in shape, are made up of two distinct structures, the cell bodies (perikarya) and the dendritic cytoplasmic processes.

Cell bodies (perikarya)

The cell bodies may be spindle-shaped or angulated or even rounded. The form of the cell bodies appears to be influenced by: (1) their location and spatial relation to the opposing hepatocytes; (2) the branching pattern growing out from the cell bodies; and (3) the dimension and number of the retinol-containing lipid droplets in the cytoplasm. These lipid droplets are recognized as clear globules in the silver-precipitated cytoplasm (Figures 7 and 8c). However, they are not always visible when silver depositions occur heavily in the cytoplasm. Following administration of excess retinol, the cell bodies are rounded up containing a large number of lipid droplets (Figure 7).

Tiny projections can be discerned on the cell bodies of stellate cells in certain animals at the light microscopic level. The structures appear to be equivalent to those characteristically observed on the perisinusoidal processes (see below) of these cells (Figure 8).

Cytoplasmic processes

Because of the branching pattern of cytoplasmic processes, the shape and size of the stellate cells in the liver differs notably from species to species (Figure 8). Generally speaking, the stellate cells in the liver of lower vertebrates are of simple form (Figure 8a). Ramifications of the cytoplasmic processes in younger animals are, similarly, not as complicated as those seen in mature ones.

Explored in full detail, at the light microscopic level the stellate cells reveal two types of processes: the 'interhepatocellular processes' and the 'subendothelial or perisinusoidal processes'. The former project from the cell body and follow their vertical course toward the nearby sinusoids through the interhepatocellular space. They penetrate hepatic cell cords as smooth, straight and thick processes (Figure 8d). The latter, which were referred to electron microscopically as 'subendothelial processes'[35,36], emit laterally from the perikaryon extending along the sinusoidal wall (Figures 5–8). In the liver of rat and rabbit, main or primary processes, while running longitudinally, throw off numbers of long slender secondary branches which encircle the sinusoid at rather regular intervals (Figures 5, 6, 8b and 8d). In the hog liver, the cytoplasmic processes, which originate at right angles to the long axis of the spindle-shaped perikaryon, encompass the sinusoid directly (Figures 4 and 8e). Some circular branches are emitted from the short longitudinal processes projected from the two poles of the elongated perikaryon.

The outstanding feature of the perisinusoidal processes is their thorny projections, i.e. the 'spines' (Figure 8). They are demonstrable by using Golgi's method. Numerous spines emit perpendicularly or obliquely from the lateral sides of flattened subendothelial processes. In spite of differing forms of stellate cells between livers of various vertebrates, they are all found, as far as have been examined so far, to have the spines in common. It is, therefore, not without solid evidence to state that the spines can be added to the characterization of the stellate cells.

Once the tip of an interhepatocellular process reaches the wall of a neighbouring sinusoid, it bursts into several perisinusoidal processes. A single stellate cell may supply interhepatocellular processes to one or more neighbouring sinusoids (Figures 5, 6, 8b, 8c and 8d). Spreading areas of individual stellate cells can amount to a length of 120 μm in rabbit liver. Stellate cells of newborn rat are small in terms of spreading distance compared with those of the adult. When retinol is given in excess, as already mentioned, the perikaryon becomes rounded, while the cytoplasmic processes seem to be slender in appearance (Figure 7).

It may be questioned whether or not any segment of the sinusoids is to be found with cytoplasmic processes of stellate cells. On this point, we observed that the cytoplasmic processes of two neighbouring stellate cells stained with Golgi's method, were closely juxtaposed

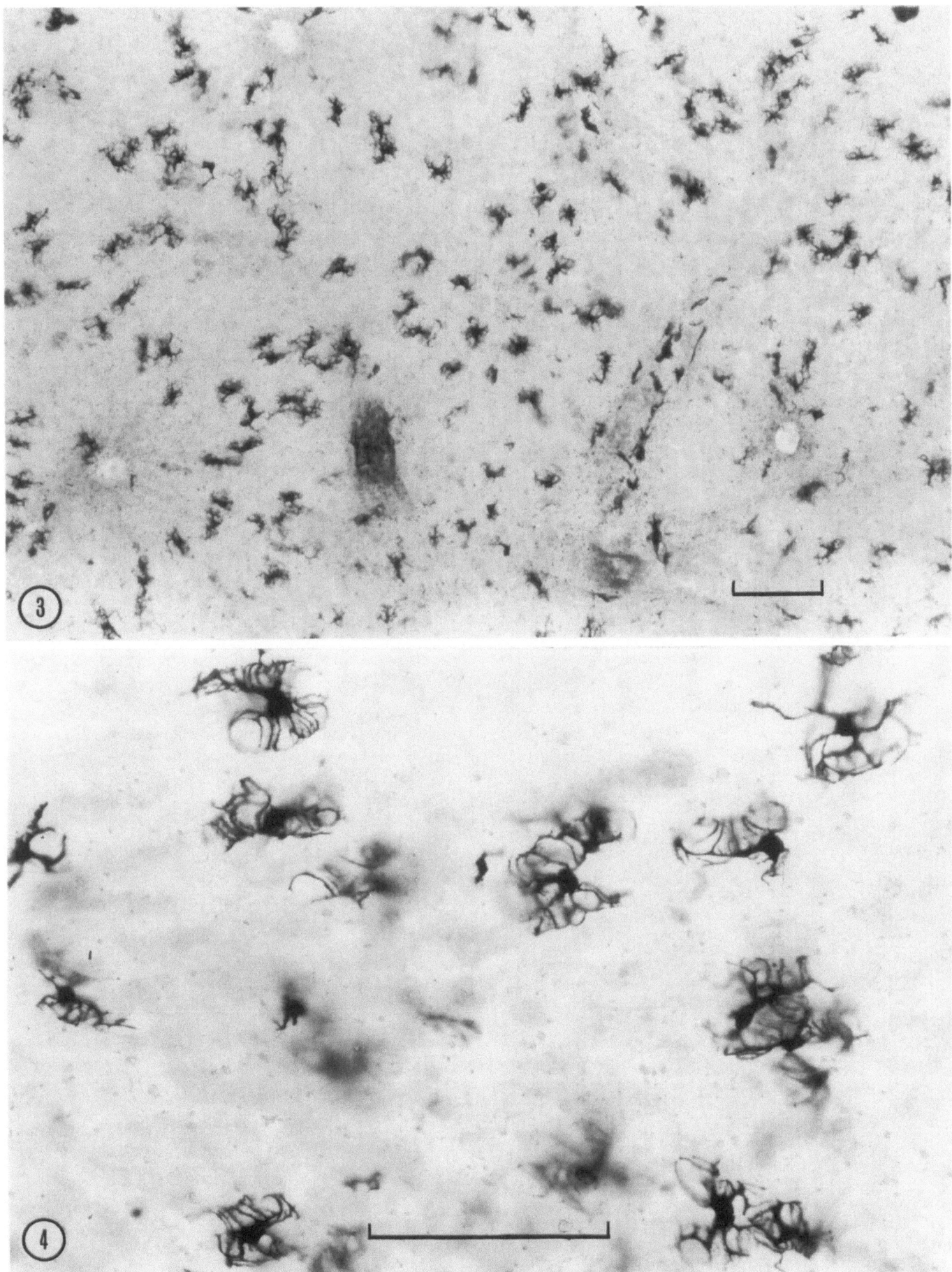

Figure 3 Low power view of a silver-impregnated preparation of a 17-day-old rat. Pericytes (stellate cells) with long cytoplasmic processes are unevenly stained. Golgi's silver method. Bar, 100 μm (×170)
Figure 4 Pericytes (stellate cells) in hog liver. Perisinusoidal processes surround sinusoids circumferentially. Golgi's silver method. Bar, 20 μm (×450)

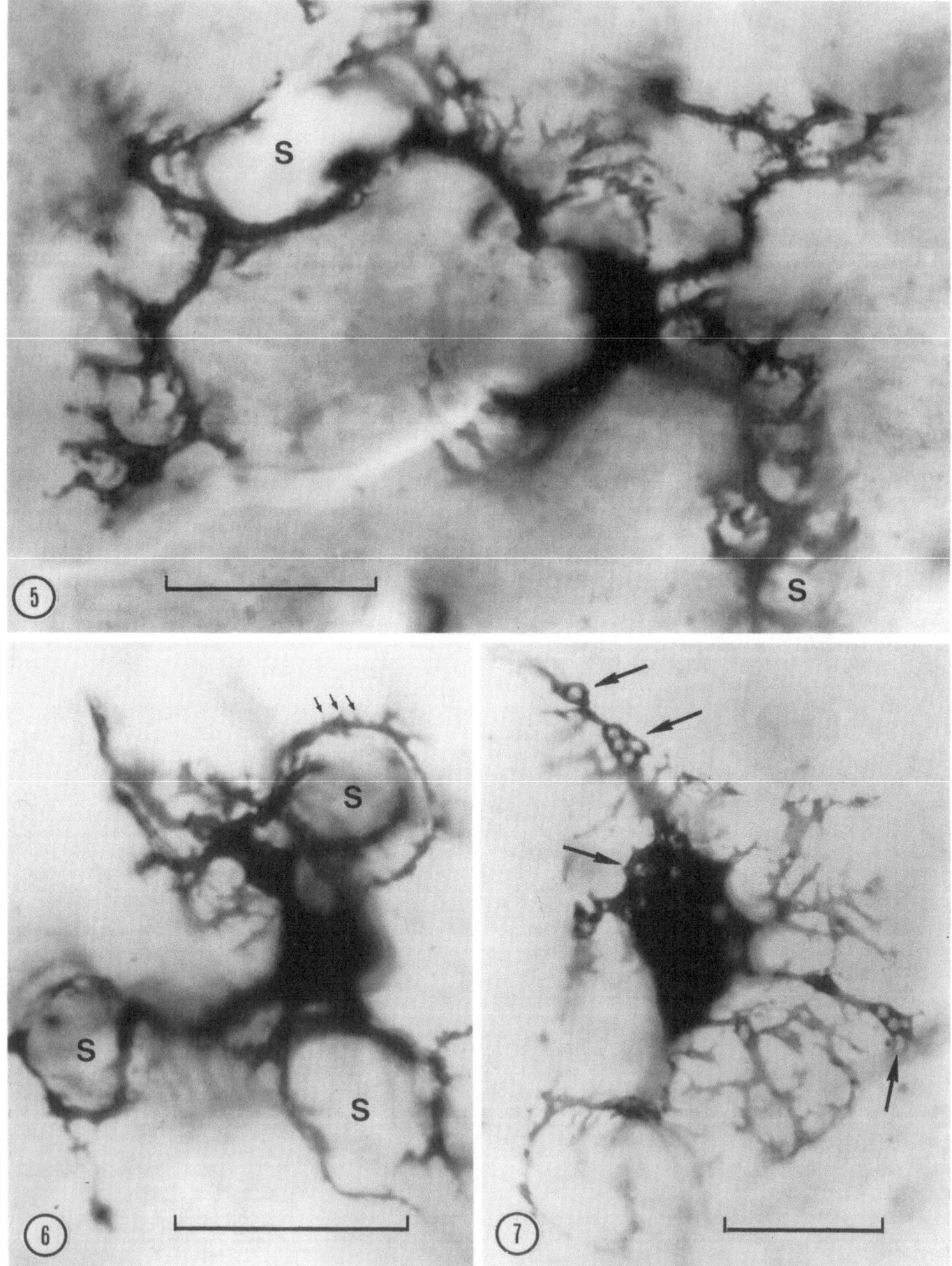

Figure 5   Dendritic branching processes extend over the wall of sinusoids (S). Golgi's silver method. Rabbit liver. Bar, 20 µm
(× 2000)
Figure 6   A pericyte of rat liver. Perisinusoidal processes with spines (arrows) encircling sinusoids (S). Golgi's silver method. Bar,
20 µm (× 2200)
Figure 7   A pericyte of the liver of a rat administered with excess retinyl palmitate (400 000 iu/kg). The cell body is abnormally
enlarged due to increased lipid droplets, while cytoplasmic processes containing a number of lipid droplets (arrows) are slender in
appearance. Golgi's silver method. Bar, 20 µm (× 1500)

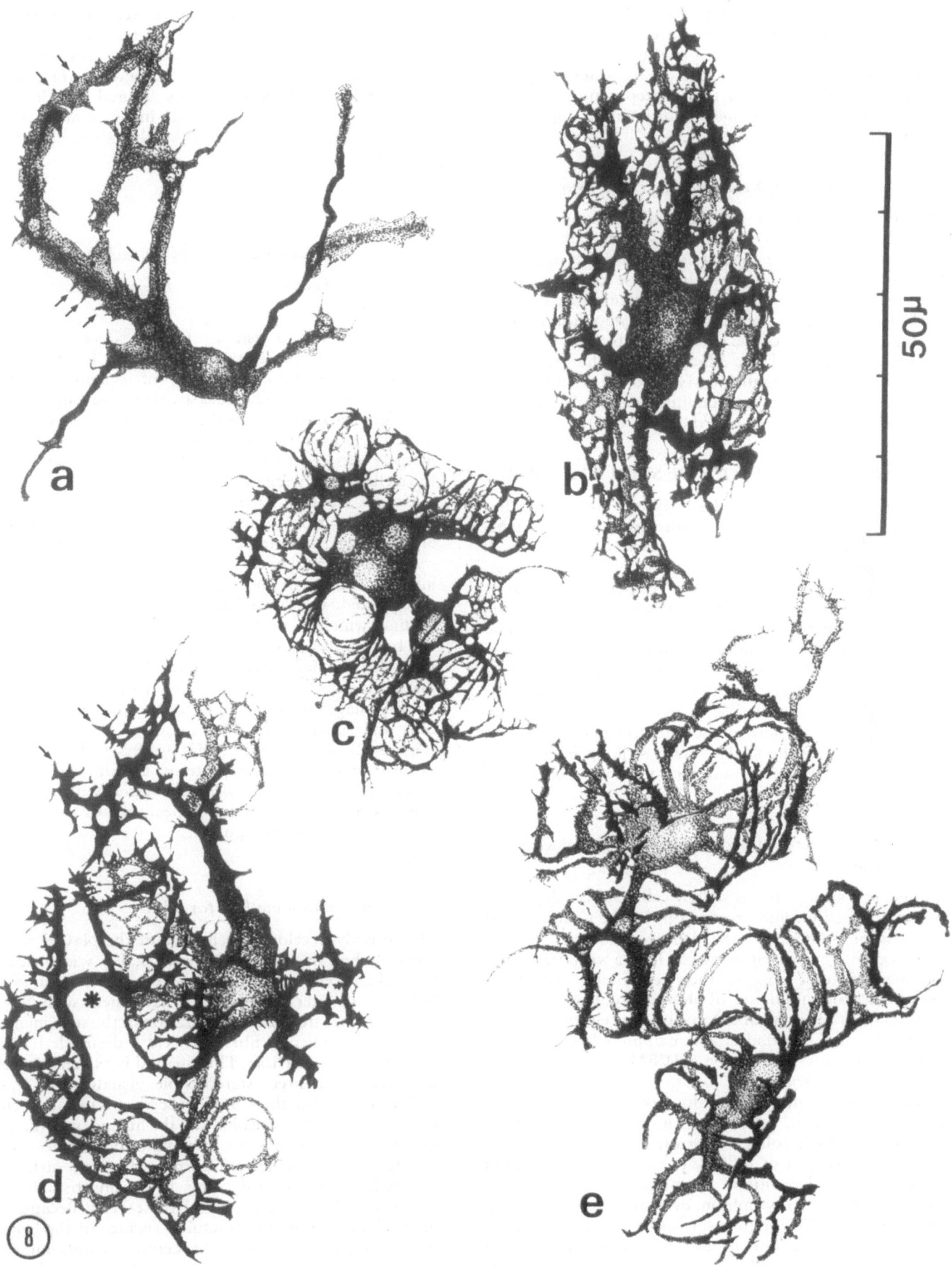

50μ

Figure 8 Drawings of pericytes (stellate cells) from livers of various vertebrates; a, lamprey (*Lampetra japonica*); b, rat; c, mouse; d, rabbit; e, hog. Arrows, spines; asterisk, interhepatocellular process (× 1300)

together, set apart by extremely narrow gaps (Figure 8e). It thus appears that the endothelial tubes along the entire length of the hepatic sinusoids are evenly encircled by the perisinusoidal processes of the stellate cells. Regular distribution of the stellate cells on the sinusoidal wall, revealed in the sinusoid-network preparations after the gold chloride reaction, may additionally support this assumption.

Myofibroblasts located around the central vein

Myofibroblasts lodged in the space surrounding the central veins are also stained by Golgi's method. They are flattened and star-shaped large cells with processes. Electron microscopy shows that these cells are characterized by the abundance of microfilaments associated with dense plaques, smooth-surfaced endoplasmic reticulum, and caveolae of the surface membrane[19]. Collagen fibrils, as well as elastic fibres, run in the vicinity of these cells. The myofibroblasts send off a number of cytoplasmic processes surrounding the central vein, some of which penetrate deep into the space of Disse.

ELECTRON MICROSCOPY OF STELLATE CELLS

During the past two decades, electron microscopy has advanced our knowledge of the ultrastructure of the perisinusoidal stellate cells in the liver, as may be traced back in the literature through review articles[2,36,37]. However, there is, as yet, no satisfactory evidence of electron microscopy studies relating to the three-dimensional morphology of the stellate cells. In electron microscopic examination, the conventional thin section does not help to disclose the key features of these cells, i.e. highly-ramified and widely-expanding, whereas these can be revealed by the use of Golgi's silver method. To cope with the problem, new methodological approaches are needed to clarify the stellate cell's striking features, as visualized by the classical method, in an electron microscopic manner.

High-voltage electron microscopy of Golgi-stained preparations

The general appearance of stellate cells has been described in detail based on light microscopy of the Golgi-stained preparations. However, the delicate structure of their processes has not been assessed. It is a very time-consuming task to reconstruct their remarkably arborizing processes from mountains of photomicrographs of serial thin sections taken with a conventional electron microscope. We therefore undertook an approach with a high-voltage electron microscope (HVEM) to survey their branching complexity.

The Golgi-stained preparations of hog liver were re-embedded in Epon, cut 4 μm thick, and examined under a JEM-1250 high-voltage electron microscope with an accelerating voltage of 1000 kV to yield a high-resolution study. Heavy depositions of metallic silver occurred innumerably in the cytoplasm, even at the most tapering ends (Figure 9). To our great surprise, we found numerous spines, which were more or less impregnated, protruding out laterally, erect or oblique, throughout the whole length of the perisinusoidal processes. To give a full

description, these spines assume the form of exceedingly attenuated processes which further break into elaborated tributaries. These hairy endings spread over the segment of the sinusoidal surface exposed between each pair of the perisinusoidal processes. The outer surface of the sinusoidal endothelium in this animal is, therefore, covered for the most part with an intricate meshwork of numerous fine processes perplexingly extended from the stellate cells.

Scanning electron microscopy of the stellate cells

Backscattered electron imaging of Golgi-stained preparations

Another attempt to visualize Golgi's silver-impregnated preparations at the electron microscopic level was done by the backscattered imaging of scanning electron microscopy (SEM). The backscattered imaging of silver-impregnated elements in the space of Disse was challenged[38]. However, since a different silver impregnation method was employed, the subendothelial processes of the stellate cells were not favourably demonstrated.

Golgi's sections, 50 μm in thickness, of rat liver were subjected to critical point-drying and were examined by SEM in the backscattered mode. The image of the stellate cells impregnated with silver revealed a high atomic number contrast in the surrounding tissue. Being heavily precipitated, the subendothelial processes with thorny outline, which lie on the other side of the endothelium, can be seen through the transparent wall of endothelium from the luminal surface (Figures 10 and 11). Lowering the accelerating voltage adequately will unmask the overlapped images of opposing semitransparent endothelial cells and subendothelial processes of the stellate cells (Figure 12). The subendothelial processes of stellate cells in rat liver show various patterns, but they are more or less angulated. They are also decorated with numerous spines which are similar in appearance to those of the hog liver as shown in Figure 9.

NaOH maceration method for SEM

The recently developed technique of the NaOH maceration method has provided a remarkably wider view of the stellate cells under SEM[39] (see also the text in the following chapter of this book). Treatment with NaOH facilitates the intercellular separation of the specimen and removes the reticular fibres to yield a desirable fracture along the space of Disse. This method is extremely useful in obtaining a direct stereoscopic visualization of the stellate cells with their long processes lying in a close relationship to the sinusoids and the hepatocytes (Figures 13 and 14). Although this technique does indeed contribute in exposing an extraordinarily wide surface of the stellate cells, it still seems to be unsatisfactory in visualizing the entire extent of these cells. Because, by this technique, only the fractured surface of the hepatic tissue is visualized under SEM, certain cytoplasmic processes, which spread deep under the sinusoid or in between the hepatocytes, are not visible.

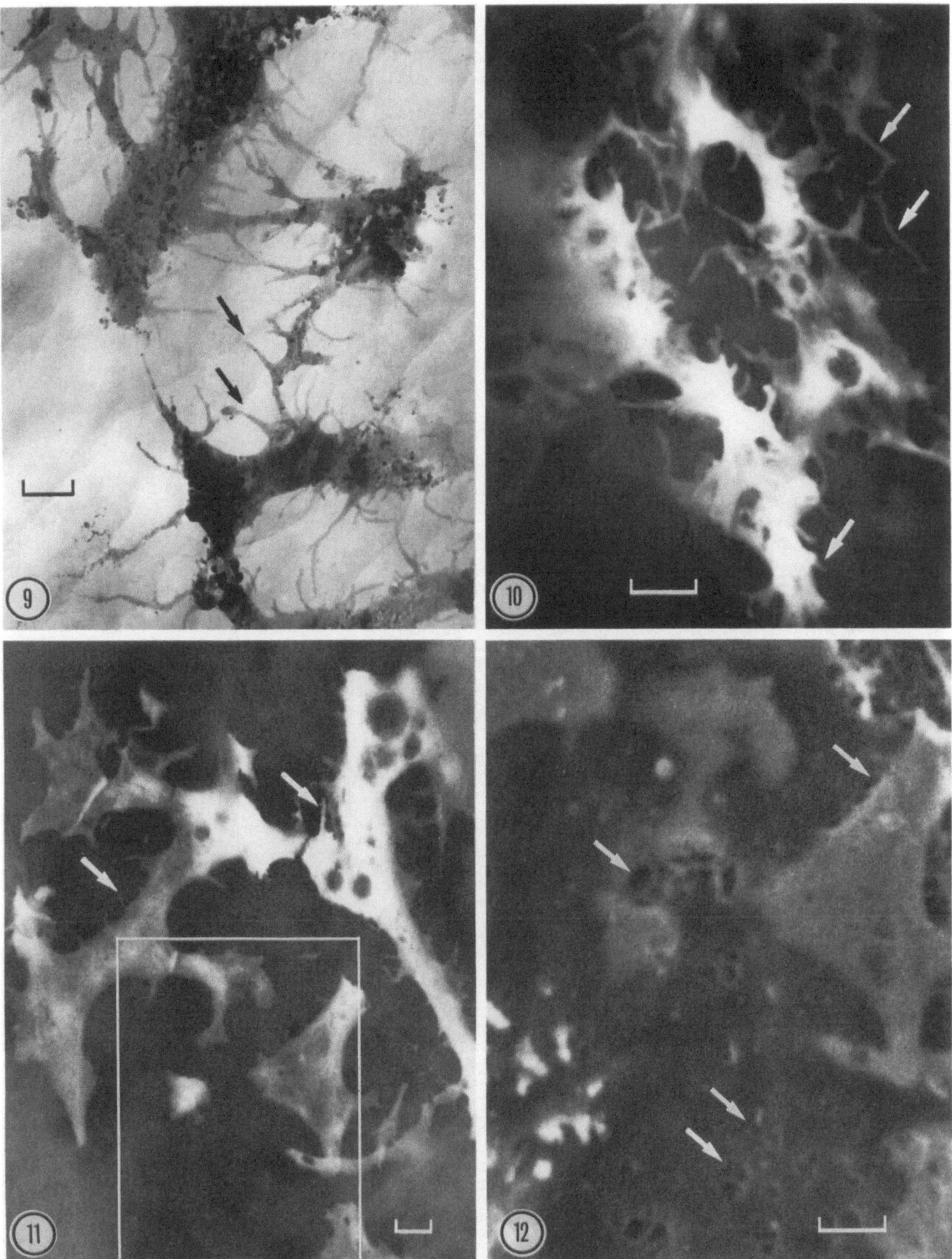

Figure 9   Electron micrograph of subendothelial processes (perisinusoidal processes) of the Golgi-stained stellate cell in hog liver. Arrows, spines. High-voltage electron microscopy with an accelerating voltage at 1000 kV. Bar, 1 μm (× 9000)

Figures 10 and 11   Backscattered electron imaging of Golgi-stained stellate cells in hog liver. Arrows, spines. SEM with an accelerating voltage at 20 kV. Bar, 1 μm (Figure 10, × 12 000; Figure 11, × 7000)

Figure 12   Backscattered electron imaging of a portion (rectangle) of Figure 11 with a lower accelerating voltage at 5 kV. Silver-stained subendothelial processes are seen through semitransparent endothelial cell. Arrows, fenestrae of the endothelial cell. Bar, 1 μm (× 13 000)

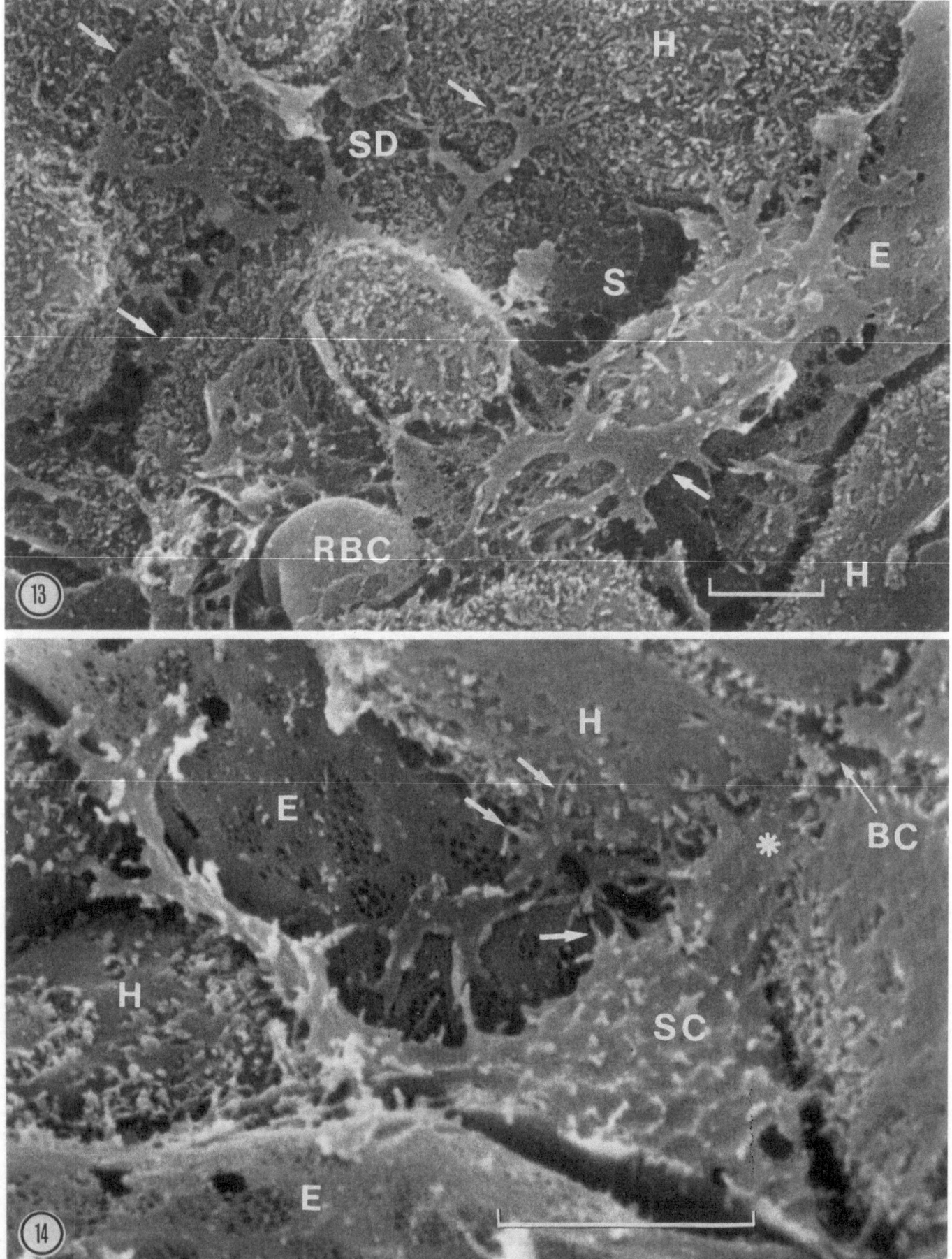

Figures 13 and 14 Scanning electron micrographs showing stellate cells (SC) of rat liver fractured after maceration with 6 mol L⁻¹ NaOH. Endothelial cells (E) of sinusoids (S) are surrounded by highly ramified subendothelial processes (arrows in Figure 13) decorated with numerous spines (arrows in Figure 14), some of which make contact with hepatocytes (H). A part of the cell body (asterisk) tapers off ahead to the vicinity of the bile canaliculus (BC). RBC, red blood corpuscle; SD, space of Disse. Bars, 5 μm (Figure 13, × 4400; Figure 14, × 9600)

DIFFERENTIATION OF STELLATE CELLS

Examination using the gold chloride method disclosed great diversity in the distribution of retinol-storing stellate cells in the body of the lamprey, *Lampetra japonica*. It is of particular interest, however, that there is definite unevenness in distribution. From available evidence concerning the distribution of the stellate cells in lower vertebrates, it is not unreasonable to conclude that the retinol-storing cells originate from the mesenchyme of the intermediate mesoderm and splanchnic mesoderm of the lateral mesoderm, while conventional fibroblasts are from the mesenchyme of the dorsal mesoderm and somatic mesoderm of the lateral mesoderm. We believe that the retinol-storing cells gradually decrease in number in the course of phylogenetic development, and accordingly, in mammals, these cells concentrate mostly in the hepatic lobules. After the administration of excess retinol, however, fibroblast-like cells inhabiting the extrahepatic splanchnic organs come to store retinol[40-44].

The pillar cells in the gill filaments of lamprey are curious in nature, since they possess both endothelial elements and contractile smooth muscle elements, and, furthermore, they also store retinol. These observed facts strongly support the concept that a number of cells in the retinol-storing cell lineages are interposed along a theoretical axis spanning between endothelial cells and smooth muscle cells[19]. The pillar cells are curious cells that possess characteristics of both endothelial cells and contractile smooth muscle cells. This aspect is backed in part by the presence of desmin in the stellate cells in liver[45].

Another piece of evidence concerning the differentiation of the stellate cells is a shift from stellate cells to myofibroblasts. The latter are located around the central vein and contain no lipid droplets in the cytoplasm under normal conditions. However, after the administration of excess retinol, they come to store it[19]. In addition, certain cytoplasmic processes of the myofibroblasts penetrate deeply into the space of Disse. Thus, it is difficult to draw a borderline between these two differently nominated cell types. Uninterrupted transformation in both directions from pericytes of the capillary walls to smooth muscle cells of arteries and veins was observed by Zimmermann[10] using Golgi's silver method. This configuration has recently been confirmed in the blood vessels of extrahepatic tissues macerated with $8 \, mol \, L^{-1} HCl$ by scanning electron microscopy[46].

RETINOL-STORAGE IN THE STELLATE CELLS

In order to determine metabolism of retinol in the liver, it is important that the different cells are obtained in a high yield. Several attempts to separate these cells by means of centrifugal elutriation of non-parenchymal cells prepared with pronase or pronase–collagenase[47], differential centrifugation in Percoll[48], and flow cytometry[49] have been made.

Chemical analysis of the lipid droplets in the isolated stellate cells shows that they are primarily involved in the storage of retinyl esters[50]. Furthermore, enzymes in retinol metabolism, i.e. retinyl palmitate hydrolase[51] and acyl-Co A:retinol acetyltransferase[52], are present in the stellate cells. Large amounts of cellular retinol-binding protein (CRBP)[52,53] and a low level of cellular retinoic acid-binding protein (CRABP)[52] are detected in both parenchymal and stellate cells. These binding-proteins appear to play a role in the intracellular transport of retinol and retinoic acid, respectively.

Evidence has been accumulated on the intercellular transport of retinol in the liver[54]. Following absorption of retinol in the intestine, it is transported in chylomicrons and their remnants in blood plasma and removed almost exclusively by the hepatic parenchymal cells[55]. In normal rats, about 50–60% of the retinoids taken up by the parenchymal cells is subsequently (after 2–4 h) transferred to the hepatic perisinusoidal stellate cells for storage[33]. The transport of retinoids from parenchymal to stellate cells appears to be mediated by binding proteins[56]. In vitamin A-deficient rats, retinol is not transferred to stellate cells but instead directed to extrahepatic tissue[54]. The amount of retinoids transferred to stellate cells could be regulated by the number of receptors for retinol-RBP on stellate cells[54].

The anatomical relationship between parenchymal cells and stellate cells *in situ* seems to be favourable for the transport of retinol to the stellate cells. The retinol-RBP complex in the blood stream or in the space of Disse, which has been released from the apposed parenchymal cells, may be taken up by the perisinusoidal processes of the stellate cells. The remarkably complex arborization of perisinusoidal processes and the abundance of minute spines are responsible for the enormously increased surface area of the stellate cells which can effectively absorb the retinol.

Another hypothesis is the direct transport of retinol-CRBP from the parenchymal cells to the stellate cells[54]. There is now, however, no conclusive morphological evidence that the stellate cells are concerned with direct transfer of retinol-CRBP from the parenchymal cells, though we frequently observe that spines or microvilli of the stellate cells are in contact with the surface of the parenchymal cells (Figures 13 and 14).

SYNTHESIS AND DEGRADATION OF COLLAGENS BY THE STELLATE CELLS

It is indisputably evident that the stellate cells produce collagens of type I, type III and Type IV *in vitro*[57-59]. In hepatic lobules, type I and type III collagens are found, by indirect immunofluorescent staining, to be distributed in perisinusoidal and interhepatocellular spaces[60]. In the rat liver, following CCl_4 intoxication, type I and type III collagens are detected in the dilated cisterns of rough endoplasmic reticulum of the stellate cells by immunoelectron microscopy[61]. After incubation of tissue blocks from the CCl_4-treated rat liver with [³H]proline, the incorporation of the radioisotope is observed over the well-developed rough endoplasmic reticulum and Golgi complex of the stellate cells[62]. Collagen synthesis by the stellate cells obtained from the CCl_4-treated rat liver is 4–6 times enhanced[59]. It is of particular interest that retinol treatment suppresses collagen synthesis in the liver[59,63]. Functional interference between retinol storage and collagen synthesis in the same cells is of paramount importance since it may lead to clinical approaches for the prevention and treatment of fibrosis and cirrhosis of human liver.

Little is known of the ultrastructure and molecular reorganization of collagens during degradation. Electron microscopic examinations of the liver and intestine in the lamprey, *Lampetra japonica*, caught during the stage of spawning migration in rivers, showed that collagen fibrils are digested and transformed to special lamellar bodies within the elongated lysosomes of the stellate cells[64]. Thus, the stellate cells, like fibroblasts, regulate collagen metabolism, producing and digesting collagens by themselves.

Acknowledgements

I should like to express my gratitude to Mr Kiyoyuki Motomatsu for skilful technical assistance and to Mr Akira Masuda for photographic work. I am equally indebted to Dr Wichai Ekataksin for checking the manuscript. Thanks are also due to Dr Osamu Matsubara, Department of Pathology, Tokyo Medical and Dental University, for providing human autopsy livers, and the members of the HVEM Laboratory of the Engineering Research Institute, University of Tokyo, for the use of its facilities. Thanks are also extended to Dr Haruki Senoo and Dr Kenji Kaneda for valuable discussions. This work was supported by a grant-in-Aid (58370001) from the Ministry of Education, Science, and Culture, Japan.

References

1. Kupffer, C. von. (1876). Ueber Sternzellen der Leber. Briefliche Mitteilung an Prof. Waldeyer. *Arch. Mikr. Anat.*, **12**, 353–358

2. Wake, K. (1980). Perisinusoidal stellate cells (fat-storing cells, interstitial cells, lipocytes), their related structure in and around the liver sinusoids, and vitamin A-storing cells in extrahepatic organs. In Bourne, G. H. and Danielli, J. F. (eds.) *International Review of Cytology*, Vol. 66, pp. 303–353. (New York: Academic Press)

3. Rothe, P. (1882). Ueber die Sternzellen der Leber. Inaug.-Dissertation Munich University

4. Wake, K. (1964). Distribution of vitamin A in the liver. In *Proceedings of The Fifth Annual General Meeting of the Japanese Histochemical Association*, p. 103

5. Wake, K. (1971). 'Sternzellen' in the liver: Perisinusoidal cells with special reference to storage of vitamin A. *Am. J. Anat.*, **132**, 429–462

6. Kupffer, C. von. (1898). Ueber Sternzellen der Leber. *Verh. Anat. Ges.*, **12** (Versammlung in Kiel), 80–86

7. Kupffer, C. von. (1899). Uber die sogenannten Sternzellen der Säugethierleber. *Arch. Mikr. Anat.*, **54**, 254–288

8. Berkley, H. J. (1893). Studies in the histology of the liver. III. The perivascular cells of the rabbit's liver. *Anat. Anz.*, **8**, 787–792

9. Dogiel, A. S. (1895). Zur Frage über die Ganglien der Darmgeflechte im den Säugetieren. *Anat. Anz.*, **10**, 517–528

10. Zimmermann, K. W. (1923). Der feinere Bau der Blut-capillaren, *Z. Anat.*, **68**, 29–109

11. Suzuki, K. (1958). A silver impregnation method in histology (Japanese text). In *The Experimental Therapy*, No. 310–320. (Osaka: Takeda Pharmaceutical Ind.)

12. Suzuki, K. (1963). The end apparatus of the vegetative nervous system. In *Proceedings of the sixteenth General Assembly of the Japan Medical Congress, Osaka*, Vol. 4, pp. 13–28

13. Ito, T. (1951). Cytological studies on stellate cells of Kupffer and fat storing cells in the capillary wall of the human liver. *Acta Anat. Nippon.*, **26**, 2

14. Ito, T. and Nemoto, M. (1956). Morphologische Studien über die 'Fettspeicherungszellen' der Leber bei verschiedenen Wirbeltieren. 1. Über die Fettspeicherungszellen der Huftiere. *Okajima Folia Anat. Jpn.*, **28**, 521–542

15. Yamagishi, M. (1959). Electron microscope studies on the fine structure of the sinusoidal wall and fat-storing cells of rabbit livers. *Arch. Histol. Jpn.*, **18**, 223–261

16. Nakane, P. K. (1963). Ito's 'fat-storing cell' of the mouse liver. *Anat. Rec.*, **145**, 265–266

17. Wake, K. (1974). Development of vitamin A-rich lipid droplets in multivesicular bodies of rat liver stellate cells. *J. Cell Biol.*, **63**, 683–691

18. Hirosawa, K. and Yamada, E. (1973). The localization of the vitamin A in the mouse liver as revealed by electron microscope radioautography. *J. Electron Microsc.*, **22**, 337–346

19. Wake, K. and Senoo, H. (1986). Morphological aspects of the differentiation of stellate cell line in the vertebrates. In Kirn, A., Knook, D. L. and Wisse, E. (eds.) *Cells of the Hepatic Sinusoid*, Vol. 1, pp. 215–220. (Rijswijk: Kupffer Cell Foundation)

20. Aterman, K. (1986). The parasinusoidal cells of the liver: A historical account. *Histochem. J.*, **18**, 279–305

21. Wisse, E., van't Noordende, J. M., van der Meulen, J. and Daems, W. Th. (1976). The pit cell: Description of a new type of cell occurring in rat liver sinusoids and peripheral blood. *Cell Tiss. Res.*, **173**, 423–435

22. Kaneda, K. and Wake, K. (1983). Distribution and morphological characteristics of the pit cells in the liver of the rat. *Cell Tiss. Res.*, **233**, 485–505

23. Kaneda, K., Dan, C. and Wake, K. (1983). Pit cells as natural killer cells. *Biomed. Res.*, **4**, 567–576

24. Dan, C., Kaneda, K. and Wake, K. (1985). A striking increase in rod-cored vesicles in pit cells (natural killer cells) and augmentation of the liver-associated natural killer activity by a streptococcal preparation (OK-432). *Biomed. Res.*, **6**, 347–351

25. Wake, K., Motomatsu, K., Senoo, H., Masuda, A. and Adachi, E. (1986) Improved Kupffer's gold chloride method for the demonstration of the stellate cells storing retinol (vitamin A) in the liver and extrahepatic organs of vertebrates. *Stain Technol.*, **61**, 193–200

26. Wake, K. (1973). Cytochemistry of the lipid droplets containing vitamin A in the liver. In Wisse, E., Daems, W. Th., Molenaar, I. and Kuijin, P. van (eds.) Electron microscopy and Cytochemistry. *Proceedings of the Second International Symposium on Electron Microscopy and Cytochemistry*, p. 279. (Amsterdam: North-Holland Publishing Co.)

27. Wake, K. (1982). The Sternzellen of von Kupffer – After 106 years. In Knook, D. L. and Wisse, E. (eds.) *Sinusoidal Liver Cells*, pp. 1–12. (Amsterdam: Elsevier Biomedical Press)

28. Yamamoto, K., Sargent, P. A., Fisher, M. M. and Youson, J. H. (1986). Periductal fibrosis and lipocytes (fat-storing cells or Ito cells) during biliary atresia in the lamprey. *Hepatology*, **6**, 54–59

29. Wake, K., Motomatsu, K. and Senoo, H. (1987). Stellate cells storing retinol in the liver of adult lamprey, *Lampetra japonica*. *Cell Tiss. Res.*, **249**, 289–299

30. Bertolini, B. (1965). The structure of the liver cells during

the life cycle of a brook-lamprey (*Lampetra zanandreai*). *Z. Zellforsch.*, 67, 297–318

31. Shin, Y. C. (1977). Some observations on the fine structure of lamprey liver as revealed by electron microscopy. *Okajima Fol. Anat. Jpn.*, 54, 25–60

32. Peek, W. D., Sidon, E. W., Youson, J. H. and Fisher, M. M. (1979). Fine structure of the liver in the larval lamprey, Petromyson marinus, hepatocytes and sinusoids. *Am. J. Anat.*, 156, 231–250

33. Blomhoff, R., Holte, K., Naess, L. and Berg, T. (1984). Newly administered ³H-retinol is transferred from hepatocytes to stellate cells in liver for storage. *Exp. Cell Res.*, 150, 186–193

34. Wake, K. and Motomatsu, K. (1986). Sinusoidal endothelial cells in rat liver made visualized individually by the Golgi method. In Kirn, A., Knook, D. L. and Wisse, E. (eds.) *Cells of the Hepatic Sinusoid*, pp. 523–524. (Rijswijk: Kupffer Cell Foundation)

35. Ito, T. and Shibasaki, S. (1968). Electron microscopic study on the hepatic sinusoidal wall and fat-storing cells in the normal human liver. *Arch. Histol. Jpn.*, 29, 137–192

36. Ito, T. (1973). Recent advances in the study on the fine structure of the hepatic sinusoidal wall. *Gumma Rep. Med. Sci.*, 6, 119–163

37. Yamada, E. (1982). Vitamin A storing cell. *Meth. Enzymol.*, 81, 834–839

38. Vonnahme, F. J. (1982). The structure and function of subendothelial processes of perisinusoidal cells in human liver disease. In Knook, D. L. and Wisse, E. (eds.) *Sinusoidal Liver Cells*, pp. 13–20. (Amsterdam: Elsevier Biomedical Press)

39. Takahashi-Iwanaga, H. and Fujita, T. (1986). Application of an NaOH maceration method to a scanning electron microscopic observation of Ito cells in the rat liver. *Arch. Histol. Jpn.*, 49, 349–357

40. Hirosawa, K. and Yamada, E. (1975). Vitamin A storing cells; An electron microscope radioautographic study. *Proceedings of The Tenth International Congress of Anatomists*, p. 482

41. Yamada, E. and Hirosawa, K. (1976). The possible existence of a vitamin A-storing cell system. *Cell Struct. Funct.*, 1, 201–204

42. Hirosawa, K. (1977). A note on autoradiography: An introduction of vitamin A-storing cells. *Acta Histochem. Cytochem.*, 10, 253–259

43. Kusumoto, Y. and Fujita, T. (1977). Vitamin A uptake cells distributed in the liver and other organs of the rat. *Arch. Histol. Jpn.*, 40, 121–136

44. Yamamoto, M. and Enzan, H. (1975). Morphology and function of Ito cell (fat-storing cell) in the liver. *Recent Adv. RES Res.*, 15, 54–75

45. Yokoi, Y., Namithisa, T., Kuroda, H., Komatsu, I., Miyazaki, A., Watanabe, S. and Usui, K. (1984). Immunohistochemical detection of desmin in fat-storing cells (Ito cell). *Hepatology*, 4, 709–714

46. Uehara, Y. and Suyama, K. (1978). Visualization of the adventitial aspect of the vascular smooth muscle cells under the scanning electron microscope. *J. Electron Microsc.*, 27, 157–159

47. Knook, D. L., Praaning-Van Dalen, D. P. and De Leeuw, A. M. (1986). Selection criteria for the choice of isolation methods for rat liver Kupffer, endothelial and fat-storing cells. In Kirn, A., Knook, D. L. and Wisse, E. (eds.) *Cells*

of the Hepatic Sinusoid, Vol. 1, pp. 445–450. (Rijswijk: Kupffer Cell Foundation)

48. Pertoft, H. and Smedsrod, B. (1986). The use of percoll gradients to purify hepatocytes and sinusoidal cells from rat liver. In Kirn, A., Knook, D. L. and Wisse, E. (eds.) *Cells of the Hepatic Sinusoid*, Vol. 1, pp. 471–472. (Rijswijk: Kupffer Cell Foundation)

49. Tanaka, Y., Hirata, R., Minato, Y., Hasumura, Y. and Takeuchi, J. (1986). Isolation and higher purification of fat-storing cells from rat liver with flow cytometry. In Kirn, A., Knook, D. L. and Wisse, E. (eds.) *Cells of the Hepatic Sinusoid*, Vol. 1, p. 473. (Rijswijk: Kupffer Cell Foundation)

50. Brouwer, A., Hendriks, H. F. J., Brekelmans, P., Buijtenhek, M. and Knook, D. L. (1986). Lipid analysis of different types of isolated liver cells and their lipid droplets. In Kirn, A., Knook, D. L. and Wisse, E. (eds.) *Cells of the Hepatic Sinusoid*, Vol. 1, pp. 175–180. (Rijswijk: Kupffer Cell Foundation)

51. Hendriks, H. F. J., Blaner, W. S., Wennekers, H. M., Brouwer, A., De Leeuw, A. M., Goodman, D. S. and Knook, D. L. (1986). Distribution of retinoids, some retinoid binding proteins and retinyl palmitate hydrolase activity in different cell types isolated from young and old rats. In Kirn, A., Knook, D. L. and Wisse, E. (eds.) *Cells of the Hepatic Sinusoid*, Vol. 1, pp. 201–205. (Rijswijk: Kupffer Cell Foundation)

52. Blomhoff, R., Rasmussen, M., Nilsson, A., Norum, K. R., Berg, T., Blaner, W. S., Kato, M., Mertz, J. R., Goodman, D. S., Eriksson, U. and Peterson, P. A. (1985). Distribution of retinoids, enzymes, and binding proteins in isolated rat liver cells. *J. Biol. Chem.*, 260, 13560–13565

53. Kato, M., Kato, K. and Goodman, D. S. (1984). Immunocytochemical studies in the localization of plasma and of cellular retinol-binding proteins and of transthyretin (prealbumin) in rat liver and kidney. *J. Cell Biol.*, 98, 1969–1704

54. Blomhoff, R. (1985), Transport and hepatic metabolism of retinol in the rat. *Inaug.-Dissertation*, Oslo University

55. Blomhoff, R., Eskild, W., Kindberg, G. M., Pryds, K. and Berg, T. (1985). Intracellular transport of endocytosed chylomicron [³H]retinyl ester in rat liver parenchymal cells. Evidence for translocation of a [³H]retinoid from endosomes to endoplasmic reticulum. *J. Biol. Chem.*, 260, 13566–13570

56. Blomhoff, R., Norum, K. R. and Berg, T. (1985). Hepatic uptake of [³H]retinol bound to the serum retinol binding protein involves both parenchymal and perisinusoidal stellate cells. *J. Biol. Chem.*, 260, 13571–13575

57. Senoo, H., Hata, R., Nagai, Y. and Wake, K. (1984). Stellate cells (vitamin A-storing cells) are the primary site of collagen synthesis in non-parenchymal cells in the liver. *Biomed. Res.*, 5, 451–458

58. Friedman, S. L., Roll, F. J. and Bissell, D. M. (1986). Collagen phenotype of rat hepatocytes in pure primary culture. In Kirn, A., Knook, D. L. and Wisse, E. (eds.) *Cells of the Hepatic Sinusoid*, Vol. 1, pp. 255–256. (Rijswijk: Kupffer Cell Foundation)

59. Shiratori, Y., Geerts, A., Ichida, T. and Wisse, E. (1986). Collagen production and Kupffer cell-modulated proliferation of fat-storing cells in culture. In Kirn, A., Knook, D. L. and Wisse, E. (eds.) *Cells of the Hepatic Sinusoid*, Vol. 1, pp. 239–244. (Rijswijk: Kupffer Cell Foundation)

60. Senoo, H., Hata, R., Nagai, Y. and Wake, K. (1986). Assembly and metabolism of collagen in the liver. In Kirn,

A., Knook, D. L. and Wisse, E. (eds.) *Cells of the Hepatic Sinusoid*, Vol. 1, pp. 227–232. (Rijswijk: Kupffer Cell Foundation)

61. Takahara, T., Kojima, T., Miyabayashi, C., Kubota, T., Matsui, S., Inoue, K., Sasaki, H. and Ooshima, A. (1986). Production of type I and type III collagens in fat-storing cells of the rat liver following carbon tetrachloride intoxication: Immunoelectron microscopic study. In *Proceedings of the Eleventh International Congress on Electron Microscopy*, Kyoto, p. 2697

62. Enzan, H. and Hara, H. (1986). Ito cells (fat-storing cells) and collagen formation in carbon tetrachloride-induced liver fibrosis. A light and electron microscopic auto-radiographic study using ^{3}H-proline as a tracer. In Kirn, A., Knook, D. L. and Wisse, E. (eds.) *Cells of the Hepatic Sinusoid*, Vol. 1, pp. 233–238. (Rijswijk: Kupffer Cell Foundation)

63. Senoo, H. and Wake, K. (1985). Suppression of experimental hepatic fibrosis by administration of vitamin A. *Lab. Invest.*, 52, 182–194

64. Wake, K., Kamino, T., Ueki, Y. and Nagai, Y. (1986). Endocytosis and degradation of collagen fibrils by vitamin A-storing cells in the liver and intestine of the lamprey. *Proceedings of the Eleventh International Congress on Electron Microscopy*, Kyoto, p. 1941

4

Scanning electron microscopy of the liver cells

G. MACCHIARELLI, P. M. MOTTA and T. FUJITA

INTRODUCTION

Seen by scanning electron microscopy (SEM), the adult mammalian liver appears to be a parenchymatous organ in which five principal types of fixed cells, each with specific morphofunctional features, are integrated to form a highly complex structure[1,2]. These cells may be classified as follows:

(1) Epithelial parenchymal cells, or **hepatocytes,** arranged in one-cell-thick laminae dispersed between the portal space and the central vein;

(2) Epithelial **biliary cells** making up the monolayered wall of the biliary ductules and biliary ducts;

(3) **Endothelial cells** which, with their large and fenestrated cytoplasmic extensions, contribute toward the structural formation of the wall of the liver capillaries (the sinusoids);

(4) **Kupffer cells,** which are the fixed macrophages within the liver sinusoids; and

(5) **Perisinusoidal cells** (stellate, fat-storing or Ito cells), commonly found within the perisinusoidal space or space of Disse.

A further type of hepatic sinusoidal cell (**pit cell**) may be observed by means of transmission electron microscopy (TEM)[3-5]. However, since these cells do not have particular surface features which render them readily differentiable from other sinusoidal cells, they will not be taken into consideration in this chapter.

In addition, by means of SEM, it is possible to study the cells of the liver's peritoneal covering, i.e. the **mesothelial cells,** which, although they are not true liver components, nevertheless have an important role in physiological and pathological processes occurring in the liver[6,7].

Although all of these cell types may be isolated and studied separately, the spatial relationship existing among them will be given special emphasis in this chapter. A precise understanding of the three-dimensional arrangement and orientation of cells within tissues is, in fact, the basis for a better appreciation of the connections between morphology and function in such a complex organ as the liver[1,2]. Nevertheless, the full comprehension of this subject has always represented a challenge to researchers.

In past centuries, many anatomists turned to the creation of diagrams in an attempt to delineate tissue architecture and cell morphology of the liver. More recently, light microscopy (LM) and TEM have revealed many of the microanatomical structures, although a view of the tissue architecture itself was realized only through the graphic representations attempted by ingenious microscopists[2]. Today, SEM, more than any other microscopic technique, may offer readily interpretable images of the disposition of cells within tissues through improvement of the two-dimensional views originally furnished by LM and TEM[7]. This has been clearly confirmed by the recent history of liver morphology studies[2]. In fact, the first publication of scanning electron micrographs of liver lobules and hepatocytes[8] represented a turning point in liver microscopy research. This and other pioneer papers[9-15] undoubtedly helped researchers to rise above previous difficulties in obtaining three-dimensional views of the liver from histological sections. However skilful plastic models, such as those by Braus and Vierling[16], Elias[17,18] and, more recently, Elias and Sherrick[19], are still considered valid.

Since Fujita's first SEM atlas[8], many technological advances have allowed us to obtain more easily a vast amount of information concerning the liver's three-dimensional microstructure, both in humans and animals, fully described in review papers[2,6,7,20-24] as well as in SEM atlases[1,25-27]. These publications have contributed significantly towards the formulation of a realistic three-dimensional view of hepatic microstructure.

The present chapter will compare the data reported in the above-mentioned literature with the most recent information available. The aim is to offer an updated overview of liver cell morphology through a series of three-dimensional diagrams and images derived from normal human and animal specimens prepared according to the most recent SEM techniques[24].

LIVER ARCHITECTURE

Spatial relationship between liver vascular components and hepatic laminae

Numerous variables may play a role in determining the lobular arrangement of the hepatic tissue unit. Factors, such as species, race, course of vessels and number of connective fibres accompanying these vessels, the level of activity in the particular area of the liver being examined, as well as individual pathological processes, may all have various significant effects on the microscopic architecture of the hepatic lobule, or acinus[1].

Since the role of the above factors will be further considered in Chapter 8; here we will simply mention the three types of glandular or tissue units, which are: (1) the classic lobule[28]; (2) the portal lobule[29]; and (3) the hepatic acinus[30]. It should be stressed that all three units share valid morphological significance, both from a physiological and pathological point of view, and that their histological demonstration may be attained through SEM. In fact, the three-dimensional SEM study of properly dissociated specimens and of vascular corrosion casts allows ready identification of the individual structures (i.e. portal vessels, terminal hepatic veins, hepatic laminae, sinusoidal lacunae) making up the histological unit and their spatial inter-relationships. Therefore, by SEM, Elias' plate theory[17-19] on the orientation of hepatic cells can be easily confirmed[2].

In mammals, the hepatic laminae are composed of one-cell-thick columns of polyhedral cells and are placed in such a way as to form a spongy structure which is perforated by a system of communicating cavities (Figures 1 and 2). It is in these cavities, the vascular lacunae, that the hepatic sinusoids are contained (Figure 2; Plate 1a)[1,20,21,24,31-35].

Hepatic laminae and vascular lacunae connect the portal spaces with the centrolobular veins (Figure 1), thus constituting the matrix of the hepatic lobule, whereas the interlobular bile ducts and central veins make up the axes of this matrix. Naturally, this system should not be considered a static one. The close spatial relationships existing between hepatic laminae and vascular lacunae confer a certain plasticity and flexibility upon the hepatic architecture. Therefore, physiological and pathological considerations aside, and looking at it from a purely morphological point of view, the hepatic lobule can assume various aspects (classic lobule, portal lobule or acinus), depending on the changes in the blood pressure gradients within the ramifications of the hepatic veins and the consequent variations of blood flow through the sinusoids[1].

Portal space and interlobular vessels

Seen by SEM, the portal space may be easily recognized by its fundamental components (portal triad) (Figure 3), both in longitudinal and transverse sections[2].

The interlobular biliary duct (Figure 3), which is connected with the bile canalicular net through the bile ductules (Figure 4), is composed of cuboidal epithelial cells. The absorptive/secretive properties of these cells are shown by the numerous microvilli that cover the cell surface towards the canalicular lumen (Figures 5 and 6)[36]. Microvilli are often arranged in longitudinal rows (Figure 5) which sometimes clearly define the polygonal shape of the epithelial cells[1,24,37]. The microvilli may also be seen dispersed all over the cell surface (Figure 6). Usually, from the centre of each cell, emerges a single long cilium which perhaps plays a role in the drainage of bile (Figure 6)[36].

The ramification of the portal vein usually appears as a large vessel (Figures 1 and 3), having a slender wall mainly formed by a few layers of smooth muscle cells. The wall of the hepatic portal veins contains numerous openings in the sinusoidal net. The inner surface shows a flat endothelium composed of irregularly polygonal cells which are occasionally elongated. At high magnification, the surfaces of these cells often present pinocytotic vesicles and small microvillous projections, difficult to distinguish from small blebs (Figure 10)[24].

The hepatic artery branch is easily distinguishable from the other components of the triad because of the considerable thickness shown by its muscular wall and the consequent reduction in luminal dimensions (Figure 3). In addition, its smooth, elongated endothelial cells, usually arranged in longitudinal columns, are endowed with pronounced cell margins that often overlap those of adjacent cells (Figure 11)[24].

Under SEM, the lymphatic vessels may be identified by their thin wall and small calibre (Figure 3). As a rule, within the portal space, there is more than a single lymph channel running parallel to the components of the portal triad[38]. As seen in vascular corrosion casts[39], the straight lymph vessels anastomose short side branches which form a network surrounding the portal tract. The terminal branches are blind-ended and are likely to have valves[39]. The lymphatic endothelial covering is composed of small polygonal cells, having a smooth, flat surface (see Chapter 7).

Connective tissue fibres are dispersed among the vascular and biliary elements of the portal space (Figures 3 and 4). Their quantity is variable, according to species and race, usually in smaller amounts in humans. These connective fibres surround the aforementioned elements and also delimit between them wide and tortuous spaces (spaces of Mall) (Figure 1) which may exert a function in the collection of interstitial fluid[1,20].

Interspersed between the connective fibres may be found nerve bundles[40,41] which, although easily recognized in TEM or LM sections, do not present characteristic superficial features that render them easily identifiable by conventional SEM[2]. Nerve terminations probably reach the perisinusoidal spaces[42] and contact hepatocytes[41,43,44] or even perisinusoidal cells[41,43]. (See Chapter 6).

SEM of vascular corrosion casts have allowed the demonstration of a capillary plexus (peribiliary plexus)[45,46] supplied by the terminal hepatic arteries which anastomose portal vein branches and sinusoids[47,48]. This structure mainly surrounds the bile duct and is likely to have a role in the control of bile production[1,45,49]. Full details of peribiliary plexus are described in Chapter 7.

Centrolobular veins

The centrolobular vein, or terminal ramus of the hepatic vein, through the interposition of sinusoids, constitutes the common drainage route of arterial and venous tributaries of the intrahepatic vascular tree. The centrolobular vein is found at the centre of the classic lobule and is drained by the sublobular veins (Figure 1). These vessels, too, present particular ultrastructural characteristics which facilitate identification by SEM (Figures 1, 7–9)[24].

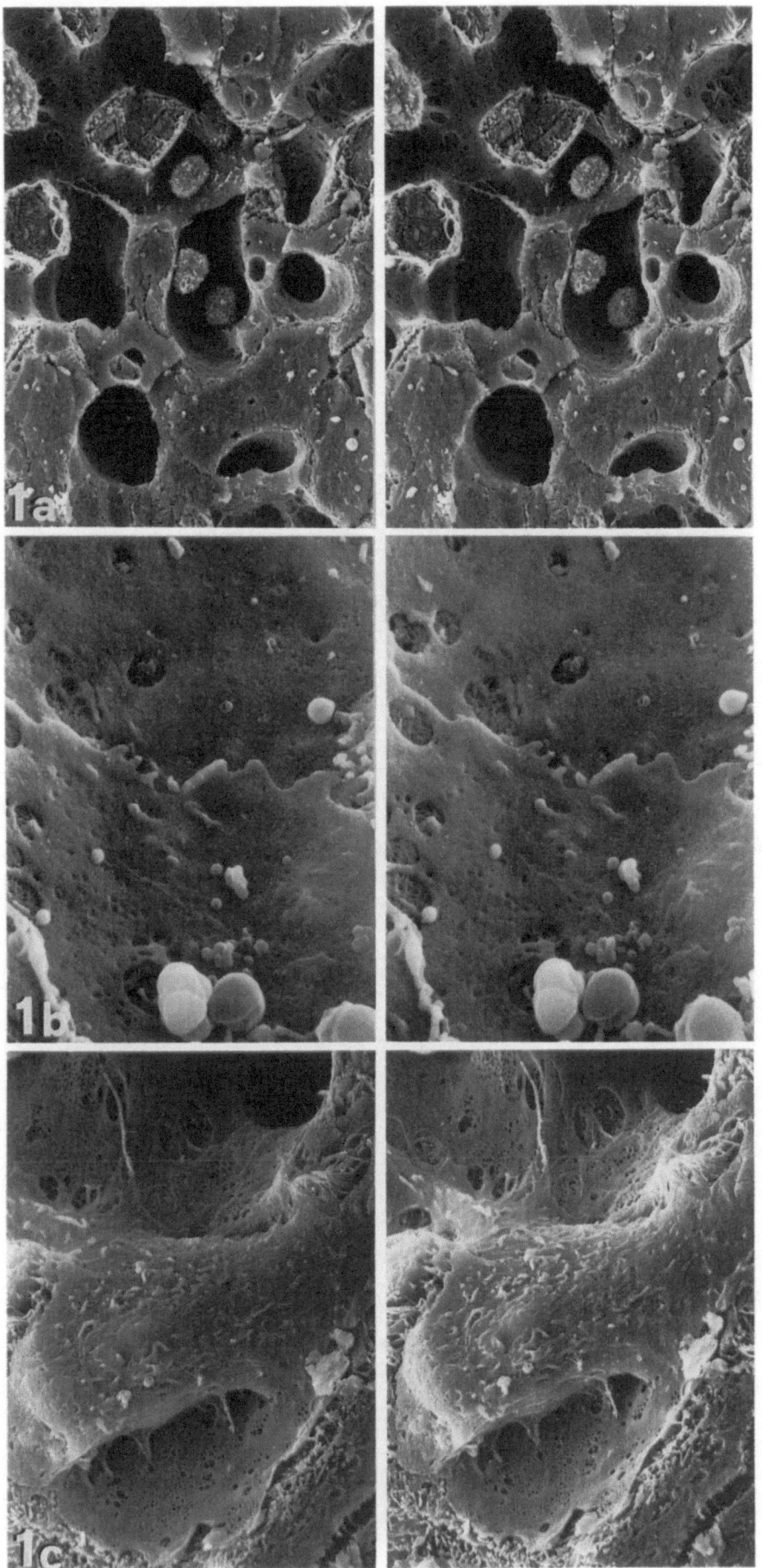

Plate 1 Vascular lacunae and sinusoidal cell: stereo pictures   a = vascular lacunae. Note the tortuous arrangement of sinusoids and the relationship between blood cells, Kupffer cell and endothelium.
   b = sinusoidal endothelium. The overlapped border of two endothelial cells is evident.
   c = Kupffer cell body. Note the small projections on the cell body and the relationship between filopodia and endothelium

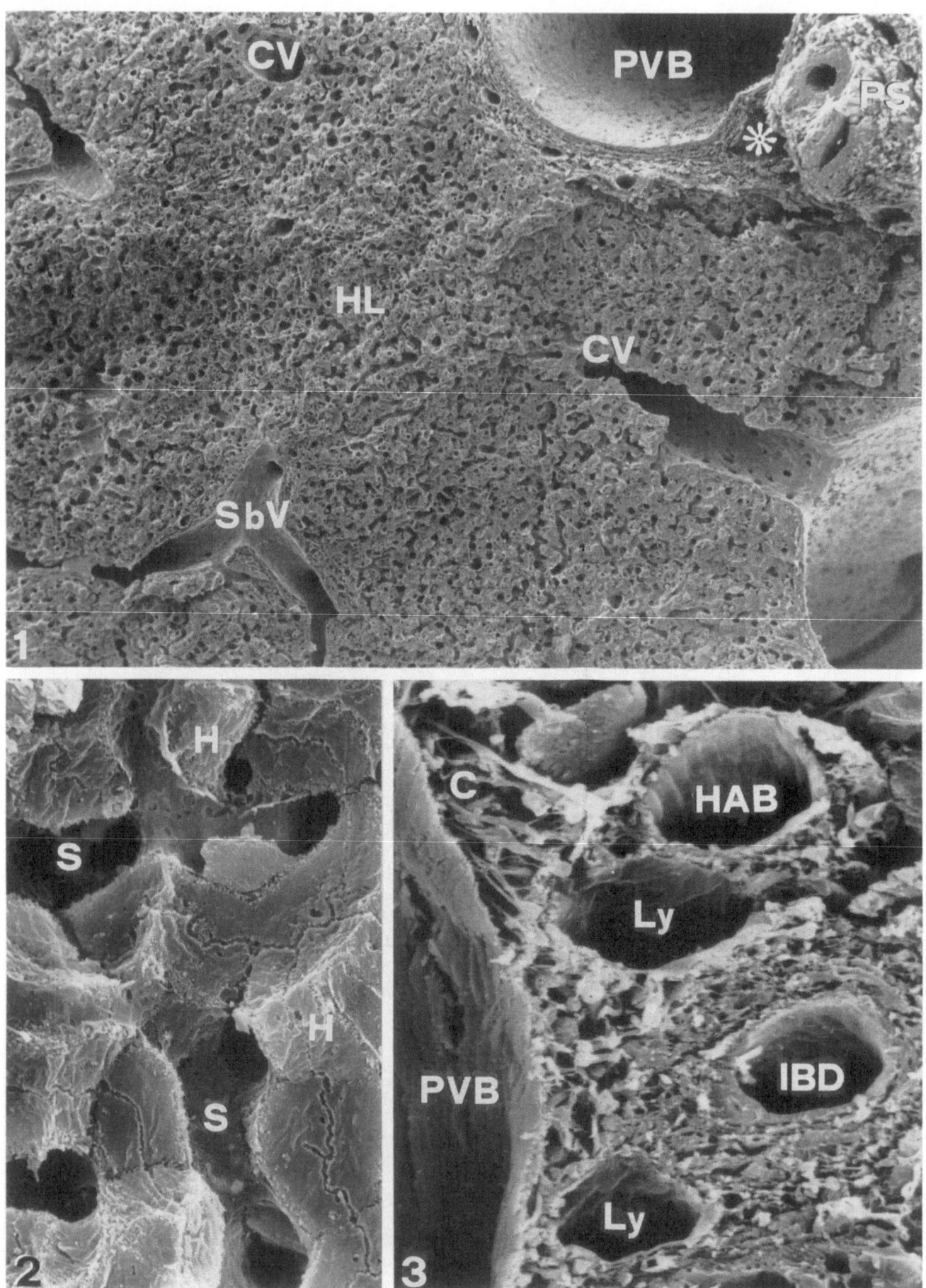

Figure 1 Liver parenchyma The spatial relationships between the vascular components of the liver lobules – portal vein branch (PVB), centrolobular vein (CV), sublobular vein (SbV), sinusoids – and the hepatic laminae (HL) are clearly shown. PS = portal space; * = space of Mall. (× 160, cat). (From Motta *et al*. 1978)[1]

Figure 2 Hepatic laminae In mammalians, the hepatocytes (H) are arranged in one-cell-thick laminae separated by the vascular lacunae which contain the sinusoids (S). (× 2000, praomys)

Figure 3 Portal space Cross-section of a portal space showing vascular and bile components. PVB = portal vein branch; HAB = hepatic artery branch; IBD = interlobular bile duct; Ly = Lymph vessels; C = connective fibres. (× 400, rat). (From Macchiarelli and Motta, 1986)[24]

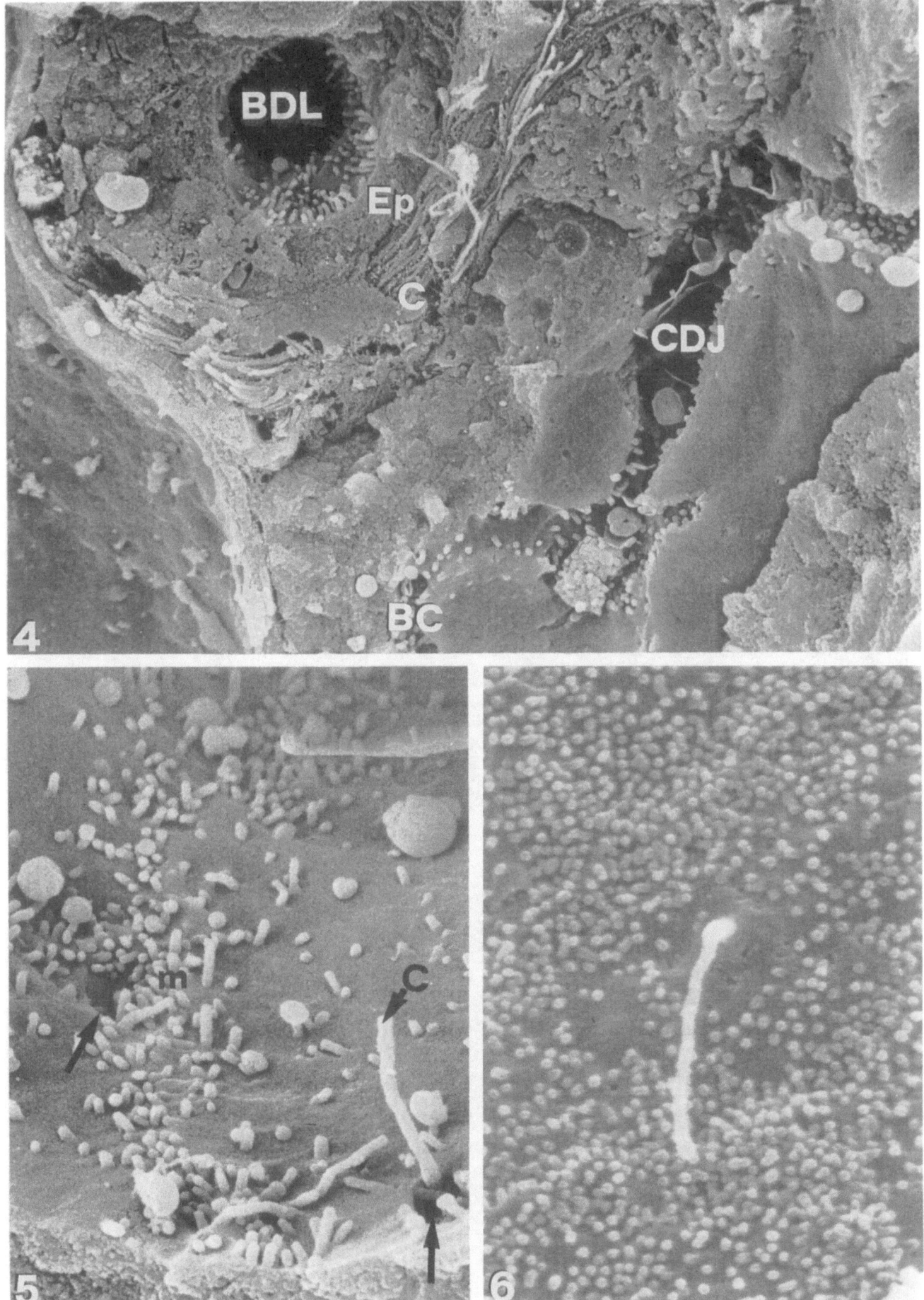

Figure 4 Bile ductule and canalicular–ductular junction The bile canaliculi (BC) through the interposition of the canalicular–ductular junction (CDJ) drain into the bile ductules (BDL) (see also Diagram 2). Note the collagen fibres (C) surrounding the epithelial cells (Ep) of the bile ductule. (× 1000, pig). (From Marinozzi *et al.*, 1977)[37]

Figure 5 Interlobular bile duct: inner surface A longitudinal row of microvilli (m) may be seen on the luminal surface of the bile duct epithelial cells. The holes (arrows) probably correspond to openings in the bile canaliculi directly connected with the interlobular bile duct. (× 30 000; pig). (From Marinozzi *et al.*, 1977)[37]

Figure 6 Interlobular bile duct: inner surface Note the large amount of microvilli dispersed over the cell. A long cilium arises from the central area of the epithelial cell. (× 30 000; praomys)

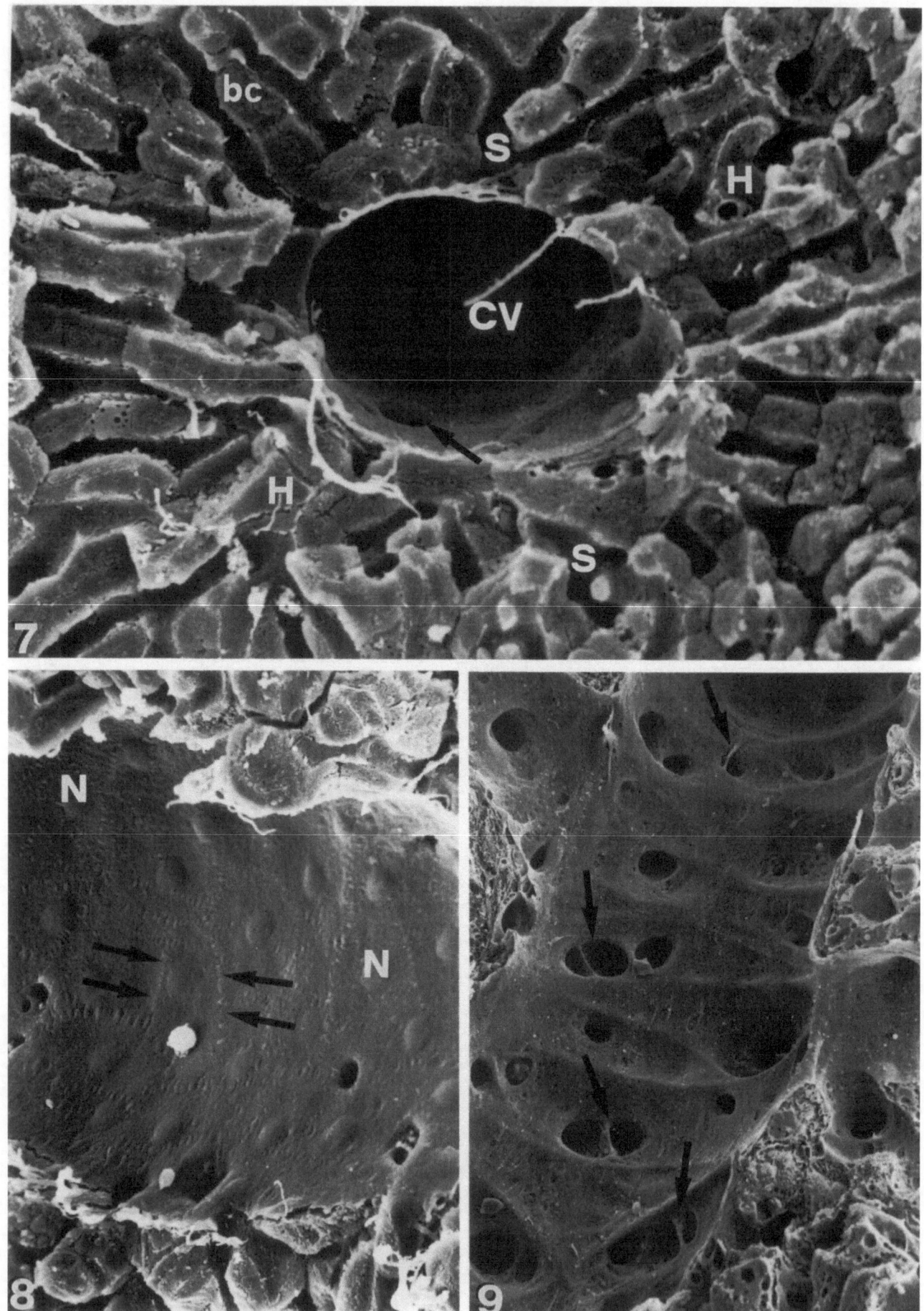

Figure 7   Centrolobular vein: cross-section   A centrolobular vein (CV) is seen at the centre of radiating laminae of hepatocytes (H). Note the thin wall of this vessel. Arrow = sinusoidal inlet; bc = bile canaliculi; S = sinusoids. (× 1500; rat) (From Macchiarelli and Motta, 1986)[24]

Figure 8   Centrolobular vein: longitudinal section   The flat endothelial cells present a central round bulge due to the nuclear protrusion. Arrows indicate cell borders; N = nuclei; * = white blood cells. (× 1000; praomys)

Figure 9   Centrolobular vein: longitudinal section   Note the numerous sinusoidal openings crossed by bridging structures (arrows). (× 900; cat)

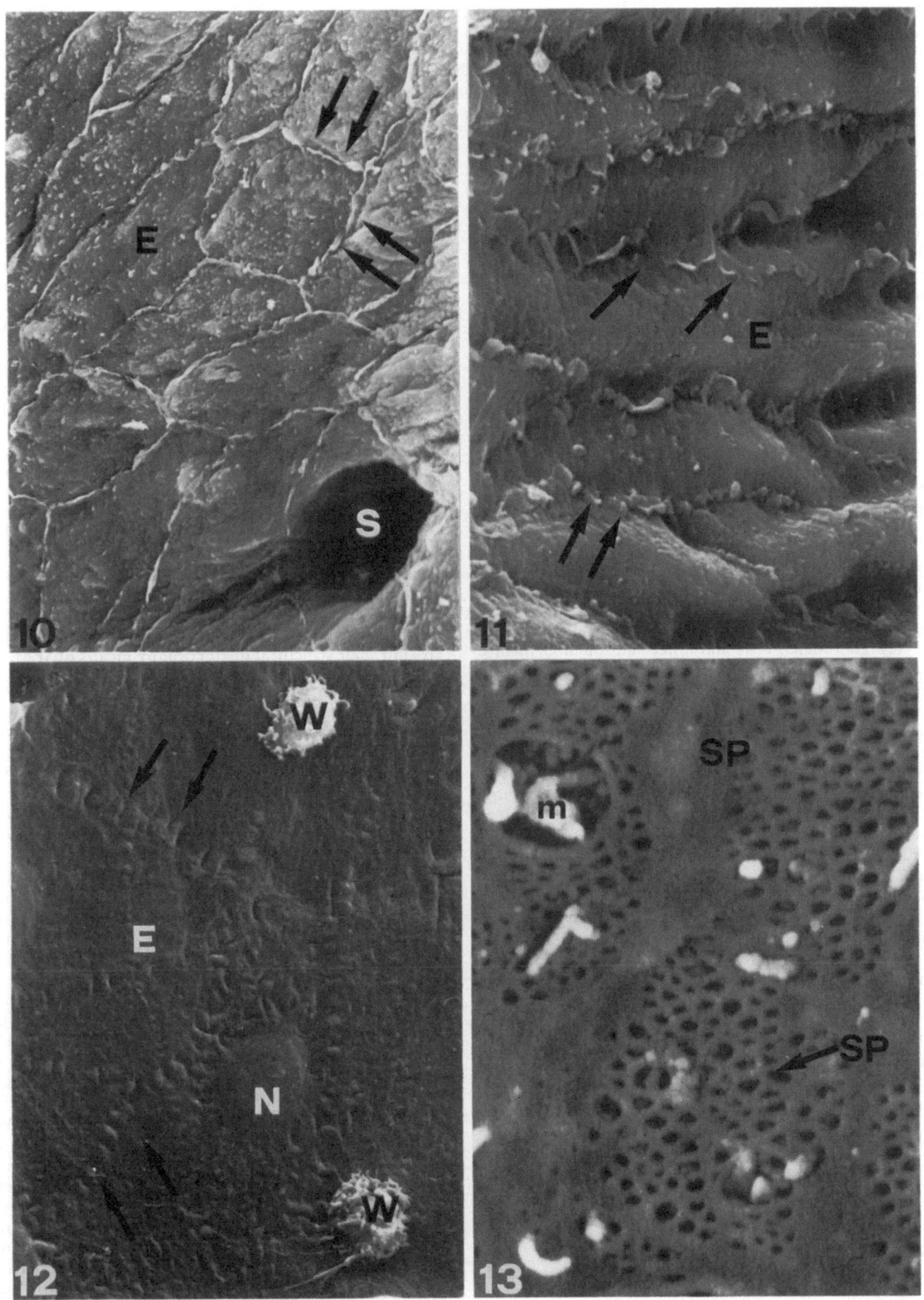

Figures 10–13 Liver endothelia The liver endothelial cells (E) change morphology from vessel to vessel. Arrows indicate cell borders. S = sinusoidal opening; N = nuclei; W = white blood cell; SP = sieve plates; m = hepatocyte's microvilli. **Figure 10** = portal vein branch (× 2500). **Figure 11** = hepatic artery branch (× 3300). **Figure 12** = centrolobular vein (× 3000). **Figure 13** = sinusoid (× 30 000). (Rat.) (From Macchiarelli and Motta, 1986)[24]

Unicellular laminae of hepatocytes, intercalated with the sinusoidal lacunae, seem to radiate outwards from the centrally placed vein (Figure 7)[1]. The vein possesses a thin wall composed of one or two layers of smooth muscle cells, and is perforated by numerous sinusoidal tributaries (Figures 8 and 9). These sinusoidal openings are often of smaller dimensions than those seen in branches of the portal vein and are sometimes crossed by connective tissue structures covered by slender evagination of fenestrated endothelium (sinusoidal bridges) (Figure 9)[35]. These bridging structures, also found within the sinusoids, perhaps play a regulatory role in sinusoidal blood flow[24]. The endothelial cells, which are round, smooth and extremely flat (Figure 8), show a central bulge due to the presence of the nucleus (Figure 12). Leukocytes or macrophages (migrating macrophages) are frequently found adherent to the surface of the endothelium (Figures 8 and 12).

LIVER SINUSOIDS

The three-dimensional structure of liver capillaries

The liver sinusoids, being the specialized hepatic capillaries where the primary role of the liver microcirculation is carried out[50], represent the speculative fulcrum of three-dimensional liver investigations. In fact, from observations of the specific spatial relationships between hepatocytes, endothelial cells and other sinusoidal elements, much basic useful knowledge relevant to the function of the 'hepatic machine' has been gleaned.

When studied in fractured samples or corroded vascular casts, sinusoids are clearly seen to anastomose the vessels of the portal space with the centrolobular veins (Figure 1) and appear to be dispersed throughout the lacunae present between the hepatocytic laminae (Figure 2; Plate 1a)[2,6,20,51,52]. Indeed, hepatic capillaries show a characteristic tortuosity; hence the term **sinusoids**. Thus, the sinusoids create a three-dimensional network of vascular and perivascular spaces which offers a huge surface for blood–hepatocyte exchanges[14,50,53].

Under SEM, the sinusoids show three fundamental sinusoidal cell types[2,4,5,54,55]: (1) endothelial cells (Figure 13; Plate 1b); (2) **Kupffer cells** (Figures 14–17; Plate 1c); and (3) **perisinusoidal cells** (Figures 18 and 19) which together form a functional system operating in the control of the exchanges between blood and hepatocytes (Diagram 1). The sinusoidal cells, in fact, due to their close spatial relationships, may co-ordinate the functions carried out within the sinusoidal spaces. These activities include:

(a) Sieving, discernment and storage of hepatocytic/blood-derived substances (endothelial sieve plates, phagocytic–immunological role of the Kupffer cells and metabolic capability of the perisinusoidal cells);

(b) Control of intrasinusoidal haemodynamics (perisinusoidal cell processes, Kupffer cell projections and intrasinusoidal bridges); and

(c) Mechanical support of the sinusoidal wall (Kupffer cells within the sinusoids; fibrogenic role of the peri-

sinusoidal cells and their flat processes in the space of Disse).

For example, the Kupffer cell projections create a large mesh within the sinusoid that forms a kind of micro-anatomical barrier for larger materials which complements the filtration of the endothelial sieve plates (Figure 13)[56], and, at the same time, allows Kupffer cells to contact blood elements or other substances in immunological responses (Figure 14)[24]. Further, Kupffer cell projections seem to form an intrasinusoidal scaffolding which may help perisinusoidal cells to maintain the sinusoidal calibre or may even contribute indirectly towards regulation of intrasinusoidal blood flow[1,57]. Functional interactions between the sinusoidal cells may also be demonstrated by experimental studies on cholesterol remnants that reach liver sinusoids. It has been suggested that endothelial cell sieve plates, in repelling larger molecules[58–61], help Kupffer cells in phagocytizing the cholesterol remnants[62]. Furthermore, the intimate relationship between Kupffer cell projections and perisinusoidal cells suggests the existence of some sort of direct exchange between these two cell types[63].

On the other hand, it is widely accepted that the sinusoidal cells may be classified morphologically into three distinct cell types. In addition, it is also well established that Kupffer cells are never formed from endothelial cells and that perisinusoidal stellate cells are distinct from liver macrophages, the latter being Kupffer cells[5]. Thus, each of these cell types possesses different features which permit their structural distinction by means of SEM.

Sinusoidal endothelium

In the liver, vascular endothelium clearly presents a variable morphology, depending upon the dimensions and functional characteristics of the vessel under examination (Figures 10–13)[24]. This phenomenon becomes all the more evident when one considers that the endothelium forms the wall of the hepatic sinusoid, where the endothelial cells, because of their position, spatial relationships and structure, play a central role in hepatic function. In fact, the sinusoidal endothelial cell, because of its particular structure, not only constitutes the wall delimiting the capillary itself, but, at the same time, acts as a regulatory barrier that selectively filters substances and molecules passing from hepatocyte to blood and vice versa[64].

By SEM, the sinusoidal endothelium is found to be flattened when the infusion pressure has been kept as low as possible during liver fixation[59,64,65]. The endothelial cells usually have a single bulge corresponding to the region of the nucleus. These cells have very variable dimensions and always possess large cytoplasmic extensions which are connected with those of the neighbouring cells. Such connections may be easily studied when the border of one cell overlaps the border of an adjacent one (Plate 1b). Numerous small openings are evenly distributed over the cytoplasmic processes (Figure 13)[14,22,32,66]. The dimensions and distribution of these openings, which are commonly called **fenestrae** and which represent the communication between the perivascular space and the capillary lumen, have been clearly demonstrated by the three-dimensional approach[12,14,20,21,32,61,64,65,67–69]. The sinusoidal fenestrae are described as openings, having a diameter of about 100 nm,

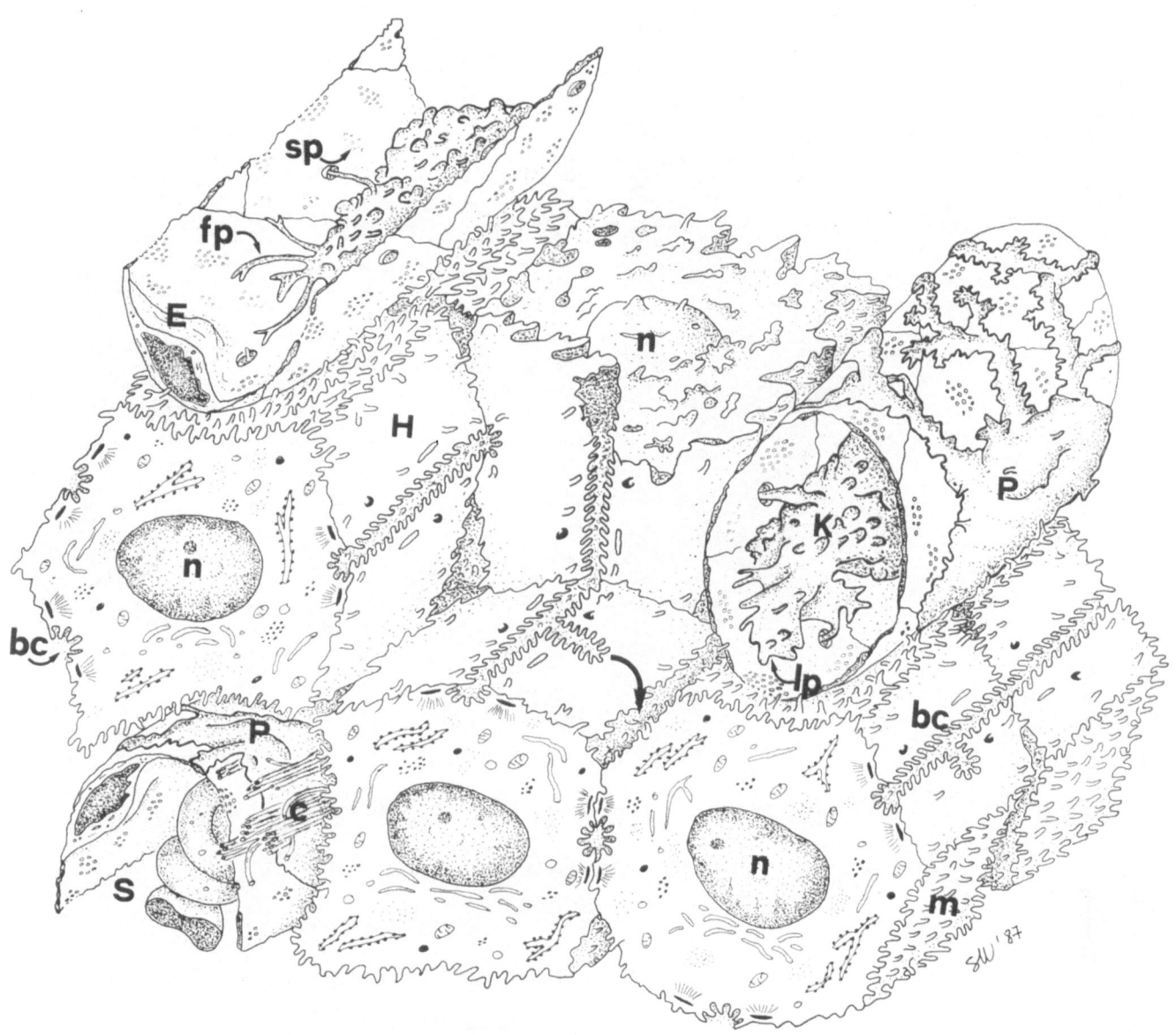

Diagram 1 Sinusoidal cells and hepatocytes The diagram shows the three principal liver sinusoidal cells (endothelial cell = E, Kupffer cell = K, and perisinusoidal cell = P) and their spatial relationship with hepatocytes (H) as seen by SEM.

Biliary facets are characterized by straight and centrally placed bile hemicanaliculi (bc) surrounded by smooth, microvilli-free areas, presenting studs and holes. Vascular facets are richly covered by microvilli (m) (the latter also extend into the interhepatocytic recesses – big curved arrow) and have close relationships with collagen–reticular fibres (c) and with the perisinusoidal cell processes. These processes, flat and branched, surround the sinusoids (S) determining the second layer of the liver capillary wall. Endothelium is flat and provided with fenestration, often clustered (sieve plates = sp) which may be crossed by the cytoplasmic prolongations of the liver macrophages. The latter, the Kupffer cells, lie on the sinusoidal endothelium and have a very close relationship with the sinusoidal wall through their filopodia (fp) and lamellipodia (lp). n = nuclei

often found clustered together, forming a characteristic structure called the **sieve plate** (Figure 13)[56]. Furthermore, isolated large fenestrae (up to 1 μm) have also been demonstrated by SEM (Figures 13 and 17)[2,24]. The latter structures, although unable to selectively sieve substances due to their wider mesh, may nevertheless be considered a physiolial expression of the endothelium's morphological dynamism. In fact, endothelium may morphologically adapt to particular conditions, such as temporary relationships with other cells[64]. Thus, the large gaps that are often found in relation to Kupffer cells (Figure 16) may be produced by the interactions between the liver macrophage and the sinusoidal wall[1,14,57]. However, the larger endothelial gaps are usually considered

either as fixation artifacts or the result of a pathological event, or even the effect of a toxic agent[1,23,54,59,70–72]. It has also been stated that dimensions and distributions of fenestrae vary in different animals[61,64] and in relation to the functional acinar area under examination, the number and diameter of fenestrae being larger in zone 3 (periportal area) than in zone 1 (central vein area)[64,69].

The sinusoidal endothelium lacks a continuous basal membrane (except in a small area of the periphery of the classic lobule)[73], permitting, through the endothelial openings, detection of the hepatocytic microvilli (Figures 13 and 17) and perisinusoidal cell processes[24]; in areas in which the flat perisinusoidal cell processes occur, the sinusoidal wall appears to be double-layered[2,32,54].

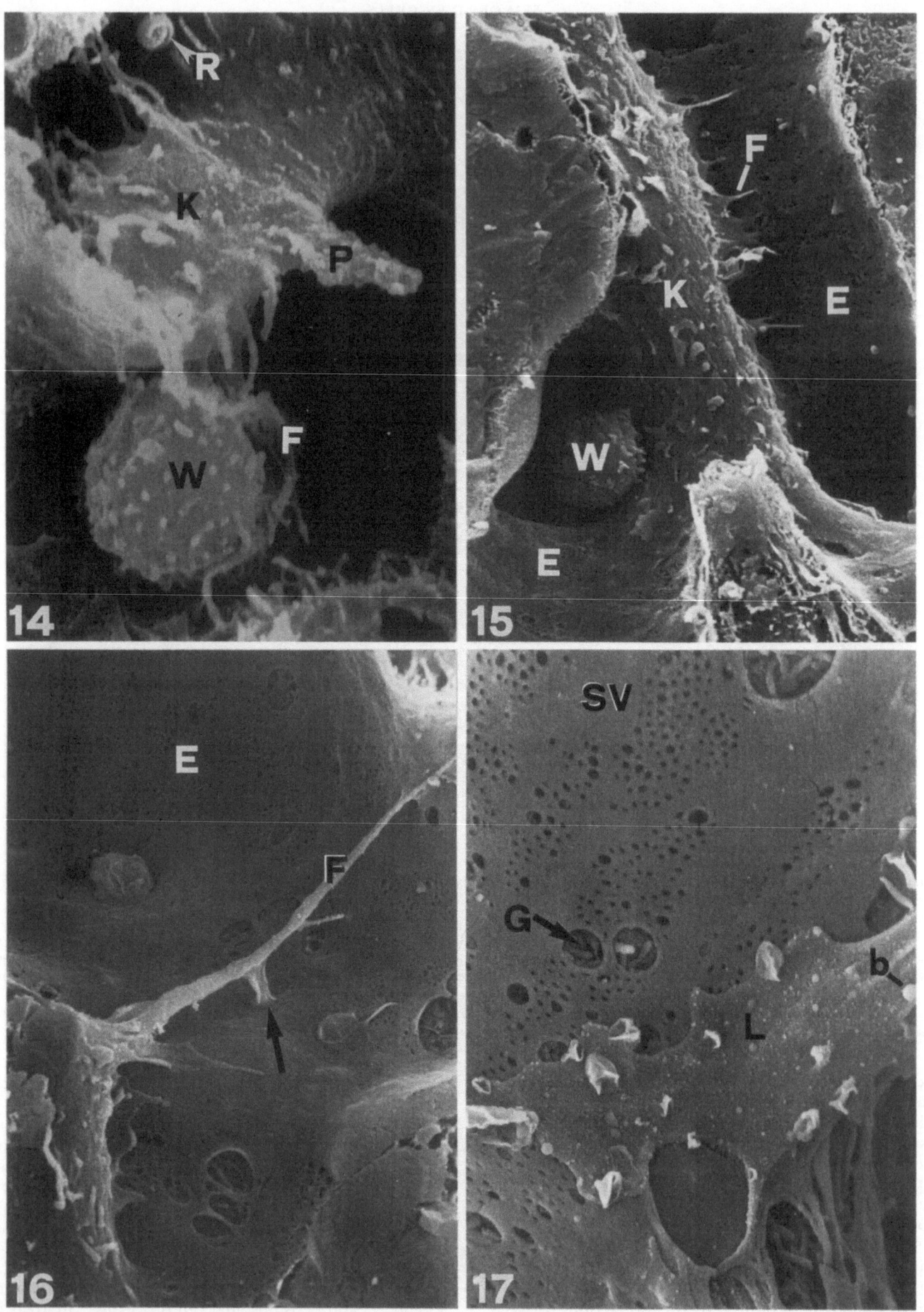

Figures 14–17 Kupffer cells Various aspects of liver macrophages are shown. **Figure 14** = a Kupffer cell (K) contacts with thin filopodia (F), a white blood element (W). Note ruffles (R) and a voluminous cytoplasmic projection (P) (×9000). **Figure 15** = a Kupffer cell body (K) lying on the endothelium (E) (×4500). **Figure 16** = a long and thin cytoplasmic filopodium (F) that contacts endothelium (E). Arrows indicate a prolongation which penetrates an endothelial fenestration (×9000). **Figure 17** = Laminar projections (lamellipodia) (L) of a Kupffer cell. b = blebs; SV = sieve plates; G = large endothelial gap (×12 000)

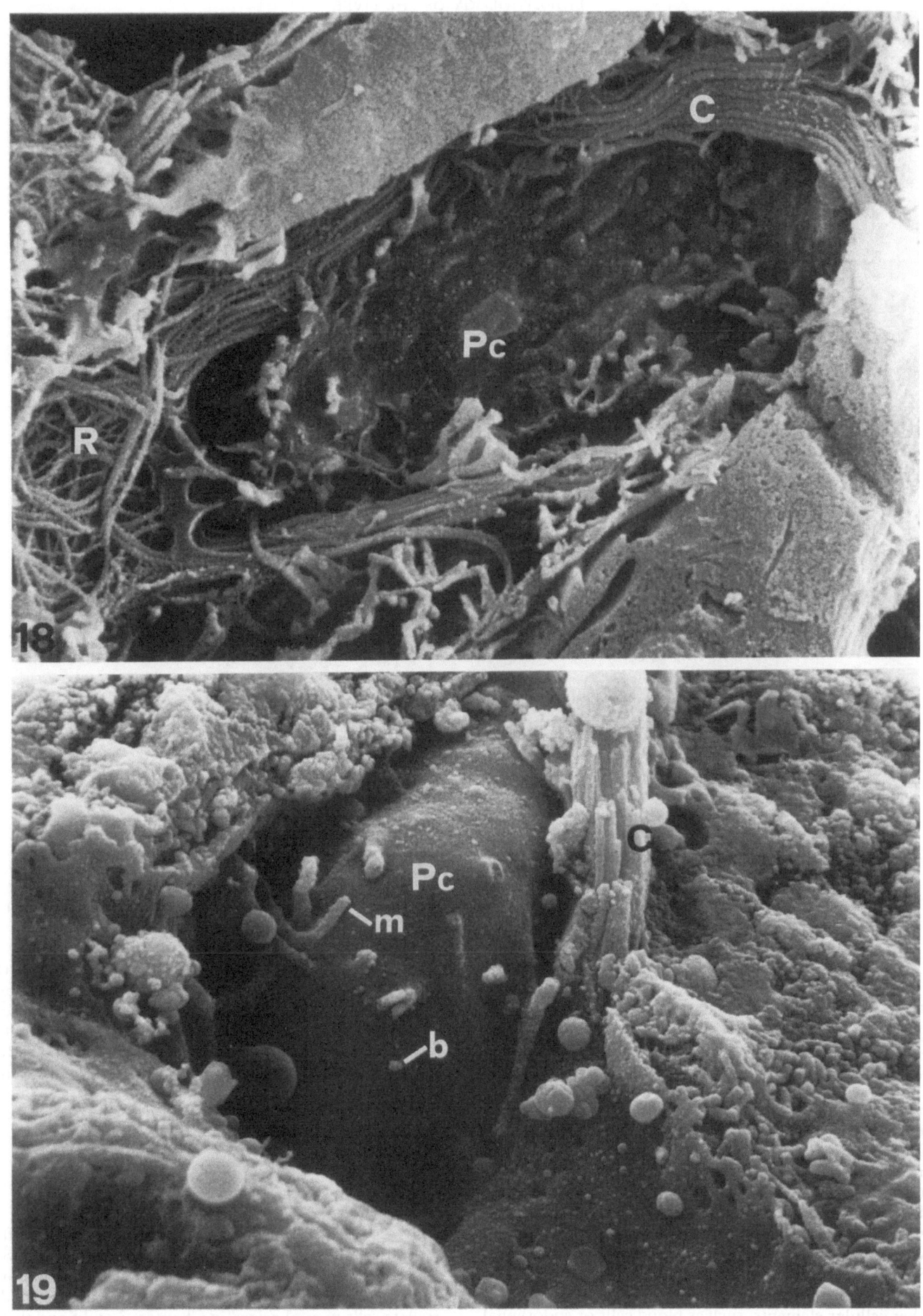

Figures 18 and 19   Perisinusoidal cell perikarya   Reticular (R) and collagen (C) fibres surround the perisinusoidal cell (Pc) perikarya.
m = microvilli; b = blebs (× 7000 (Figure 18) and × 16 000 (Figure 19))

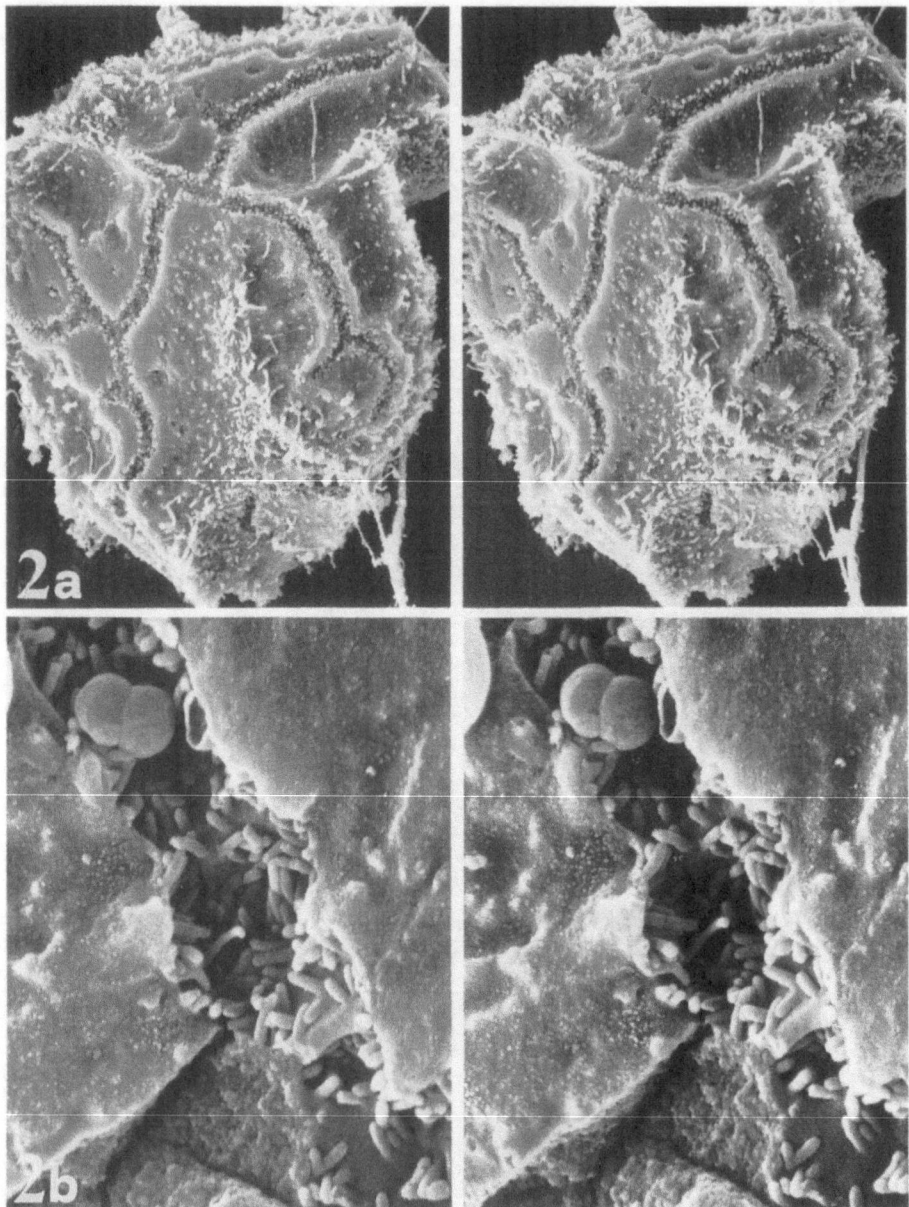

Plate 2 Hepatocytes and bile ductules: stereo pictures   a = isolated hepatocyte; b = bile canaliculus with microvilli arising from its bed

Kupffer cells

Stereo SEM pictures provide an excellent view of the three-dimensional aspect and the distribution of the Kupffer cells within the liver sinusoids[1,57] (Plate 1a,c). Kupffer cells are characterized by a large and irregularly rounded body that often lies over the luminal surface of the endothelium (Figure 2; Plate 1c). Their size, shape and surface features are strictly dependent upon the activity state of the cell. Usually, on the cell surface are present various numbers of blebs, holes, microvilli, ruffles and thin filopodia[12,14,20,32,57,74] which are dynamic features of the macrophages[2,57] (Figures 14 and 15; Plate 1c). During cell activation, these structures become more evident and long cytoplasmic projections of different sizes (Figures 15 and 16) and lamellipodia (Figure 17) are seen arising from the cell body. Such projections may reach other cellular elements, such as blood cells or endothelial cells. It has been suggested that the position of the Kupffer

cells within the sinusoid may produce changes in the fenestration pattern of the endothelium[24,74]. Furthermore, cell contacts between endothelial cells and Kupffer cells can be frequently seen by both SEM and TEM[74,75]; the latter also showed junctional complexes between Kupffer and endothelial cells similar to those commonly found between endothelial cells[76]. Nevertheless, no cell membrane fusions between these two cell types have been clearly demonstrated by SEM.

Perisinusoidal cells

The history of perisinusoidal cells is so fascinating, as well as so rich in misconceptions, that, even today, after more than 100 years since the first description by von Kupffer, most of the enigmas of these cells remain unresolved[2,55,63,77]. However, the debate about perisinusoidal stellate cells is emphasized in Chapters 3 and 5 and therefore it will not be repeated here.

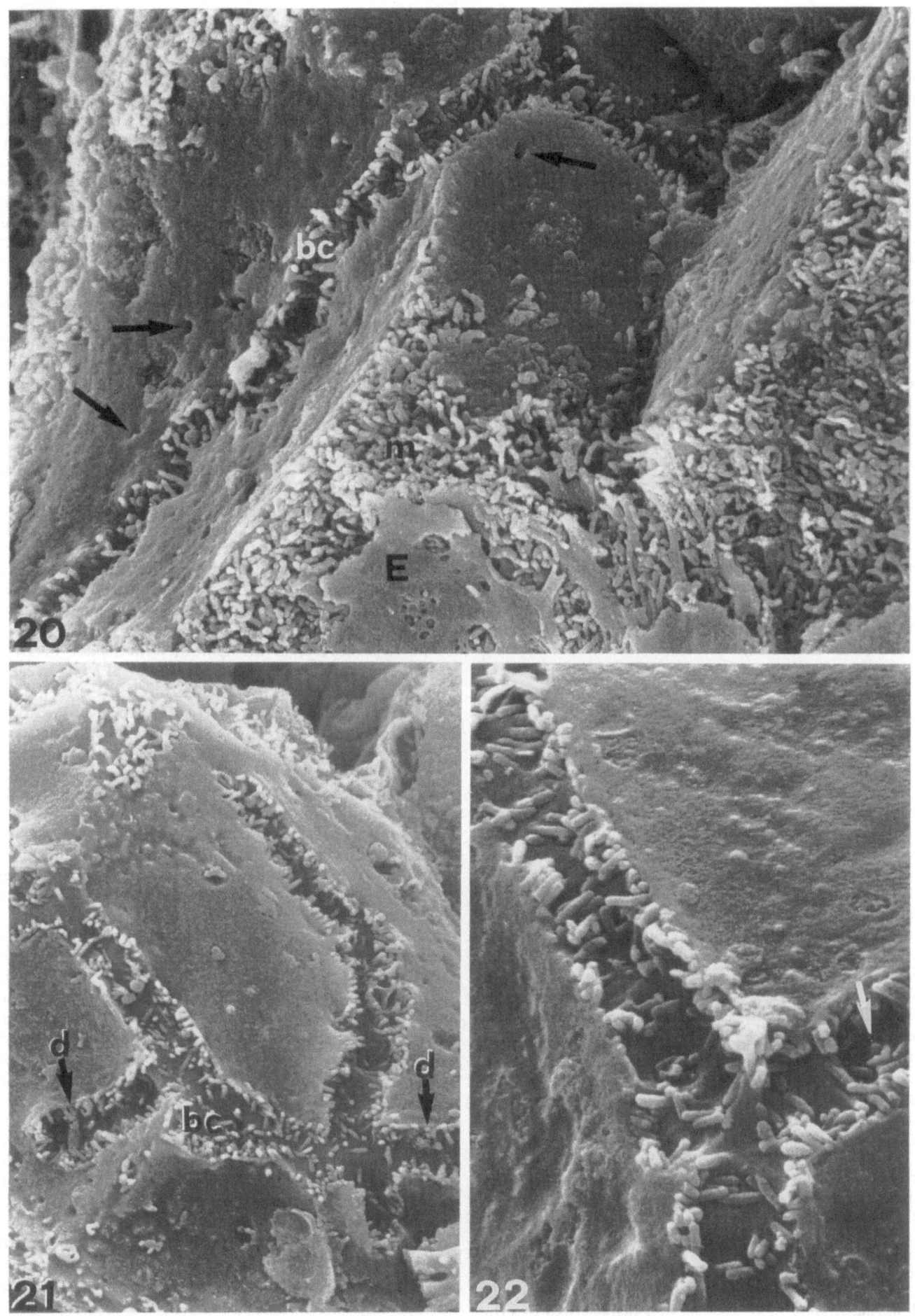

Figure 20 Mammalian hepatocyte Note the vascular facet rich in microvilli (m). E = endothelium; bc = bile canaliculus; arrows indicate small holes in the junctional complex between adjacent hepatocytes (× 9000)

Figures 21 and 22 Biliary facets of hepatocytes Periportal area. Note the large calibre of the bile canaliculi (bc) and of the bile canalicular diverticula (d + arrows). At high magnification it is possible to detect the microvilli of the canalicular bed (see also Plate 2b); arrow indicates an intracellular sacculation (× 5000 (Figure 21) and × 20 000 (Figure 22))

Although LM and TEM have permitted a morphological and histochemical differentiation of the cells populating the space of Disse, leading to an heterogeneous nomenclature for these elements*, SEM showed only cells having homogeneous morphological features. Thus, in terms of SEM, we must classify these elements by their position within the liver perivascular space and we will simply call them perisinusoidal cells.

As seen three-dimensionally, the perisinusoidal cells are structurally distinct in two areas: the area containing the nucleus (perikaryon) and the cytoplasmic processes[63,79,80] (see Chapters 3 and 5). The perikarya are usually intermingled in a fine network of reticular fibres and are surrounded by a variable amount of collagen bundles (Figures 18 and 19)[1,2,81]. The body is rounded or ovoid in shape[2,63,79] and may have rare microvillous projections[63] (Figure 19) and a single long cilium[1,24,55,82]. The cytoplasmic processes have different sizes and shapes. They are usually flattened (laminar dendritic processes)[1,2] and surround the sinusoids (subendothelial processes)[63], forming in certain areas a second layer of the sinusoidal wall[7,32,54,81]. In addition, it has been demonstrated that subendothelial processes have secondary and tertiary flat branches which contact neighbouring perisinusoidal cells or even Kupffer cell cytoplasmic prolongations penetrated within the space of Disse through the endothelial fenestrae[63]. It has been recently suggested that the topographical arrangement of perisinusoidal cell processes may play a role in the mechanical support of the sinusoidal wall[63] and of the parenchymal cells (hepatoskeletal system)[79].

THE HEPATOCYTE

The lobule or acinus is commonly described as the basic histofunctional unit of the liver, containing all the elements required to accomplish hepatic functions. However, when studying the morphology of the liver parenchymal cell, it can be noted that the hepatocyte itself contains all the structural elements necessary to carry out all the functions of the liver[50,83].

In fact, when critical point-dried liver samples are adequately dissociated, it is possible to collect isolated hepatocytes, which are often connected to sinusoidal elements, and study them by stereo SEM[2] (Plate 2a). By this technique, hepatic parenchymal cells appear to be polyhedral structures possessing numerous facets (six or more sides are usually described)[1,50], characterized by specific morphofunctional features. These features are dependent upon the relationship existing between a given facet and the neighbouring structure, such as an adjacent hepatocyte or a sinusoidal cell (Diagram 1). Given the morphological diversity of its facets, the hepatocyte can

behave as an amphicrine unit. In fact, the hepatocyte is capable of simultaneously secreting bile into the bile canaliculi (exocrine function), elaborating a plasma filtrate derived from the interstitial spaces and producing substances destined for the sinusoids (endocrine function). Therefore, such functional polarity must correspond to a morphological polarity[84], allowing us to classify the hepatocyte facets into two groups: those facing the sinusoids are said to constitute the **vascular pole** of the cell, whereas those in contact with adjacent hepatocytes, therefore delimiting the bile canaliculus, are said to make up the **biliary pole** of the cell[1,85].

The vascular facets are easily visible in isolated hepatocytes (Plate 2a) or, in non-dissociated tissue, through artifactual breaks in the endothelium[1,24] (Figure 20). These flat surfaces are covered by a large number of microvilli[2] (25–50 microvilli/μm^2 of cell surface)[20] that are generally short (0.5 μm) and have a diameter of approximately 0.1 μm. In addition, larger microvilli may be seen emerging from the edges of the vascular facet (i.e. the interface between the vascular facets and the biliary facets) as well as from the peripheral parts of the biliary facet (Plate 2a). This type of dispersion of the microvilli, in effect, creates a sort of absorptive carpet which lines the walls of the interstitial spaces. The latter consist of the spaces of Disse and their extensions in the interhepatocytic recesses. In fact, according to the original description furnished by Disse[86], in the liver, the interstitial space is the area between the vascular facet of the hepatocyte and the endothelium (space of Disse); however, it has been clearly shown by SEM[2,14] (Diagram 1) that the interstitial space also extends into the non-adherent areas between the biliary facets of two facing hepatocytes. This area can be called the **interhepatocytic recess**[87]. From the present morphological evidence, it seems reasonable to suggest the existence of a labyrinthine system of spaces surrounding the hepatocytes and sinusoids which facilitates interstitial fluid drainage[2,6].

When liver samples are fractured, dissociation usually occurs between the biliary facets, thus revealing longitudinal grooves formed by the bile hemicanaliculi (Figures 20–22). The hemicanaliculus, which is one of the two halves of the bile canaliculus, runs down the centre of the entire facet (Figure 20) and usually ranges between 0.5 and 2.5 μm in width, being largest near the portal area[2,10,13,33,87,88] (Figure 21). In these preparations, the bile hemicanaliculi appear to be in clear continuity with those of neighbouring cells. They are usually straight and unbranched (Figure 20) but they may also be tortuous and possess a few short branches mostly near the portal area (Figures 21 and 22). They are bordered by two dense columns of short microvilli which are also seen arising from the canalicular bed, especially in stereo pictures (Plate 2b). At high magnification, in the bed of wider canaliculi, sacculations and diverticula may be discovered (Figure 22). The latter structures may correspond to the so-called 'intracellular bile canaliculi' already described in the past[2]. At the sides of the bile grooves, it is possible to detect a narrow smooth area, about 0.4 μm in width. These smooth bands probably correspond to the area of the junctional attachment between two adjacent hepatocytes. On these bands, in addition, a few studs and holes, which are part of the junctional complex, can be seen[87] (Figure 22).

---

* The cells housed in the perisinusoidal space of Disse are indifferently called Ito cells, fat-storing cells, vitamin A storing cells, stellate cells, perisinusoidal stellate cells, fibroblast-like cells, interstitial cells and lipocytes. In addition, in the space of Disse, other cellular types, such as fibroblasts, pit cells, pericytes and others have been described[2,4,5,24,50,54,55,77,78]. However, it seems reasonable to consider a principal type of perisinusoidal cell having vitamin A storage capacity, characterized by cytoplasmic lipid inclusions, and playing a role in fibrogenesis under pathological and experimental conditions.

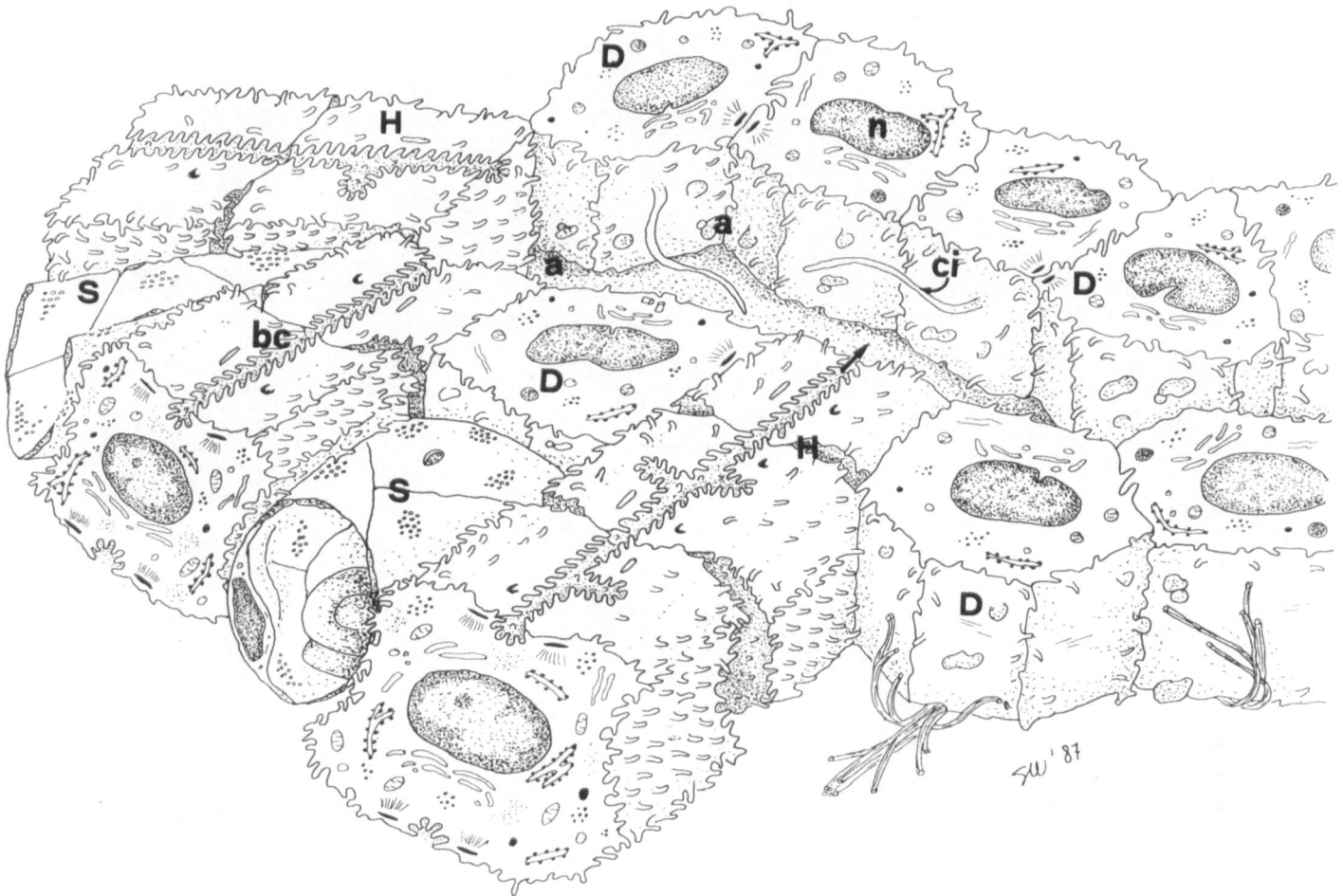

Diagram 2 The canalicular-ductular junction The picture represents the pathway of the bile drainage within the bile ductule. Periportal hepatocytes (H) are placed near the ductular epithelial cells (D) and possess large bile canaliculi (bc). They converge towards the bile ductule forming an ampullary dilatation (a). Bile canaliculi may also reach the ductule isolated (straight arrow). The inner surface of ductular epithelial cells is similar to that of interlobular bile duct but presents few microvilli and isolated cilia (ci). These cells rest on a thin basal lamina which is usually surrounded by collagen fibres. S = sinusoid, n = nuclei

THE CANALICULAR-DUCTULAR JUNCTIONS AND THE BILE DUCTULES

Although direct connection between bile canaliculi and interlobular bile ducts may occasionally be seen[1] (Figure 5), as a rule, the bile canaliculi join the bile ducts through the interposition of the bile ductules, also named **cholangioles** or **canals of Hering**[89]. These connections can be studied three-dimensionally in favourable cross-sections of the periportal space area (Figure 4). In fact, SEM studies have fully explained the relationship existing between bile canaliculi and interlobular ducts[1,15,20,21,23,37,90] which was only partially detected in LM and TEM sections[91-94].

As mentioned above, the biliary surfaces of the hepatocytes situated near the portal space area show larger bile canaliculi (up to 2.5 μm in width)[6] (Figures 21 and 23). In this area, several bile canaliculi may be seen converging toward the ductules of Hering, forming the canalicular–ductular junction[37]. Two kinds of canalicular–ductular junction may be observed by means of SEM[36,90] (Figures 4, 23 and 24; Diagram 2). Usually, bile canaliculi, prior to reaching the junction, form a characteristic dilatation, corresponding to the 'preductular ampulla' recognized in LM and TEM sections. Otherwise, bile canaliculi are also seen joining the ductules without any sacculation or ampullary dilatation.

The hepatocytes surrounding the portal space area may be connected with cuboid epithelial cells, similar to those of the interlobular bile ducts (Figure 23), to form the roots of the ductules of Hering. The wall of the ductules of Hering is formed by a monolayer of cuboid epithelial cells resting on a thin basal lamina and surrounded by collagen fibres (Figure 23). The internal (luminal) surface of the epithelial cells is almost totally covered by thin microvilli. In addition, long cilia may be seen arising from the centre of a few cells[15] (Figure 23). Their presence has been related to a cynetic role for the propulsion of the bile. Furthermore, if a chemoreceptor function of the cilia exists, control of bile quality and quantity may be influenced by these structures, in association with the bile-secretion regulatory activity of the peribiliary plexus[1,2].

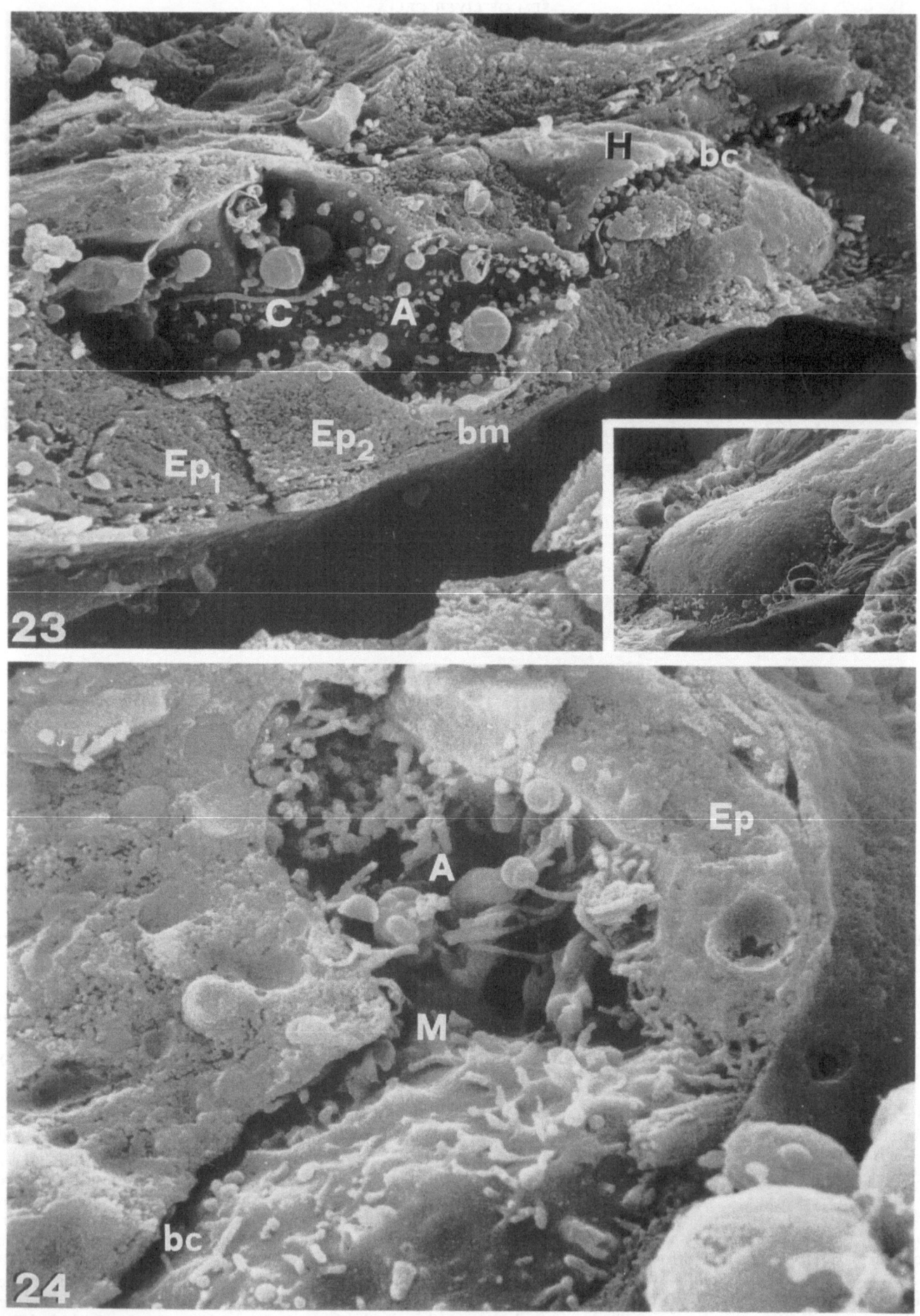

Figures 23 and 24 Canalicular ductular junction   bc = bile canaliculus; A = ampulla; C = cilium; Ep = epithelial cells; H = hepatocyte; m = microvilli; bm = basal membrane. In the insert of Figure 23, the outer wall of a bile ductule (canal of Hering) is seen. Note the smooth surface due to the presence of a basal lamina. Collagen fibres surround the ductule

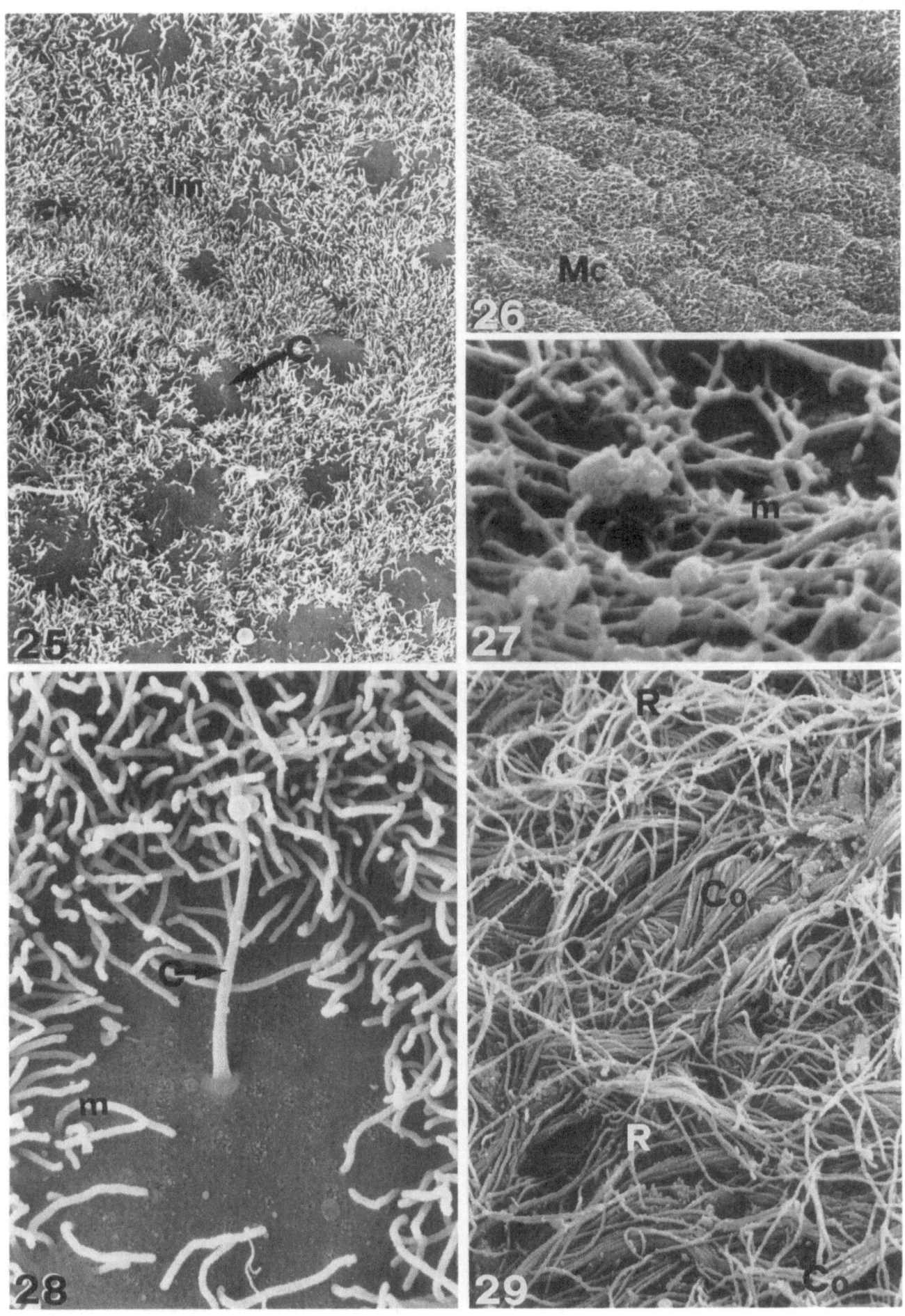

Figures 25–29 **The mesothelial cover and the Glisson's capsula**   m = microvilli; C = cilia; Mc = mesothelial cells; R = reticular fibres; Co = collagen fibres. (From Motta *et al*. 1977; and Macchiarelli and Motta, 1986)[1,24]

THE MESOTHELIAL COVERING MEMBRANE AND THE FIBROUS CAPSULA

The mesothelial cells contribute to the formation of the liver's peritoneal covering. They may be scanned easily once the residual of the serosal exudate has been removed by carefully washing during preparation of the samples[24] (Figure 25). These cells have a regular polygonal shape (Figure 26). Their body is usually flat and is often covered by numerous microvilli of variable length and size, often ranging between 1 and 2 μm, showing strands of granules adhering to their surface[1,6,24] (Figure 27). Not infrequently, especially in the cat and in humans, but rarely in rodents, a single cilium is seen emerging from a microvilli-free area in the centre of the cell[1] (Figure 28). The cilia may appear to be rudimentary (ciliogenesis) or completely formed (mature cilia), with a characteristic ball-shaped top that seems to be floating within the periserosal spaces[1,2]. It has to be emphasized that some chemoreceptor capability can be presumed for these structures.

The large number of microvilli, usually present on the surface of the mesothelial cells, demonstrates that these cells are actively involved in absorption and secretion of the fluids of the periserosal spaces[94-97]. These fluids play a role in ionic and nutrient exchange occurring in these spaces, and may also act as an antifriction film, protecting the surface of the mesothelial cells[95]. In addition, it might be thought that the motile property of the cilia, if any, would be useful in facilitating the drainage of the serosal exudate[2].

The mesothelial cell covering membrane, through the interposition of the basal lamina, lies upon a layer of connective fibres, mostly arranged in bundles[1,94]. As seen by SEM, in humans, such a connective layer appears to be arranged in an irregular net formed of fibres of various sizes (collagen–reticular) (Figure 29), among which it is also possible to detect small vessels and fusiform cell elements resembling fibroblasts and/or smooth muscle cells[2].

These connective fibre bundles follow the biliary and vascular ramifications within the parenchyma, clearly delimiting, in a few species (pig, camel), the lobular architecture of the liver[1].

Further, the thinnest argyrophilic ramifications of these bundles (reticular fibres) reach the perisinusoidal spaces, creating a sort of large net scaffolding for the hepatic laminae and the vascular lacunae[1,2,50,94]. It is supposed that, in those animals which lack this connective net (cod), the perisinusoidal stellate cells form, with their cytoplasmic prolongations, a substitute supporting structure for the hepatic cells[79].

Acknowledgements

The authors wish to thank Dr Stefania A. Nottola (Department of Anatomy, University of Rome 'La Sapienza') for her valuable artistic work (Diagrams 1 and 2), and Dr Sharon Greene for helping with the manuscript. C.N.R. and M.P.I. provided funds for this work.

References

1. Motta, P., Muto, M. and Fujita, T. (1978). *The Liver. An Atlas of Scanning Electron Microscopy.* (Tokyo/New York: Igaku Shoin)
2. Motta, P. M. (1984). The three-dimensional microanatomy of the liver. *Arch. Histol. Jpn.,* **47**, 1–30
3. Kaneda, K. and Wake, K. (1983). Distribution and morphological characteristics of the pit cells in the liver of the rat. *Cell Tiss. Res.,* **233**, 485–505
4. Bradfield, J. W. B. (1984). Liver sinusoidal cells. *J. Pathol.,* **142**, 5–6
5. Kirn, A., Knook, D. L. and Wisse, E. (1986). *Cells of the Hepatic Sinusoid,* Vol. 1. (Rijswijk: The Kupffer Cell Foundation)
6. Motta, P. M. (1977). The three-dimensional fine structure of the liver as revealed by scanning electron microscopy. *Int. Rev. Cytol. Suppl.,* **6**, 347–397
7. Motta, P. M., Fujita, T. and Nishi, M. (1982). Scanning electron microscopy of the mammalian liver. In Motta, P. M. and DiDio, L. J. A. (eds.) *Basic and Clinical Hepatology,* pp. 31–50. (The Hague/Boston/London: Martinus Nijhoff)
8. Fujita, T., Tokunaga, J. and Inouè, H. (1971). *Atlas of Scanning Electron Microscopy in Medicine,* pp. 20–21. (Tokyo: Igaku-Shoin Ltd.)
9. Bierring, F. and Skaaring, P. (1973). Scanning electron microscopy of liver. *JEOL News,* **11e**, 16–17
10. Brooks, S. E. H. and Haggis, G. H. (1973). Scanning electron microscopy of rat's liver. Application of freeze-fracture and freeze-drying techniques. *Lab. Invest.,* **29**, 60–64
11. Tanaka, K. and Iino, A. (1973). Demonstration of fibrous components in hepatic interphase nuclei by high resolution scanning electron microscopy. *Exp. Cell. Res.,* **81**, 40–46
12. Itoshima, T., Kobayashi, T., Shimada, Y. and Murakami, T. (1974). Fenestrated endothelium of the liver sinusoids of the guinea-pig as revealed by scanning electron microscopy. *Arch. Histol. Jpn.,* **37**, 15–24
13. Miyai, K., Wagner, R. M. and Richardson, A. L. (1974). Preparation of liver for combined SEM and TEM study. *Scanning Electron Microsc.,* I, 283–290
14. Motta, P. and Porter, K. R. (1974). Structure of rat liver sinusoids and associated tissue spaces as revealed by scanning electron microscopy. *Cell. Tiss. Res.,* **148**, 111–125
15. Motta, P. and Fumagalli, G. (1974). Scanning electron microscopy demonstration of cilia in rat intrahepatic bile ducts. *Z. Anat. Entwickl-Gesch.,* **145**, 223–226
16. Braus, E. and Vierling, H. (1930). In Clara, M., Herschel, K. and Ferner, H., (eds.), *Atlas der Normalen Mikroskopischen Anatomie des Menschen,* 1974, (Leipzig: JA Barth)
17. Elias, H. (1949). A re-examination of the structure of the mammalian liver. I. Parenchymal architecture. *Am. J. Anat.,* **84**, 311–334
18. Elias, H. (1949). A re-examination of the structure of the mammalian liver. II. The hepatic lobule and its relation to the vascular and biliary system. *Am. J. Anat.,* **85**, 379–465
19. Elias, H. and Sherrick, J. C. (1969). *Morphology of the Liver.* (New York: Academic Press)
20. Grisham, J. W., Nopanitaya, W., Compagno, J. and Nagel, A. E. H. (1975). Scanning electron microscopy of normal rat liver: the surface structure of its cells and tissue components. *Am. J. Anat.,* **144**, 295–322
21. Grisham, J. W., Nopanitaya, W. and Compagno, J. (1976).

Scanning electron microscopy of the liver: a review of methods and results. In Popper, H. and Schaffner, F. (eds.), *Progress in Liver Diseases*, Vol. V, pp. 1–23. (New York: Grune & Stratton Inc.)

22. Motta, P. M. (1981). Three-dimensional architecture of the mammalian liver. A scanning electron microscopy review. In DiDio, L. J. A., Motta, P. M. and Allen, D. J. (eds.) *Three Dimensional Microanatomy of Cell and Tissue Surfaces*, pp. 33–50. (Amsterdam: Elsevier/North Holland Inc.)

23. Motta, P. M. (1982). Scanning electron microscopy of the liver. In Popper, H. and Schaffner, F. (eds.) *Progress in Liver Diseases*, Vol. VII, pp. 1–16. (New York: Grune & Stratton Inc.)

24. Macchiarelli, G. and Motta, P. M. (1986). The three-dimensional microstructure of the liver. A review by scanning electron microscopy. *Scanning Electron Microsc.* III, 1019–1038

25. Motta, P. M., Andrews, P. M. and Porter, K. R. (1977). *Microanatomy of Cell and Tissue Surfaces. An Atlas of SEM*, pp. 105–115. (Philadelphia: Lea & Febiger)

26. Kessel, R. G. and Kardon, R. H. (1979). *Tissues and Organs. A Text Atlas of Scanning Electron Microscopy*, pp. 112–121. (San Francisco CA: WH Freeman)

27. Fujita, T., Tanaka, T. and Tokunaga, J. (1981). *Scanning Electron Microscopic Atlas of Cells and Tissues*, pp. 144–157. (Tokyo: Igaku-Shoin Ltd)

28. Kiernan, F. (1833). The anatomy and physiology of the liver. *Philos. Trans. R. Soc. London*, 123, 711–770

29. Mall, F. P. (1906). A study of the structural unit of the liver. *Am. J. Anat.*, 5, 227–308

30. Rappaport, A. M., Borowy, Z. J., Lougheed, W. M. and Lotto, W. N. (1954). Subdivision of hexagonal liver lobules into a structural and functional unit. Role in hepatic physiology and pathology. *Anat. Rec.*, 119, 11–34

31. Muto, M. (1975). A scanning electron microscopic study on endothelial cells and Kupffer cells in rat liver sinusoids. *Arch. Histol. Jpn.*, 37, 369–386

32. Muto, M., Nishi, M. and Fujita, T. (1977) Scanning electron microscopy of human liver sinusoids. *Arch. Histol. Jpn.*, 40, 137–151

33. Vonnahme, F. J. (1981). A scanning electron microscopic study of the liver of the monkey Macaca Speciosa. II. Intra- and extrahepatic biliary system. *Cell. Tiss. Res.*, 215, 207–214

34. Vonnahme, F. J. and Muller, O. (1981). A scanning electron microscopic study of the liver of the monkey Macaca Speciosa. I. Vascular system of the hepatic lobule. *Cell. Tiss. Res.*, 215, 193–205

35. Wisse, E., De Zanger, R. B., Jacobs, R. and McCuskey, R. S. (1983). Scanning electron microscope observations on the structure of portal veins, sinusoids and central veins in rat liver. *Scanning Electron Microsc.*, III, 1441–1452

36. Itoshima, T., Yoshino, K., Yamamoto, K., Ohata, W., Kubota, M., Ukida, M., Ito, T., Hirakawa, H., Munetomo, F. and Shimada, Y. (1977). Scanning electron microscopy of the bile ductule. *Gastroenterol. Jpn.*, 12, 476–482

37. Marinozzi, G., Muto, M., Correr, S. and Motta, P. (1977). Scanning electron microscope observations of intrahepatic biliary tree. I, canaliculo–ductular junction. Bile ductules and ducts. *J. Submicrosc. Cytol.*, 9, 127–143

38. Niiro, G. K. and O'Morchoe, C. C. (1986). Pattern and distribution of intrahepatic lymph vessel in the rat. *Anat. Rec.*, 215, 351–360

39. Yamamoto, K. and Phillips, M. J. (1986). Three-dimen-sional observation of the intrahepatic lymphatics by scanning electron microscopy of corrosion casts. *Anat. Rec.*, 214, 67–70

40. Skaaring, P. and Bierring, F. (1977). Further evidence for the existence of intralobular nerves in the rat liver. *Cell. Tiss. Res.*, 177, 287–290

41. Ueno, T., Noguchi, K., Abe, H. and Tanikawa, K. (1986). Electron microscopic study on the innervation of the normal human liver. In Imura, T., Maruse, S. and Suzuki, T. (eds.) *Electron Microscopy 1986. Proceedings of the XI International Congress on Electron Microscopy*, Vol. IV, pp. 2929–2930. (Kyoto)

42. Skaaring, P. and Bierring, F. (1976). On the intrisic innervation of normal rat liver. Histochemical and scanning electron microscopical studies. *Cell. Tiss. Res.*, 171, 141–155

43. Ohata, M. (1984). Electron microscope study on the innervation of guinea-pig liver – Proposal of sensory nerve terminals in the hepatic parenchyme. *Arch. Histol. Jpn.*, 47, 149–178

44. Akiyoshi, H. and Ichihara, K. (1986). Ultrastructural studies of the liver innervation in guinea pig. In Imura, T., Maruse, S. and Suzuki, T. (eds.) *Electron Microscopy 1986. Proceedings of the XI International Congress on Electron Microscopy*, Vol. IV, pp. 2931–2932. (Kyoto)

45. Murakami, T., Itoshima, T. and Shimada, Y. (1974). Peribiliary portal system in the monkey liver as evidenced by the injection replica scanning electron microscope method. *Arch. Histol. Jpn.*, 37, 245–260

46. Ohtani, O. and Murakami, T. (1978). Peribiliary portal system in the rat liver as studied by the injection-replica scanning electron microscope method. *Scanning Electron Microsc.*, II, 241–245

47. Nopanitaya, W., Grisham, J. W., Aghajanian, J. G. and Carson, J. L. (1978). Intrahepatic microcirculation: SEM study of the terminal distribution of the hepatic artery. *Scanning Electron Microsc.*, II, 837–842

48. Ohtani, O. and Murakami, T. (1985). The blood supply of the liver and the pancreas: scanning electron microscopy of vascular cast and intravital microscopy of living tissues. In *XII International Congress of Anatomy, London, Abstract book*, p. 522. (Cambridge: Book Production Consultants)

49. Ohtani, O., Murakami, T. and Jones, A. L. (1982). Microcirculation of the liver, with special reference to the peribiliary portal system. In Motta, P. M. and DiDio, L. J. A. (eds.) *Basic and Clinical Hepatology*, Vol. II, pp. 85–96. (The Hague: Martinus Nijhoff)

50. Fawcett, D. W. (1986). *Bloom and Fawcett – A Textbook of Histology*, 11th Edn. (Philadelphia: W. B. Saunders Company)

51. Kardon, R. H. and Kessel, R. G. (1980). Three-dimensional organization of the hepatic microcirculation in the rodent as observed by scanning electron microscopy of corrosion cast. *Gastroenterology*, 79, 72–81

52. Ohtani, O. (1981). Microcirculation studies by the injection-replica method with special reference to the portal circulations. In Allen, D. J., Motta, P. M. and DiDio, L. J. A. (eds.) *Three Dimensional Microanatomy of Cells and Tissue Surfaces*, pp. 51–70. (Amsterdam: Elsevier/North Holland)

53. Motta, P. M. (1975). A scanning electron microscopic study of the rat liver sinusoid: endothelial and Kupffer cells. *Cell. Tiss. Res.*, 164, 371–385

54. Wisse, E. and Knook, D. L. (1977). *Kupffer Cells and Other Liver Sinusoidal Cells.* (Amsterdam: Elsevier/North Holland Biomedical Press)

55. Knook, D. L. and Wisse, E. (1982). *Sinusoidal Liver Cells.* (Amsterdam: Elsevier/North Holland Biomedical Press)

56. Wisse, E. (1970). An electron microscopic study of the fenestrated endothelial lining of rat liver sinusoids. *J. Ultrastruct. Res.*, 31, 125–150

57. Motta, P. M. (1979). The location of Kupffer cells in the liver of different mammals. A three dimensional analysis by scanning electron microscopy. *Verb. Anat. Ges.*, 73, 827–830

58. Fraser, R., Bosanquet, A. G. and Day, W. A. (1978). Filtration of chylomicrons by the liver may influence cholesterol metabolism and atherosclerosis. *Atherosclerosis*, 29, 113–123

59. Fraser, R., Bowler, L. M., Day, W. A., Dobbs, B., Johnson, H. D. and Lee, D. (1980). High perfusion pressure damages the sieving ability of sinusoidal endothelium in rat livers. *Br. J. Exp. Pathol.*, 61, 222–228

60. De Zanger, R. B. and Wisse, E. (1982). The filtration effect of rat liver fenestrated sinusoidal endothelium on the passage of (remnant) chylomicrons to the space of Disse. In Knook, D. L. and Wisse, E. (eds.) *Sinusoidal Liver Cells*, pp. 69–76. (Amsterdam: Elsevier)

61. Wright, P. L., Smith, K. F., Day, W. A. and Fraser, R. (1983). Small liver fenestrae may explain the susceptibility of rabbits to atherosclerosis. *Arteriosclerosis*, 3, 344–348

62. Werb, Z. (1983). How the macrophage regulates its extracellular environment. *Am. J. Anat.*, 166, 237–256

63. Takahashi-Iwanaga, H. and Fujita, T. (1986). Application of an NaOH maceration method to a scanning electron microscopic observation of Ito cells in the rat liver. *Arch. Histol. Jpn.*, 49, 349–357

64. Wisse, E., De Zanger, R. B., Charles, K., Van Der Smissen, P. and McCuskey, R. S. (1985). The liver sieve: considerations concerning the structure and function of endothelial fenestrae, the sinusoidal wall and the space of Disse. *Hepatology*, 5, 683–692

65. Wisse, E., De Wilde, A. and De Zanger, R. (1983). Perfusion fixation of human and rat liver tissue for light and electron microscopy: a review and assessment of existing methods with special emphasis on sinusoidal cell and microcirculation. In Preul, J., Barnard, T. and Haggis, H. G. (eds.) *The Science of Biological Specimen Preparations for Microscopy and Microanalysis*, pp. 31–38. (Chicago IL: SEM Inc, AMF O'Hare)

66. Montesano, R. and Nicolescu, P. (1978). Fenestrations in endothelium of rat liver sinusoids revisted by freeze-fracture. *Anat. Rec.*, 190, 861–870

67. Wisse, E., De Zanger, R. and Roland, J. (1983). Scanning EM observations on rat liver sinusoids relevant to microcirculation and transport processes. *J. Clin. Electron. Microsc.*, 16, 427–430

68. Wright, P. L., Smith, K. F., Day, W. A. and Fraser, R. (1983). Hepatic sinusoidal endothelium in sheep: an ultrastructural reinvestigation. *Anat. Rec.*, 206, 385–390

69. Vidal-Vanaclocha, F. and Barbera-Guillem, E. (1985). Fenestration patterns in endothelial cells of rat liver sinusoids. *J. Ultrastruct. Res.*, 90, 115–123

70. Nopanitaya, W., Lamb, J. C., Grisham, J. W. and Carson, J. L. (1976). Effect of hepatic venous outflow obstruction on pores and fenestrations in sinusoidal endothelium. *Br. J. Exp. Pathol.*, 57, 604–609

71. Wisse, E. and Knook, D. L. (1979). The investigation of sinusoidal cells: a new approach to the study of liver function. In Popper, H. and Shaffner, P. (eds.) *Progress in Liver Diseases*, Vol. VI, pp. 153–171. (New York: Grune & Stratton Inc.)

72. Mak, K. M. and Lieber, C. S. (1984). Alterations in endothelial fenestrations in liver sinusoids of baboons fed alcohol: a scanning electron microscopic study. *Hepatology*, 4, 386–391

73. Burkel, E. W. and Low, F. N. (1966). The fine structure of rat liver sinusoids, space of Disse and associated tissue space. *Am. J. Anat.*, 118, 769–784

74. Motta, P. (1977). Kupffer cells as revealed by scanning electron microscopy. In Wisse, E. and Knook, D. L. (eds.) *Kupffer Cells and Other Liver Sinusoidal Cells.* (Amsterdam: Elsevier/North Holland Biomedical Press)

75. Tamaru, T. and Fujita, H. (1978). Electron-microscopic studies on Kupffer's stellate cells and sinusoidal endothelial cells in liver of normal and experimental rabbits. *Anat. Embryol.*, 154, 125–942

76. Ito, T., Tanuma, Y. and Shibasaki, S. (1980). Junctions between Kupffer cells and hepatic sinusoidal endothelium. A review. *Okajimas Folio Anat. Jpn.*, 57, 145–158

77. Wake, K. (1980). Perisinusoidal stellate cells (fat-storing cells, interstitial cells, lipocytes), their related structure in and around the liver sinusoids, and vitamin A-storing cells in extrahepatic organs. *Int. Rev. Cytol.*, 66, 303–353

78. Ito, T. (1951). Cytological studies on stellate cells of Kupffer and fat-storing cells in the capillary wall of the human liver. *Acta Anat. Nippon.*, 26, 42–74

79. Fujita, H., Tatsumi, H., Ban, T. and Tamura, S. (1986). Fine-structural characteristics of the liver of the cod (*Gadus morhua macrocephalus*), with special regard to the concept of a hepatoskeletal system formed by Ito cells. *Cell. Tissue Res.*, 244, 63–67

80. Shibasaki, S., Aoki, T. and Taira, K. (1986). Profiles of Ito cells in the rat liver: a scanning and thin-section electron microscopic study. In Imura, T., Maruse, S. and Suzuki, T. (eds.) *Electron Microscopy 1986. Proceedings of the XI Congress on Electron Microscopy*, Vol. IV, pp. 2925–2926. (Kyoto)

81. Fraser, R., Day, W. A. and Fernando, N. S. (1986). Review: the liver sinusoidal cells. Their role in disorders of the liver, lipoprotein metabolism and atherogenesis. *Pathology*, 18, 5–11

82. Tobe, K., Tsuchiya, T., Itoshima, T., Nagashima, H. and Kobayashi, T. (1985). Electron microscopy of fat-storing cells in liver diseases with special reference to cilia and cytoplasmic cholesterol crystals. *Arch. Histol. Jpn.*, 48, 435–441

83. Schaffner, F. and Popper, H. (1985). Structure of the liver. In Berk, W. S. *Bockus Gastroenterology*, 4th Edn., Vol. VI, pp. 2625–2658. (Philadelphia: W. B. Saunders Co.)

84. Evans, W. H. (1980). A biochemical dissection of the functional polarity of the plasma membrane of the hepatocyte. *Biochim. Biophys. Acta*, 604, 27–64

85. Jones, A. L. and Spring-Mills, E. (1983). The liver and gallbladder. In Weiss, L. (ed.) *Histology. Cell and Tissue Biology*, pp. 708–748. (New York: Elsevier Science Publishing Co. Inc.)

86. Disse, J. (1890). Über die Lymphbahnen der Säugethierleber. *Arch. Mikrosk. Anat.*, 36, 203–224

87. Motta, P. and Fumagalli, G. (1975). Structure of rat bile

canaliculi as revealed by scanning electron microscopy. *Anat. Rec.*, **182**, 499–514

88. Nopanitaya, W. and Grisham, J. W. (1975). Scanning electron microscopy of mouse intrahepatic structures. *Exp. Mol. Pathol.*, **23**, 441–458

89. Hering, E. (1867). Uber den bau der Wirbelthierleber. *Arch. F. Mikr. Anat.*, **3**, 88–114

90. Itoshima, T., Kiyotoshi, S., Kawaguchi, K., Yoshino, K., Munetomo, F., Ohta, W., Shimada, Y. and Nagashima, H. (1980). Scanning electron microscopy of rat bile canalicular–ductular junction. *Scanning Electron Microsc.*, **III**, 373–378

91. Lettule, M. (1915). Les capillicules biliaires du foie humain. Leur repartition a l'interieur du lobule hepatique et leur modes d'abouchement dans les canaux perii-lobulaires. *J. Physiol. Pathol. Gen.*, **1**, 789–801

92. Daems, W. T. (1961). The microanatomy of the smallest biliary pathway in mouse liver tissue. *Acta Anat.*, **46**, 1–24

93. Steiner, J. W. and Carruthers, J. S. (1961). Studies on the fine structure of the terminal branches of the biliary tree. I. The morphology of normal bile canaliculi, bile preductules – ducts of Hering – and bile ductules. *Am. J. Anat.*, **38**, 639–649

94. Tanikawa, K. (1979). *Ultrastructural Aspects of the Liver and Its Disorders*. (Tokyo: Igaku-Shoin)

95. Andrews, P. M. and Porter, K. R. (1973). The ultrastructural morphology and possible functional significance of mesothelial microvilli. *Anat. Rec.*, **177**, 409–426

96. Barberini, F., Carpino, F., Renda, T. and Motta, P. M. (1977). Etude au microscope électronique à balayage du péritoine du rat. *Anat. Anz.*, **142**, 486–496

97. Barberini, F., Correr, S. and Motta, P. M. (1987). The peritoneum. In Motta, P. M. and Fujita, H. (eds.) *Ultrastructure of the Digestive Tract*, Chap. 15, pp. 243–259. (Norwell, Mass: Martinus Nijhoff Publishing)

5

The three-dimensional fine structure of Ito cells and hepatocytes studied by a maceration method

H. TAKAHASHI-IWANAGA and T. FUJITA

INTRODUCTION

The Ito cell[1] is a stellate cell housed in the perisinusoidal space of Disse. The Ito cell is known to have a vitamin A storing ability[2-6], and to share fibrogenetic functions with fibroblasts[7-11].

Ito and Nemoto (1952)[12] assumed that the Ito cells might send out cytoplasmic processes along the sinusoidal wall based on the fusiform shapes of the cells sandwiched between the hepatocytes and the sinusoidal endothelium. However, these investigators failed to visualize the three-dimensional shapes of the Ito cells, because, at that time, there were no methods for selectively staining these cells.

Transmission electron microscope (TEM) studies[8,13-15] revealed that the Ito cells extend several attenuated processes beneath the sinusoidal endothelium. Numerous profiles of the Ito cell processes were demonstrated by TEM studies, suggesting a complicated branching pattern. Several investigators assumed that these subendothelial Ito cell processes might protect the sinusoidal wall mechanically and have a contractile ability with which they could regulate the calibre of the sinusoid[16,17]. However, it has been difficult to conceive of the three-dimensional extensions of these processes from fragmental TEM images.

On the other hand, early investigators reported on perisinusoidal cells stained by various metal impregnation methods. Von Kupffer (1876)[18] showed numerous 'Sternzellen' (stellate cells) impregnated with gold outside the liver sinusoid. A century later, Wake (1971)[5] (see also Chapter 13) re-evaluated the gold impregnation study and stated that the 'Sternzellen' in the initial report by von Kupffer[18], but not those in his later papers, are identical to the Ito cells. The gold-impregnated Ito cells, as shown by von Kupffer[18] and by Wake[5] extend from one to five, horn-like processes with very few branches. These processes appeared far less numerous and simpler in shape than expected from the TEM studies.

Zimmermann (1923)[19] observed flattened cells, surrounding the sinusoid with their branching processes, by means of Golgi–Kopsch's impregnation method, and referred to these cells as 'Perizyten' of the liver. Based on their perisinusoidal location, it was assumed that the 'Perizyten' corresponded to the Ito cells[17]. The question of whether the 'Perizyten' might be identical to the Ito cells remains to be settled.

In order to fill these gaps between the TEM and the light microscopic findings concerning the three-dimensional structure of the Ito cells, scanning electron microscopy (SEM) seems to be a useful method. Notwithstanding, there is great difficulty in viewing the entire shape of these cells by SEM. By routine specimen preparation procedures, the hepatocytes and the sinusoidal endothelium are rarely separated from each other. Moreover, the Ito cells are covered with reticular fibres in the space of Disse.

Recently, T-Iwanaga and Fujita[20] showed that treatment of liver tissue with NaOH effectively removed reticular fibres and that this treatment also facilitated separation between the hepatocytes and the sinusoidal wall, thus exposing numerous Ito cells along the sinusoids.

This paper describes the three-dimensional fine structure of Ito cells observed by SEM using the NaOH maceration method. Furthermore, SEM also reveals pericytes of central veins and smooth muscle cells surrounding sublobular veins. In addition, this paper makes mention of the hepatocytes, which are isolated by the maceration method. The isolated hepatocytes reveal their three-dimensional shapes and fine surface structures.

METHODOLOGY

Most SEM studies were restricted to the free or fractured surfaces of cells until Evan et al.[21] discovered a new method for the removal of collagen and basement membrane which embed these cells and make their surface view obscure. These investigators treated SEM specimens with HCl, and then with collagenase, succeeding in exposing the cell surfaces. Many researchers have applied this HCl-digestion method, or modifications of it, to various tissues e.g., small vessels[22,23], seminiferous tubules[24], peripheral nerve tissue[25-27] and some exocrine glands[28-30].

Recently, several kinds of chemical agents have been utilized in order to disintegrate the cellular and intercellular elements obscuring the objects of interest. Miller et al.[31] recommended KOH treatment, combined with enzyme digestion, for the exposure of vascular beds of intestine. Shimada *et al.*[32] used NaClO in their SEM study on the Purkinje fibres in the heart. For our own SEM observation of the liver, we applied an NaOH maceration method which will be described below.

Animals are anaesthetized with sodium pentobarbital and perfused through the ascending aorta with Locke's solution, followed by 2.0% glutaraldehyde in 0.1 mol L^{-1} phosphate buffer, pH 7.3. The liver is excised and cut into small cubes, about 2 mm on each side, and immersed in the same fixative for 3 h or more at room temperature. The tissue pieces are rinsed in phosphate buffer (pH 7.3) and placed in 6 N NaOH for 20–30 min at 60°C. After the NaOH maceration, the tissue is rinsed in the phosphate buffer and conductive-stained by the tannin–osmium method of Murakami[33]. The osmicated tissue blocks are dehydrated through a graded series of ethanol, transferred to isoamyl acetate and critical point dried using liquid CO$_2$. The dried tissue pieces are pricked with a thin needle and fractured into several fragments. The tissue fragments are evaporation-coated with gold–palladium and examined in an SEM. This paper mainly describes the rat liver treated with this NaOH maceration technique.

THREE-DIMENSIONAL STRUCTURE OF ITO CELLS

Ito cells are found all over the hepatic lobules of the rat at regular intervals of 30–55 μm (Figure 1). These cells possess a round and flattened cell body which is located in the perisinusoidal spaces of Disse, or in the parasinusoidal spaces described by Motta *et al.*[34]. The latter are deep recesses between adjacent hepatocytes continuous with the former. The surfaces of the hepatocytes against both of these spaces are densely covered with microvilli. Eight to ten cell processes, also flattened, radiate from a margin of each cell body and surround the sinusoid. The Ito cells in the central portion of the hepatic lobule occasionally send out some processes to the central vein (Figure 2).

Ito cell processes show a characteristic pattern of branching in their course along the sinusoid or on the central vein. Some of their processes, here called major processes, are longer and thicker than the others, accordingly called minor processes. The major processes arising from each cell vary in number from one to four, and measure 2–3 μm in width at the proximal portion, becoming thinner towards the distal portion. They are extended longitudinally along the sinusoid for length of 15–20 μm, and are occasionally bifurcated at a fork of the sinusoid. The major processes issue many secondary branches bilaterally and at right angles, these measuring 0.5–1.0 μm in width (Figures 3 and 4). Each of these side branches pursues a semicircular course along the sinusoidal wall and, together with its counterpart extending on the opposite side, surround almost the entire circumference of the sinusoid. The outlines of the side branches are double serrated as they extend short tertiary processes of 0.5 μm width, which bear thorn-like processes of the fourth order of various lengths. The minor processes issuing directly from the cell body correspond to the side or secondary branches of the major processes in their manner of surrounding the sinusoid circularly and in their double serrated contours.

The 'Sternzellen', gold-impregnated and observed by von Kupffer[18] and Wake[5] under the light microscope, showed fewer cell processes than the Ito cells observed under the SEM, probably because only the proximal trunks of their major processes were impregnated. SEM strongly suggests that the 'Perizyten' of Zimmermann[19] correspond to the Ito cells, because these cells coincide with each other in their perisinusoidal location, in their flattened shape and in the branching pattern of their processes. Zimmermann successfully revealed the tertiary processes of his cells, though he was unable to see the processes of the fourth order or thorns which are disclosed by SEM.

The side branches of the major processes, and the minor processes themselves, are disposed at regular intervals, circularly surrounding the sinusoid along its whole circumference (Figures 1, 3 and 4). This finding supports the assumption by Tanuma and Ito[17] that the subendothelial processes of the Ito cells may reinforce the sinusoidal wall. SEM observations provide no information with regard to the possible contractility of the Ito cell processes, a proposition by Gemmell and Heath[16] and by Tanuma and Ito[17]. However, a force which might be generated by contraction of the circular processes of the Ito cells would be effectively transferred to the circumference of the sinusoid.

The Ito cell processes only rarely cross or overlap each other, keeping their entire surface area in contact with the sinusoidal endothelium which is perforated by numerous fenestrations (Figures 3 and 4). This location of the Ito cell processes appears to favour the uptake of vitamin A from the blood.

The surfaces of the body and processes of the Ito cells show sparse short microvilli on the aspect facing the hepatocytes. Small rounded elevations, corresponding to lipid droplets, occasionally occur on the perikarya or on the major processes (Figure 4). Such cytoplasmic elevations often emit an excessive amount of secondary electrons and are recognized as bright spots because the lipid droplets are impregnated with osmium more strongly than the surrounding cytoplasm.

The Kupffer cells or their parts are often found protruding into Disse's space (Figure 4). They are readily distinguishable from Ito cells as their processes branch less frequently and as their surfaces are densely covered with microprojections of various size and shape. The Kupffer cells usually interpose between the sinusoidal endothelium and the processes of the Ito cells, which are often enfolded by microprojections of the Kupffer cells.

PERIVASCULAR CELLS OF THE CENTRAL VEINS AND THE SUBLOBULAR VEINS

The basal surfaces of the central veins and sublobular veins are exposed after treatment with NaOH (Figures 5–9). The central veins, which vary in diameter from 20 to 80 μm, are perforated by numerous round openings, measuring 5–10 μm in diameter (Figures 5 and 8). These openings are disposed at intervals of 12–30 μm and considered to be orifices of sinusoids which pour into the veins. On the other hand, the sublobular veins measure more than 120 μm in diameter, showing less frequent perforations than the central veins (Figure 9). Some of their perforations are about 10 μm in diameter and are assumed to be sinusoidal openings. Others measure 25–

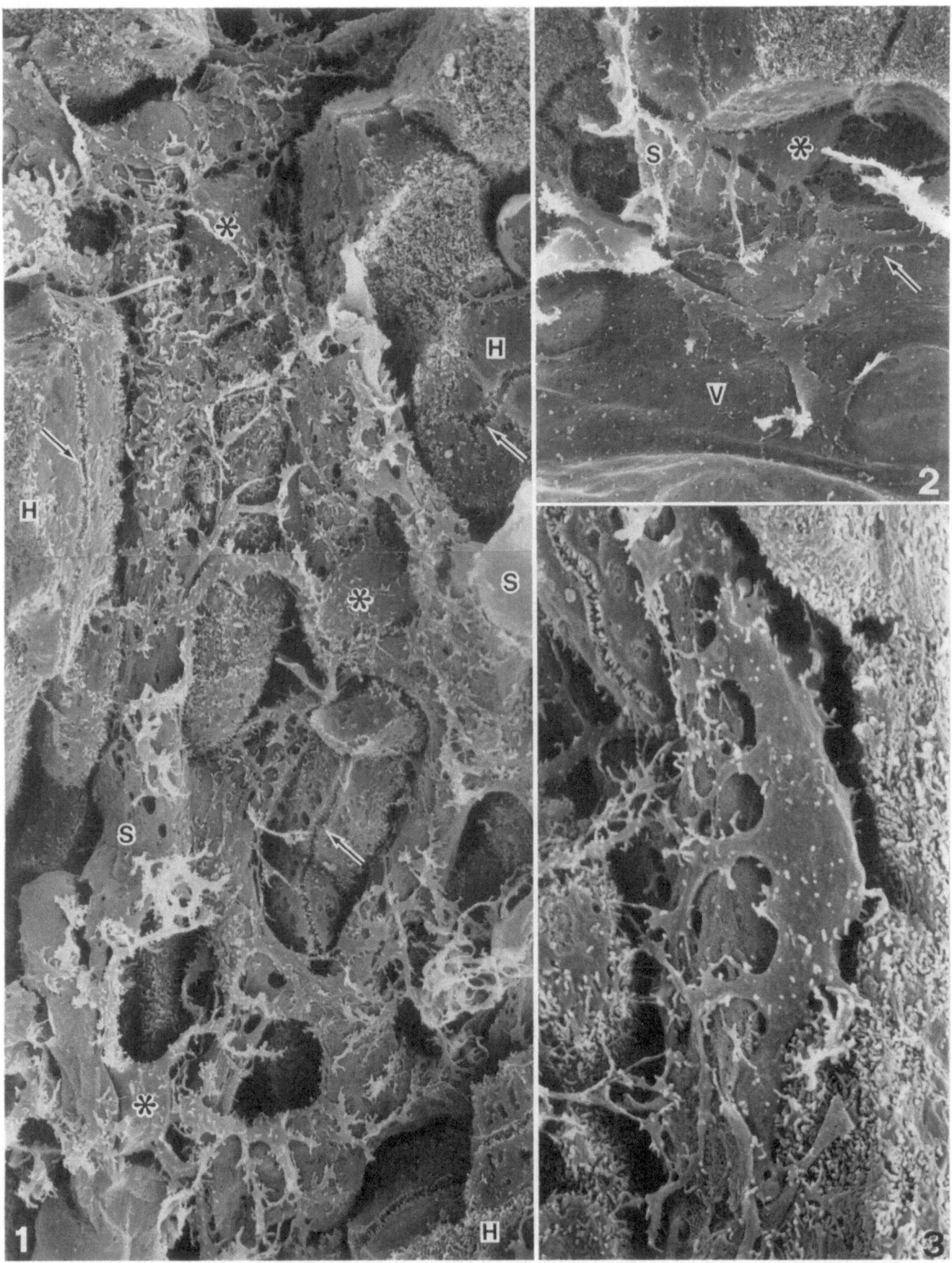

Figure 1 Low magnification view of Ito cells from rat liver treated with NaOH. Their cell bodies (asterisks) are disposed at regular intervals and radiate cytoplasmic processes, which circularly surround a sinusoidal capillary (S). Hepatocytes (H) show microvillous surfaces which confront the space of Disse, and smooth surfaces where adjoining hepatocytes are connected with each other. Arrows: bile canaliculi. × 2000

Figure 2 An Ito cell (asterisk) located in a central portion of a hepatic lobule. One of its processes (arrow) is extended along a basal surface of a central vein (V). S: sinusoid. × 1500

Figure 3 An Ito cell in a perisinusoidal space extending two major processes in opposite directions. × 3400

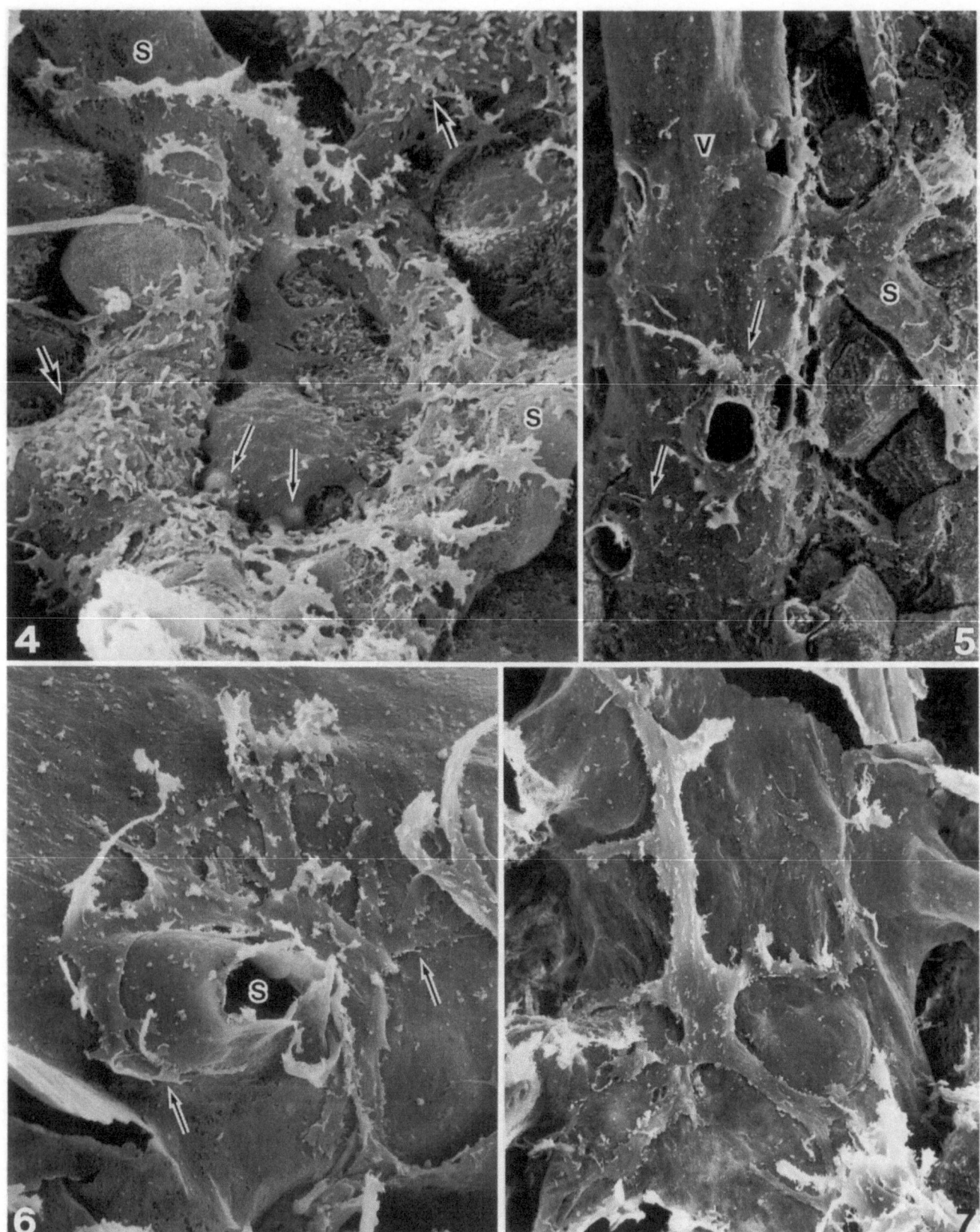

Figure 4 An Ito cell which is situated in a parasinusoidal space issues one major process. Round elevations (small arrows) are recognized as bright spots on the cell body. Sinusoidal endothelium (S) shows small fenestrations arranged in clusters. Large arrows: extrasinusoidal Kupffer cells. (Takahashi-Iwanaga and Fujita[20]) × 2800

Figure 5 Basal aspect of a small central vein (V) exposed by the NaOH maceration method. Pericytes (arrows) surround sinusoidal openings with their crescent cell bodies and radiate numerous cell processes. S: a sinusoid. × 960

Figure 6 A crescent pericyte which surrounds a sinusoidal opening (S) of a medium-sized central vein measuring about 50 μm in diameter. The pericyte extends numerous processes with serrated contours (arrows) along the basal surfaces of the central vein and the sinusoid. × 2300

Figure 7 A pericyte located between sinusoidal openings of a medium-sized central vein. Its cell processes are less numerous than those of the crescent pericytes around the sinusoidal openings and show rather smooth contours. × 1700

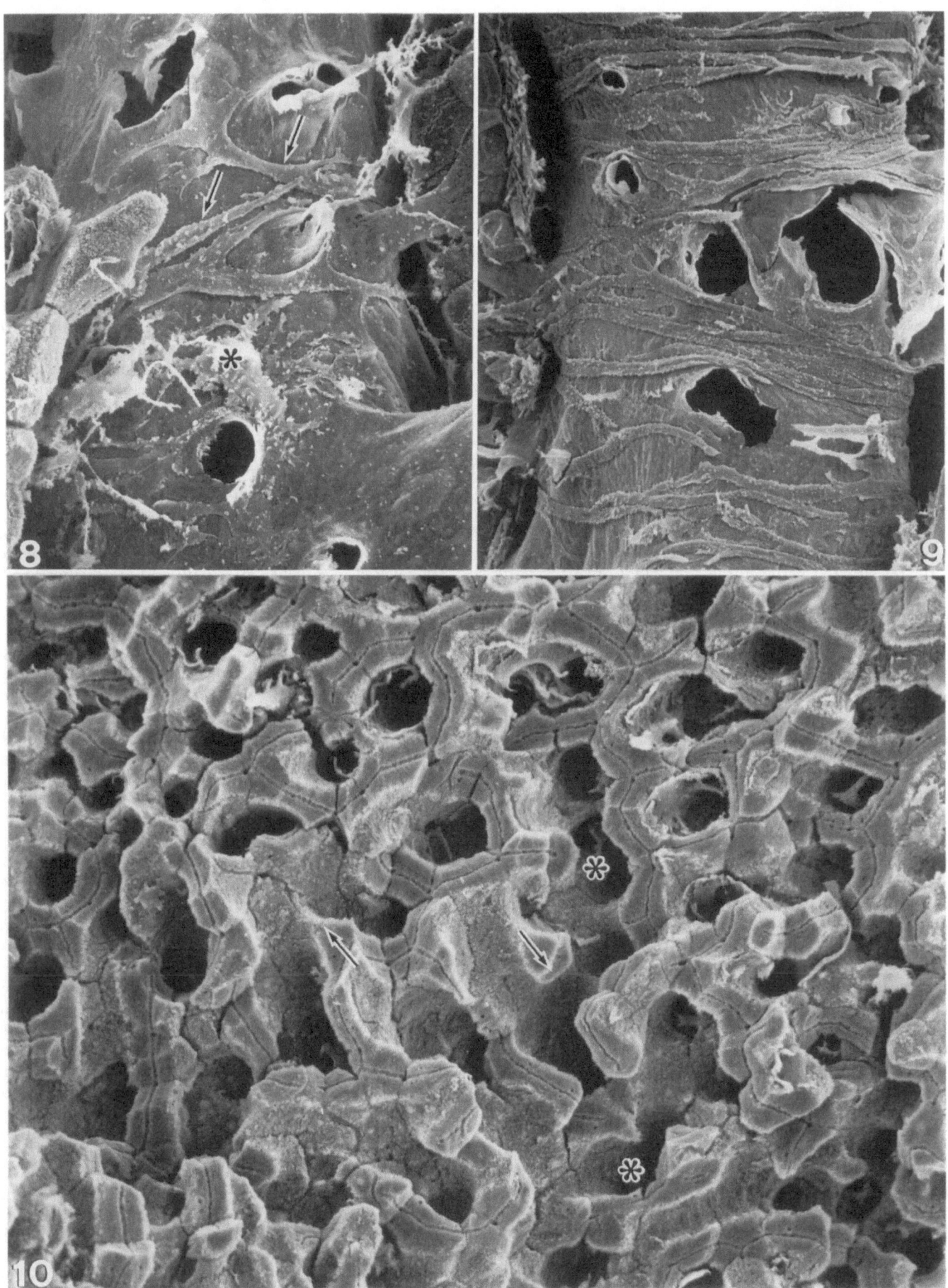

Figure 8 Basal aspect of a large central vein. It reveals elongated pericytes (arrows) which are oriented at right-angles to the long axis of the vein. A crescent pericyte with numerous serrated processes (asterisk) is found surrounding a sinusoidal opening. × 960

Figure 9 A sublobular vein revealing round openings of central veins and sinusoids. A network of smooth muscle cells circularly surrounds the sublobular vein. × 370

Figure 10 Anastomosing plates of hepatocytes exposed by NaOH maceration. Tubular spaces for sinusoidal capillaries run between the liver plates, showing crooked courses (asterisks) and oblique anastomoses with each other (arrows). × 670

40 μm in diameter and correspond to the openings of central veins. The central veins and the sublobular veins are sparsely surrounded by pericytes or smooth muscle cells.

On the small central veins which measure 20–30 μm in diameter, pericytes are usually found surrounding the sinusoidal openings with their crescent cell bodies, which are flattened, measuring 5–8 μm in width and about 20 μm in length (Figure 5). These pericytes radiate numerous attenuated processes along the basal surfaces of the central veins and sinusoids. Cytoplasmic processes arising from each cell are 8–10 in number and measure 1.5–2.0 μm in width and 6–20 μm in length. These cell processes extend short branches and thorns, which are rather sparse in comparison with those of the Ito cell processes. Some processes, measuring about 20 μm in length, send out several side branches bilaterally at right-angles in the same manner as observed at the major processes of the Ito cells.

On the central veins of medium size, measuring 30–50 μm in diameter, pericytes are located both around and between the sinusoidal openings (Figures 6 and 7). The pericytes surrounding the sinusoidal openings are identical to the crescent pericytes of the small central veins in their numerous processes with branches. However, the pericytes situated between the sinusoidal openings issue cytoplasmic processes which are smaller in number and have fewer branches or thorns than those of the crescent pericytes. Their processes measure 2–5 μm in width and 20–30 μm in length and run in straight courses.

In the case of large central veins, measuring 50–80 μm in diameter, most pericytes show elongated cell bodies and processes, which are oriented at right-angles to the long axis of the vein (Figure 8), not unlike the way in which smooth muscle cells circularly surround the sublobular veins. Contours of the processes of these pericytes are almost straight lines with very few branches or thorns. Beside these cells, a small number of crescent pericytes with numerous serrated processes occur around the sinusoidal openings.

The sublobular veins are surrounded circularly by smooth muscle cells which are elongated in shape and have an almost constant width of 3–5 μm, showing occasional bifurcations (Figure 9). Neighbouring cells are connected with each other in some areas of their sides to form a network which enshrouds the vein. The crescent pericytes are not found at the sublobular vein.

The cresent pericytes surrounding the sinusoidal openings of the central veins are similar in appearance to the Ito cells because both of them radiate numerous subendothelial processes with flattened shapes and serrated contours. It is worth while mentioning that the endothelia of the central veins are reported to show sparse fenestrations for short distances around the sinusoidal openings, as does the sinusoidal endothelium[34,35]. The question of whether the crescent pericytes might possess vitamin A storing ability remains to be elucidated.

Motta et al.[34] pointed out, in their SEM study, that the lumina of some sinusoidal openings are reduced in diameter by bulging endothelial cells. The crescent cell bodies of the pericytes which surround the sinusoidal openings may possibly be involved in these endothelial bulgings. Knisely[36] proposed 'outlet sphincters' which

might be situated at the sinusoidal openings. Contractile ability of the crescent pericytes remains to be investigated.

ISOLATED HEPATOCYTES

Elias[37], in 1949, assumed a theoretical pattern of a three-dimensional arrangement of liver plates which forms tubular spaces for sinusoidal capillaries running straight and parallel to each other (Figures 1–33 in Elias and Sherrick[38]). These spaces communicate with each other through round windows perforating the liver plates. He schematically proposed four types of polyhedral hepatocytes composing the theoretical liver plates (Figures 49, 50, 52, 53 in Elias[37]). However, SEM reveals that the architecture of liver plates is not as regular as that of theoretical ones, as Elias himself predicted. The tubular spaces which course between the real liver plates are crooked in shape and anastomosed 'obliquely'[37] with each other (Figure 10). So it is expected that hepatocytes actually show more variable and more complex shapes than the four basic types proposed by Elias.

The hepatocytes isolated by the NaOH maceration method are polyhedral in shape, measuring 20–25 μm in length and 17–20 μm in width (Figure 11). Most hepatocytes possess about eight facets, two or three of which are covered with dense microvilli and are assumed to be sinusoidal facets where the cells encounter Disse's space. The other facets, which are smooth and have narrow grooves of bile hemicanaliculi, are referred to as intercellular facets through which the hepatocytes are attached to each other (Figures 12 and 13). (See also Chapter 4.)

The real hepatocytes observed by SEM are irregularly distorted and possess no axis of symmetry. Elias depicted, in his model of liver plates, all sinusoidal facets of the hepatocytes as regular hexagons, while those of real cells are irregular pentagons, hexagons or, sometimes, large heptagons. Elias assumed that the hepatocytes might show rectangular or pentagonal facets on the intercellular aspects. However, real hepatocytes are usually connected with each other by trapezoid facets of various sizes. SEM also reveals intercellular facets of triangular (Figure 14), pentagonal and hexagonal shape.

Fine surface structures of isolated hepatocytes are preserved very well, in spite of the rigorous treatment with NaOH (Figures 12 and 13).

The microvilli on the sinusoidal facets measure about 0.13 μm in diameter and about 0.6 μm in length (Figure 13). They are tilted in random directions and are often curved into arches. Similar microvilli occur sparsely on the external margins of the intercellular facets, showing microvillous zones measuring 2–3 μm in width (Figures 12 and 14). These zones of neighbouring hepatocytes form a recess of the Disse's space designated by Motta et al.[34] as the 'parasinusoidal space'.

Wedge-shaped areas which are covered with microvilli often extend from the sinusoidal facets to the intercellular facets (Figures 12 and 13). In these areas, the parasinusoidal spaces form conical diverticula between the hepatocytes. The wedge-shaped extensions of the sinusoidal facets are usually found at the cell ridges where two intercellular facets meet. Occasionally, two extensions from opposite sides are fused with each other to form a narrow channel traversing an intercellular facet. Here, the parasinusoidal space penetrates through a liver plate,

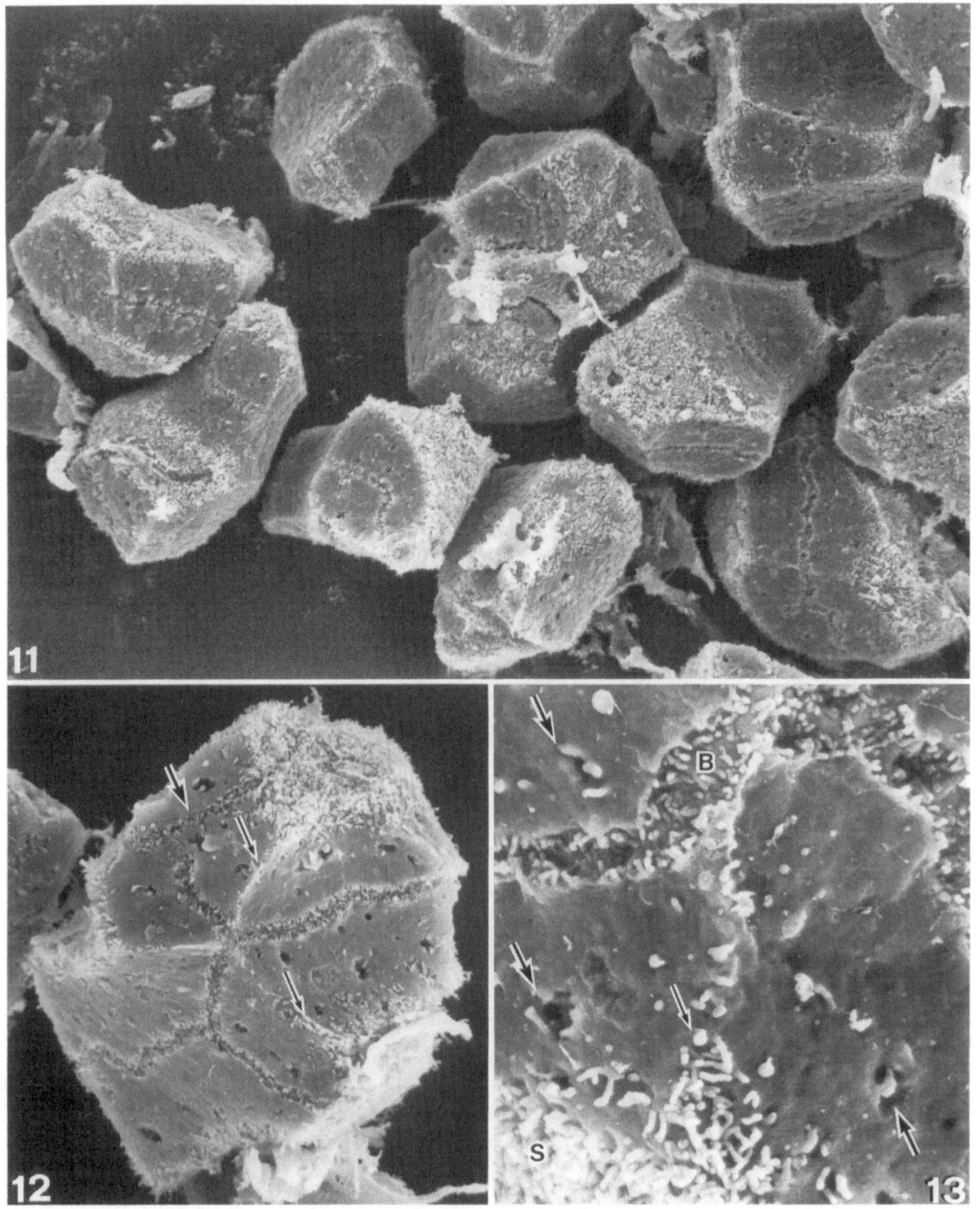

Figure 11 Hepatocytes isolated from each other after maceration with NaOH. The cells are irregularly polyhedral in shape, showing sinusoidal facets covered with microvilli and intercellular facets which are smooth and traversed by narrow grooves of bile hemicanaliculi. × 1500

Figure 12 An isolated hepatocyte. Its sinusoidal facet sends out wedge-shaped extensions which enter intercellular facets along cell ridges (small arrows). Similar extensions from opposite facets are fused with each other to form a narrow channel (large arrow) which traverses an intercellular facet. × 3200

Figure 13 High magnification of a hepatocyte. Its sinusoidal facet (S) is covered with microvilli and issues a wedge-shaped extension (small arrow). Its intercellular facets show small pits (large arrows) which have two or three microprojections. B: bile hemicanaliculus covered with numerous cylindrical microvilli. × 9100

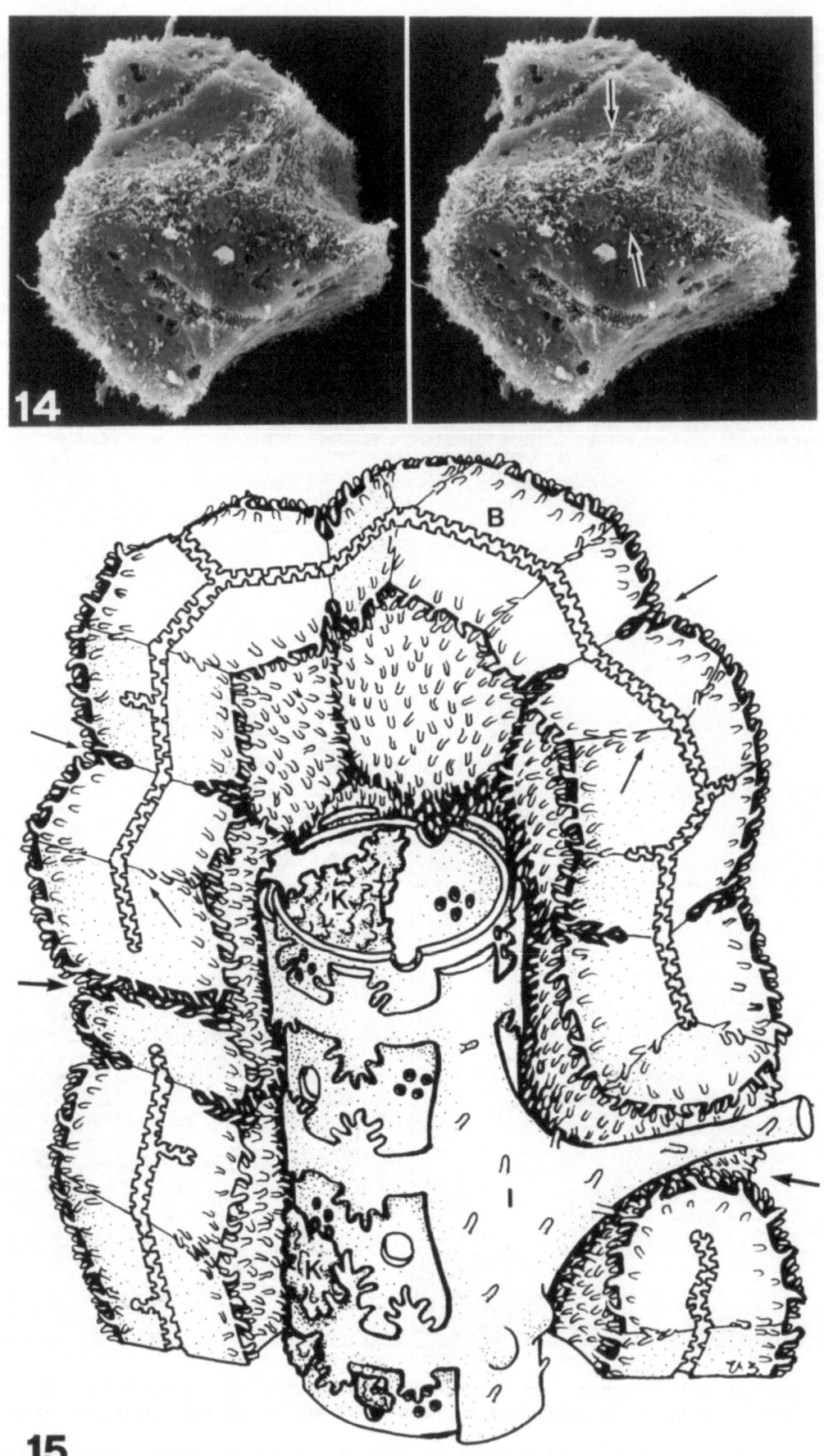

Figure 14   An isolated hepatocyte revealing two triangular facets on its intercellular aspects (in stereo). External margins of these intercellular facets have sparse microvilli (arrows). ×2600

Figure 15   A three-dimensional schematic view of the liver plate. Hepatocytes show sinusoidal facets covered with microvilli and smooth intercellular facets traversed by a bile canaliculus (B). The external margins of the intercellular facets have sparse microvilli, forming a parasinusoidal space, an intercellular recess of Disse's space. The parasinusoidal space reveals numerous conical diverticula (small arrows) along the ridges of the hepatocytes, and occasionally forms narrow channels (large arrows) which pass through the liver plate. I: an Ito cell. K: Kupffer cells

as described by Motta et al.[34] (Figure 15). Although these wedge-shaped areas provide access to the bile canaliculi, leaving only short distances of no more than 1 μm, no connection is found between them.

The grooves of the bile hemicanaliculi, measuring 0.5–1.0 μm in width, course in the central area of the intercellular facets (Figure 14). They are often extended in zigzag courses, and sometimes send out lateral branches (Figure 15). The bile canaliculi have cylindrical microvilli, measuring about 0.11 μm in diameter and 0.2–0.4 μm in length (Figure 13). Bile canaliculi show intracellular diverticula which have microvilli, as reported by Motta et al.[34]

Each intercellular facet shows several round pits, measuring 0.3–1.3 μm in diameter (Figures 12 and 13). Two or three microvilli or microplicae are found at their orifices. These pits are presumed to be involved in the interdigitation between adjoining hepatocytes. Fujita et al.[39] demonstrated, by SEM, knob-like protrusions and corresponding pits on the intercellular surfaces of human hepatocytes.

Acknowledgement

The authors wish to thank Mr K. Adachi for his technical assistance.

References

1. Ito, T. (1951). Cytological studies on stellate cells of Kupffer and fat storing cells in the capillary wall of the human liver (Japanese abstract). Acta Anat. Nipon., 26, 42

2. Nakane, P. K. (1963). Ito's 'fat-storing cell' of the mouse liver. Anat. Rec., 145, 265–266

3. Bronfenmajer, S., Schaffner, F. and Popper, H. (1966). Fat-storing cells (lipocytes) in human liver. Arch. Pathol., 82, 447–453

4. Kobayashi, K. and Takahashi, Y. (1971). Effect of the administration of large doses of vitamin A on the fine structure of rat liver with special reference to changes in the fat-storing cell. Arch. Histol. Jpn., 33, 421–443

5. Wake, K. (1971). 'Sternzellen' in the liver: Perisinusoidal cells with special reference to storage of vitamin A. Am. J. Anat., 132, 429–462

6. Hirosawa, K. and Yamada, E. (1973). The localization of the vitamin A in the mouse liver as revealed by electron microscope radioautography. J. Electron Microsc., 22, 337–346

7. Schnack, H., Stockinger, L. and Wewalka, F. (1966). Die Bindegewebszellen des Disseschen Raumes in der menschlichen Leber bei Normalfällen und pathologischen Zuständen. Wien. Klin. Wochenschr., 78, 715–724

8. Ito, T. and Shibasaki, S. (1968). Electron microscopic study on the hepatic sinusoidal wall and the fat-storing cells in the normal human liver. Arch. Histol. Jpn., 29, 137–192

9. McGee, J. O'D. and Patrick, R. S. (1972). The role of perisinusoidal cells in hepatic fibrogenesis. An electron microscopic study of acute carbon tetrachloride liver injury. Lab. Invest., 26, 429–440

10. Kawanami, O. (1973). Electron microscopic study of mammalian liver with periodic acid methenamine silver stain – Basement membrane structure and fibrogenesis in space of Disse. Acta Pathol. Jpn., 23, 717–738

11. Tanikawa, K. (1975). Ultrastructure of hepatic fibrosis and fat-storing cells. In Popper, H. and Becker, K. (eds.) Collagen Metabolism in the Liver, pp. 93–99. (New York: Stratton Intercontinental Medical Book Corp.)

12. Ito, T. and Nemoto, M. (1952). Über die Kupfferschen Sternzellen und die 'Fettspeicherungszellen' ('fat-storing cells') in der Blutkapillarenwand der menschlichen Leber. Okajima's Fol. Anat. Jpn., 24, 243–258

13. Yamagishi, M. (1959). Electron microscope studies on the fine structure of the sinusoidal wall and fat-storing cells of rabbit livers. (Japanese text with English abstract). Arch. Histol. Jpn., 18, 223–261

14. Schnack, H., Stockinger, L. and Wewalka, F. (1967). Adventitious connective tissue cells in the space of Disse and their relation to fiber formation. Rev. Int. Hepatol., 17, 855–860

15. Wisse, E. (1970). An electron microscopic study of the fenestrated endothelial lining of rat liver sinusoids. J. Ultrastruct. Res., 31, 125–150

16. Gemmell, R. T. and Heath, T. (1972). Fine structure of sinusoids and portal capillaries in the liver of the adult sheep and the newborn lamb. Anat. Rec., 172, 57–70

17. Tanuma, Y. and Ito, T. (1978). Electron microscope study on the hepatic sinusoidal wall and fat-storing cells in the bat. Arch. Histol. Jpn., 41, 1–39

18. Kupffer, C. von (1876). Über Sternzellen der Leber. Briefliche Mittheilung an Prof. Waldeyer. Arch. Mikrosk. Anat., 12, 353–358

19. Zimmermann, K. W. (1923). Der feinere Bau der Blutcapillaren. Z. Anat. Entw.-Gesch., 68, 29–109

20. Takahashi-Iwanaga, H. and Fujita, T. (1986). Application of an NaOH maceration method to a scanning electron microscopic observation of Ito cells in the rat liver. Arch. Histol. Jpn., 49, 349–357

21. Evan, A. P., Dail, W. G., Dammrose, D. and Palmer, C. (1976). Scanning electron microscopy of cell surfaces following removal of extracellular material. Anat. Rec., 185, 433–446

22. Uehara, Y. and Suyama, K. (1978). Visualization of the adventitial aspect of the vascular smooth muscle cells under the scanning electron microscope. J. Electron Microsc., 27, 157–159

23. Shimada, T. (1981). Lymph and blood capillaries as studied by a new SEM technique. Biomed. Res., 2, 243–238

24. Hamasaki, M. and Murakami, M. (1979). SEM observation of the contractile cell of Japanese monkey seminiferous tubules treated with HCl-collagenase. J. Electron Microsc., 28, 154–157

25. Fujiwara, T. and Uehara, Y. (1980). Scanning electron microscopy of myenteric plexus: a preliminary communication. J. Electron Microsc., 29, 397–400

26. Desaki, J. and Uehara, Y. (1981). The overall morphology of neuromuscular junctions as revealed by scanning electron microscopy. J. Neurocytol., 10, 101–110

27. Matsuda, S. and Uehara, Y. (1984). Prenatal development of the rat dorsal root ganglia. A scanning electron-microscopic study. Cell Tissue Res., 235, 13–18

28. Nagato, Y., Yoshida, H. and Uehara, Y. (1980). A scanning electron microscope study of myoepithelial cells in exocrine glands. Cell Tissue Res., 209, 1–10

29. Williams, J. M. and Daniel, C. W. (1983). Mammary ductal elongation: differentiation of myoepithelium and basal lamina during branching morphogenesis. Dev. Biol., 97, 274–290

30. Takahashi, H. (1984). Scanning electron microscopy of the rat exocrine pancreas. Arch. Histol. Jpn., 47, 387–404

31. Miller, B. G., Woods, R. I., Bohlen, H. G. and Evan, A. P. (1982). A new morphological procedure of viewing microvessels: a scanning electron microscopic study of the vasculature of small intestine. *Anat. Rec.*, **203**, 493–503

32. Shimada, T., Nakamura, M., Kitahara, Y. and Sachi, M. (1983). Surface morphology of chemically-digested Purkinje fibers of the goat heart. *J. Electron Microsc.*, **32**, 187–196

33. Murakami, T. (1974). A revised tannin–osmium method for non-coated scanning electron microscope specimens. *Arch. Histol. Jpn.*, **36**, 189–193

34. Motta, P., Muto, M. and Fujita, T. (1978). *The Liver. An Atlas of Scanning Electron Microscopy.* (Tokyo: Igaku-Shoin, Ltd.)

35. Grisham, J. W., Nopanitaya, W., Compagno, J. and Nagel, A. E. H. (1975). Scanning electron microscopy of normal rat liver. The surface structure of its cells and tissue components. *Am. J. Anat.*, **144**, 295–322

36. Knisely, M. H. (1947). The structure and mechanical functioning of the living liver lobules of frogs and Rhesus monkeys. *Proc. Inst. Med. Chicago*, **16**, 286–305

37. Elias, H. (1949). A re-examination of the structure of the mammalian liver. II. The hepatic lobule and its relation to the vascular and biliary system. *Am. J. Anat.*, **85**, 379–456

38. Elias, H. and Sherrick, J. C. (1969). *Morphology of the Liver.* (New York and London: Academic Press)

39. Fujita, T., Tanaka, K. and Tokunaga, J. (1981). *SEM Atlas of Cells and Tissues.* (Tokyo: Igaku-Shoin Ltd.)

6

The innervation of the liver

W. G. FORSSMANN, B. BRÜHL and S. ITO

INTRODUCTION

According to recent studies, the innervation of the gastrointestinal organs, including the large digestive glands, appears to be organized in a rather hierarchical system[1,2] of which, however, not many details are well known. Similarly, the liver exhibits a so-called **intrinsic nervous system**, which is built up by neurones located within the hilus region of this organ. These neurones of the liver are found associated with the hepatic nerve plexus at the hilus surrounding the entering blood vessels, mainly the hepatic arteries. The hepatic nerves of sympathetic or parasympathetic origin may modulate the activity of the intrinsic liver nerves, and, probably, important local circuits may be formed by the intrinsic ganglia and their intraparenchymatous fibres. The nerves within the liver may also stem directly from sympathetic or vagal connections[3-8], then constituting the so-called **extrinsic liver innervation**. They belong to the primary liver nerves running with the vagus nerve or the thoracic sympathetic branches: these nerves are mainly afferent and possibly efferent in nature. This concept of liver innervation can be postulated from a number of review publications[9-11].

ORGANIZATION OF THE EXTRINSIC LIVER INNERVATION

The extrinsic neurones for liver innervation have to be divided into those forming efferent[12-16] and those forming afferent[17-23] pathways. These neurones are classified in superordinate regulatory groups of neurones located in many areas of the brain stem[3-8] – the modulatory centres – (see Figure 1) which terminate at the perikarya of efferent neurones in the primary liver nerve nuclei, forming a medullospinal system – **the primary centres**. These connections have been traced by retrograde transport after application of HRP. The primary centres actually known are seen in Figure 1, showing the **efferent connections** to the liver by the pathways of the vagus nerve and the medullospinal tract of the sympathetic fibres. It is not known which of these efferent nerves from the vagal and sympathetic primary centres contribute directly to the intrahepatic plexus (see below). The **afferent connections** from liver receptors are the primary

sensory endings of the spinal ganglia or of the inferior vagal (nodose) ganglia. No significant ultrastructural studies of afferent liver innervation have been published so far except one paper by Ohata[24]. Only a few nerve terminals have been shown to exhibit receptor-ending qualities[17-23]; however, their nature is unknown.

ORGANIZATION OF THE INTRINSIC LIVER INNERVATION

The afferent liver nerves running to the sympathetic and parasympathetic sensory neurones are organized in the same way as in other viscera: probably their receptor endings are only found in the intrahepatic connective tissue. Some of them are found close to the liver hilus, containing a myelin sheath and can be well discerned from amyelinic afferent or efferent nerves. The afferent myelinic nerve fibres may be located in different nerve bundles surrounded by a proper perineuronal sheath (see also reference 25). The nature of amyelinic fibres, which are, in most cases, efferent, cannot be distinguished by electron microscopy. Topographically, the efferent intrahepatic nerves form a plexus around the blood vessels called the **plexus perivasculosus** intrahepaticus and, in the parenchyma of the liver lobules, the **plexus parenchymatosus** intrahepaticus (Figures 2–4). Most of the perikarya of these nerves are located in the ganglia of the liver hilus[25,26]: all those of the plexus parenchymatosus seem to be axons of intrinsic ganglia because they are not affected when a combined vagotomia–sympathectomia of the liver is carried out (Figures 19–22). The efferent liver nerves of the plexus perivasculosus may also originate from the hepatic branches of the vagus or coeliac ganglia. The ultrastructure of the ganglia of the hilus has not been studied; in the dog liver, however, we have seen a similar organization of the clusters of perikarya as in other viscera. The ganglionic agglomerations exhibit different types of neurones which are surrounded by a neuropil and numerous synaptic interconnections are observed. This may be relevant for intrahepatic circuits, or the synaptic connections are those formed by vagal or sympathetic efferent fibres from the primary centres.

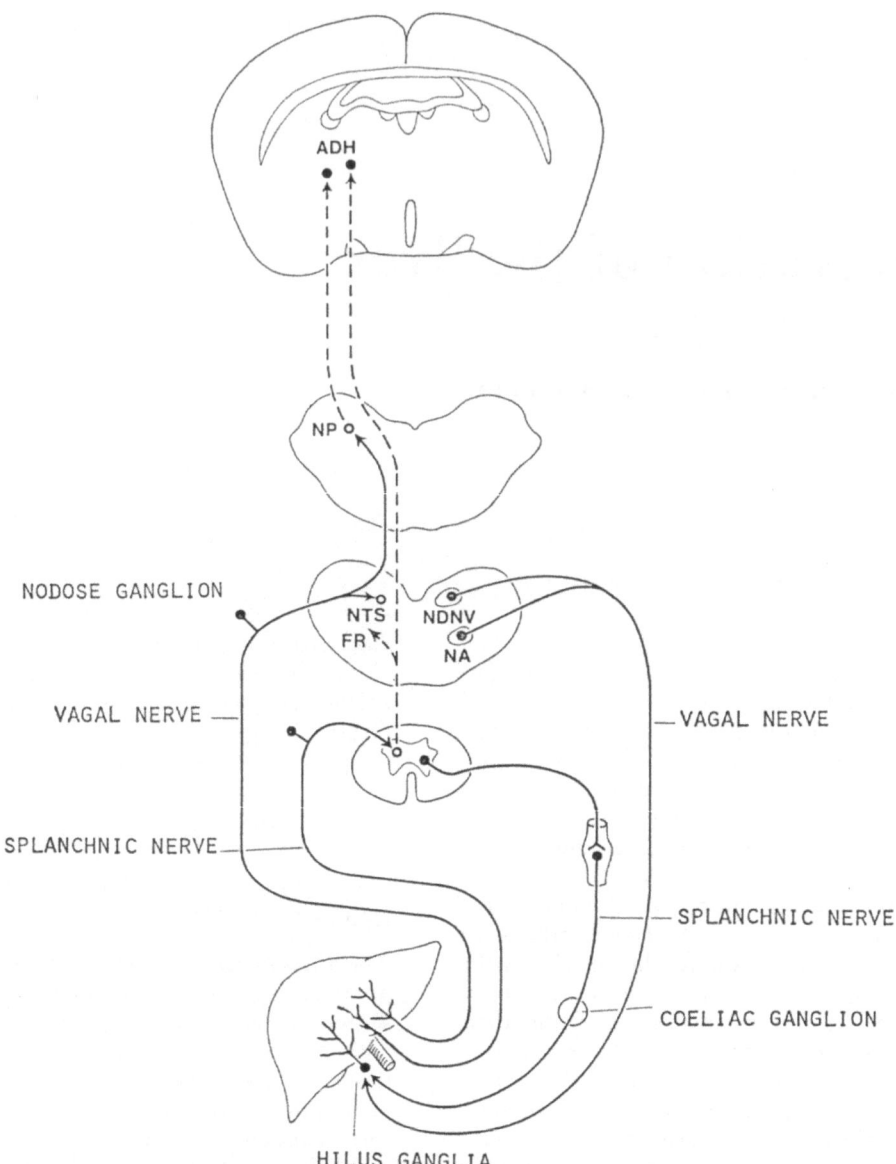

Figure 1   Schematic drawing of the autonomic innervation of the liver   The functional circuit of liver innervation according to our actual knowledge includes: (1) modulatory nuclei of the upper brain stem, such as the dorsal hypothalamic area (ADH) and the nuclei parabrachiales (NP), (2) the primary centres of the medulla oblongata et spinalis including the dorsal nucleus of the vagal nerve (NDNV), the nucleus ambiguus (NA), the reticular formation (FR), and the nucleus solitarius (NTS), (3) the peripheral pathways via the vagus nerve and sympathetic nerves, and (4) the intrinsic innervation by hilus ganglionic cells and their intrahepatic extension, such as the intrahepaticus perivascular and the intrahepatic parenchymatous plexus. (Modified from refs. 1 and 2)

HISTOCHEMICAL NATURE OF INTRAHEPATIC NERVES

The histochemical nature of liver nerves was studied using the techniques of enzyme histochemistry for acetyl-cholinesterase, fluorescence microscopy and autoradiography for catecholamines, as well as immunohisto-chemistry for neuropeptides[27-35] (Figures 2–5, 15 and 16). The most effective method was the fluorescence induction by paraformaldehyde vapours or glyoxylic acid for the adrenergic nerves which are seen in the entire intrahepatic plexus[35]. Also, some small intensely fluorescent cells (SIF cells) are seen in the hilus ganglia. Acetylcholinesterase is confined to the intrinsic ganglia and the perivascular plexus. The immunohistochemistry for neuropeptides

showed that vasoactive intestinal polypeptide (VIP), neurotensin (NT), substance P (SP) an neuropeptide Y (NPY) are seen in both intrahepatic plexus; however, their exact relation to the classical neurotransmitters is unknown. It can be deduced from neuropeptide immuno-histochemistry that in the liver all nerves of the plexus parenchymatosus are of adrenergic nature and, at the same time, they exhibit a co-storage of catecholamines with the vasoactive intestinal polypeptide (VIP).

Histochemistry of liver nerves using the fluorescence method revealed that the distribution of intra-parenchymatous nerves is quite different according to the species examined: catecholamine-fluorescent nerves are not detected in the parenchyma of rat or mouse liver, whereas human, monkey, cat, guinea pig, rabbit and dog

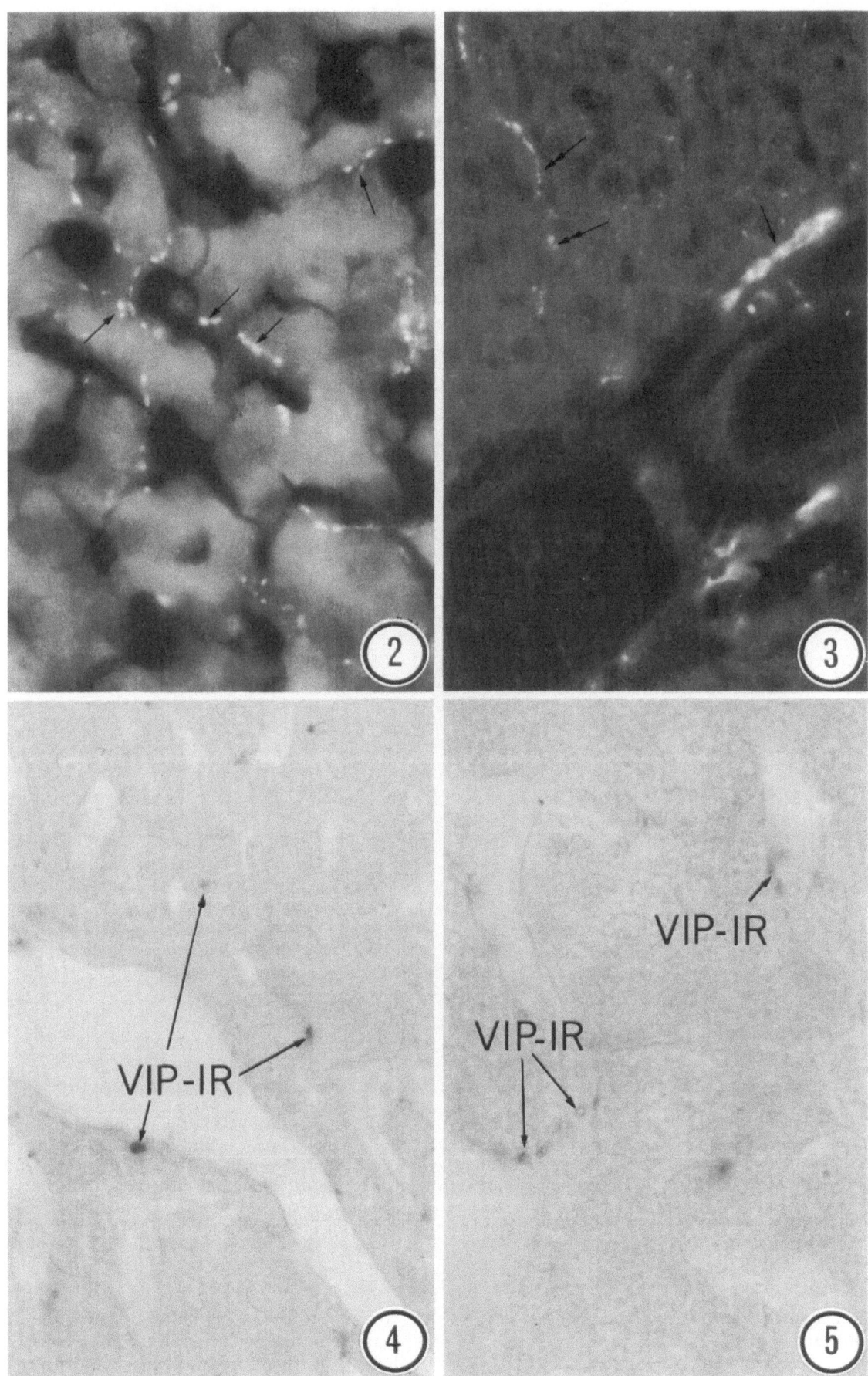

Figures 2–5 Histochemical demonstration of liver nerves by fluorescence and immunohistochemical light microscopy Fluorescence and immunohistochemical analysis of liver innervation shows a catecholaminergic and a peptidergic intrahepatic innervation. In Figure 2, the extensive intraparenchymatous plexus of catecholamine-fluorescent nerves (arrows) in the dog liver is seen (×470). Figure 3 shows the strongly fluorescent catecholaminergic nerves in the perivascular plexus of the portal trias (arrows) and some filigrane intralobular nerves (double arrows) of the plexus intraparenchymatosus of the rabbit liver (×330). Figure 4 demonstrates the immunohistochemical localization of vasoactive intestinal polypeptide (VIP-IR) in liver nerves in the area of the portal trias in the monkey (*Tupaia belangari*) liver (×470). As seen in Figure 5, VIP-IR nerves are also localized in the hepatic parenchyma (arrows) of a monkey liver (*Tupaia belangari*) (×850).

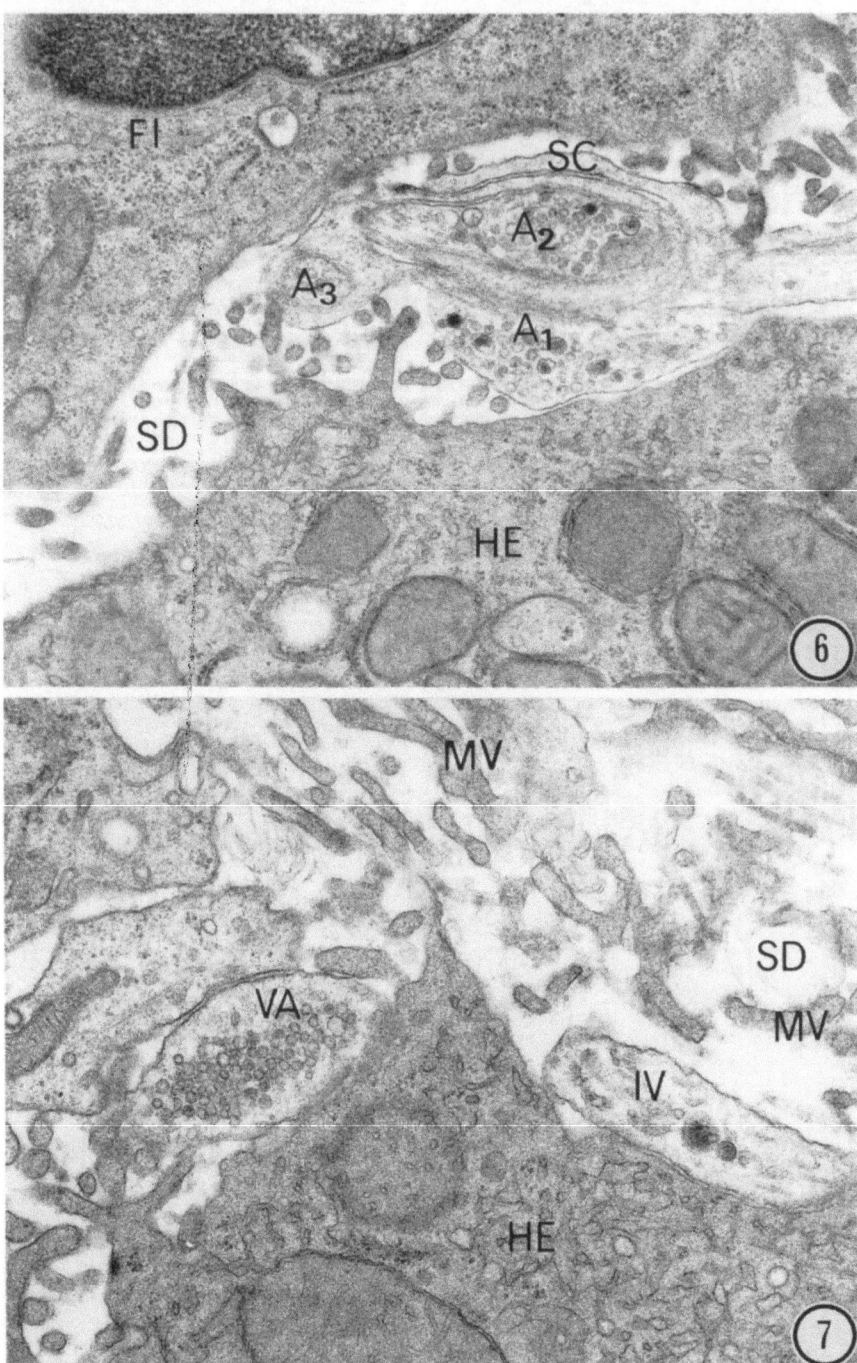

Figures 6–7   Intrahepatic nerves of the guinea pig   In Figure 6, a bundle of axons (A_1-A_3) in the periportal area is observed, one of which forms a neurohepatic contact (A_1) while the others are still surrounded by a satellite cell (SC). Note the heteromorphic synaptic vesicles in the varicosities, the hepatocyte (HE) and the fibrocyte (FI) in the space of Disse (SD) $(\times 31\,700)$. Figure 7 is an electron micrograph of a guinea pig liver taken in a more centrolobular region exhibiting a liver nerve with its intervaricosity (IV) and the vesicle containing varicosity (VA). Note that vesicles of the empty or small dense-cored type appear. Note further the hepatocyte (HE) in contact with the nerve and the space of Disse (SD) with the hepatocyte microvilli (MV) $(\times 37\,200)$

hepatic parenchymas are rich in adrenergic nerves[35] (also from unpublished results).

ULTRASTRUCTURE OF INTRAHEPATIC NERVES

In the early years of electron microscopy, reports of liver nerves were very scarce, probably because research was mainly done on the rat liver where a few nerves are confined to the interlobular tissue or the portal hepatic vessels, but hardly any seen in the parenchyma. Until the late 1970s, therefore, the existence of liver nerves in the parenchyma was controversial among electron microscopists. Thereafter, a number of papers appeared showing the ultrastructural features of liver nerves in several species[36–43]. Species variation is now well known to occur in different mammals with respect to the dis-

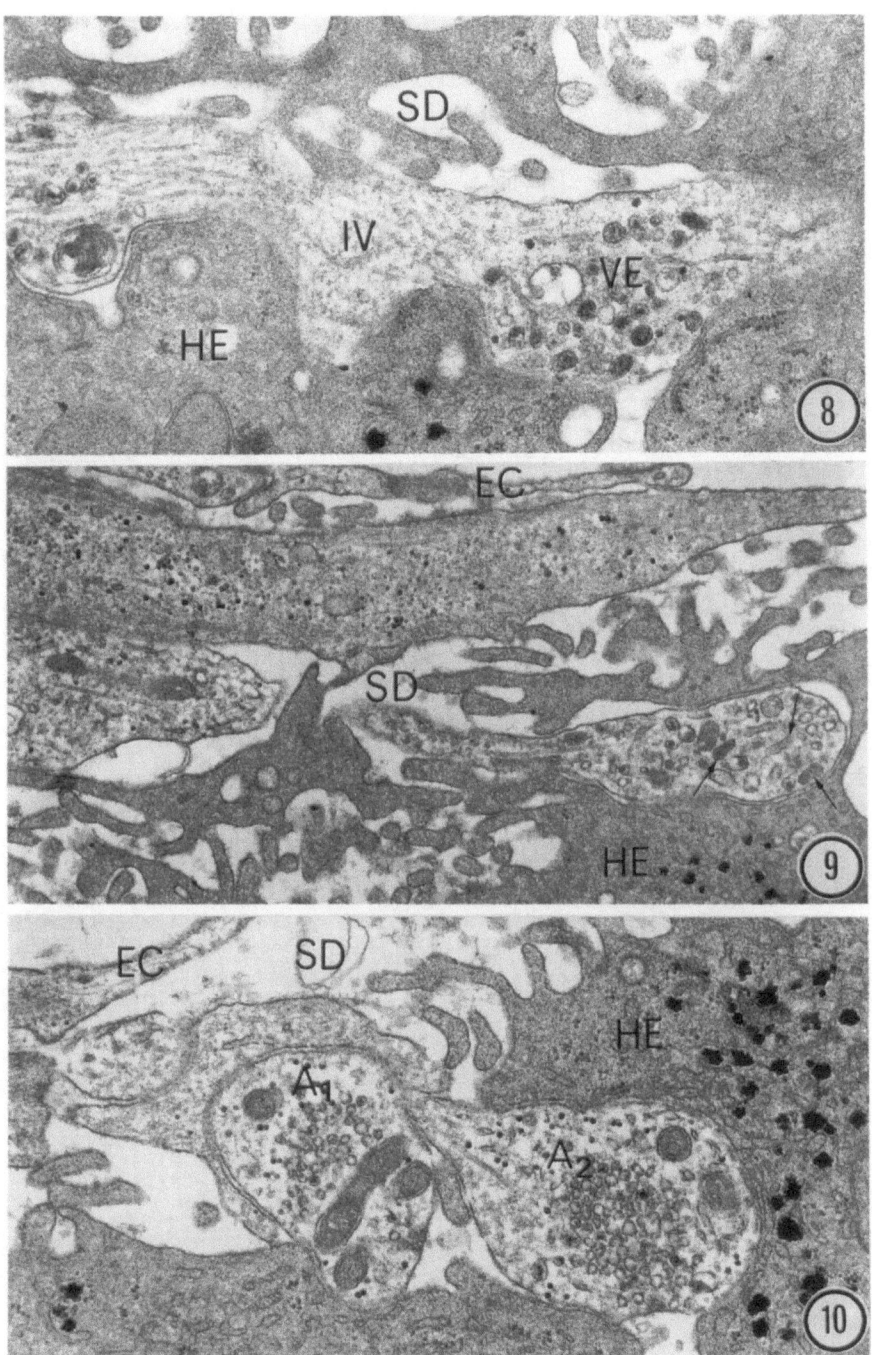

Figures 8–10 Intrahepatic nerve endings in rabbit liver parenchyma Different nerve endings according to the vesicle content are seen in rabbit liver here. Figure 8 exhibits heteromorphous dense-cored vesicles (VE), and an intervaricose (IV) region of the axon is seen ($\times 38\,200$). In Figure 9, some elliptic vesicles (arrows) are found ($\times 30\,000$). The axons (A₁ and A₂) seen in Figure 10 contain mostly small dense-cored vesicles ($\times 35\,500$). Hepatocyte (HE), endothelial cells (EC), space of Disse (SD)

tribution pattern and composition of transmitter vesicles within the terminals and varicosities (Figures 6–14).

In general, the nerves of the **perivascular plexus** are composed of bundles of axons which are surrounded by cytoplasmic extensions of satellite cells. These are, as a rule, located around branches of the hepatic artery. Larger vessels are accompanied by numerous bundles which follow the segmental and subsegmental branches to reach the periportal triads. Within the transsections, it can be seen that the intervaricose axonal segments are variable in diameter. Also in the perivascular plexus, clusters of synaptic vesicles are seen to form varicosities. In the varicosities, different vesicle types are observed, most frequently empty vesicles but also dense-cored vesicles of different core sizes and structures (Figures 6–14). Some of the endings exhibit morphological characteristics

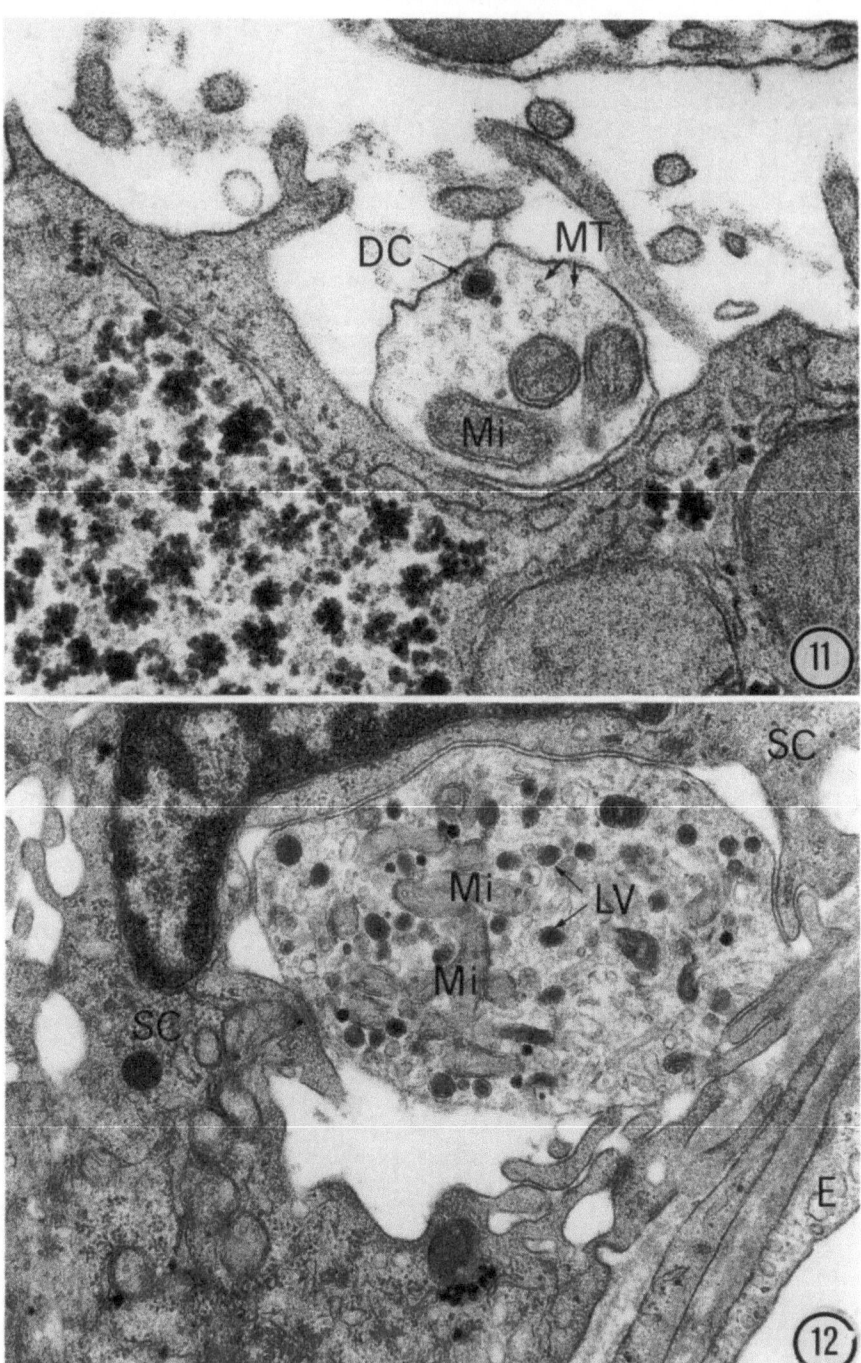

Figures 11–12   Intrahepatic nerves of cat liver   Figure 11 shows a nerve–hepatocyte contact in cat liver. The axon contains some mitochondria (Mi), microtubuli (MT), and a dense-cored vesicle (DC). This is an electron micrograph taken from the deep hepatic lobule (× 69 600). In Figure 12, a large nerve ending close to the periportal region is seen. The surrounding cell (SC) is not a hepatocyte. The vascular wall of a portal vein branch with its endothelium (E) is also closely related to this varicosity, containing numerous mitochondria (Mi) and heteromorphous large dense-cored vesicles (LV). This may be an afferent nerve ending (× 38 200)

of afferent endings (Figures 12–15); however, a definite identification of sensory endings in the liver and their specific functional implication is completely unproven.

As the nerves enter the hepatic lobules, forming the **plexus parenchymatosus**, smaller bundles are seen which, in the initial segment, may be gathered by a satellite cell, but soon the nerves lose their relationship with glial cells and usually run as single axons along the space of Disse. The intervaricosities are very small and located in grooves

of the hepatocytes exhibiting a simple ultrastructure. The hepatocyte membrane and the intervaricosity are separated by a regular 2 nm interspace and only microtubules and, rarely, mitochondria or single vesicles are observed. The axons may form several segments of short, swollen-like varicosities where clusters of synaptic vesicles are found. The varicosities – sometimes real endings – are most frequently seen in indentations of hepatocytes where small leaflet-like cytoplasmic extensions cover the thick-

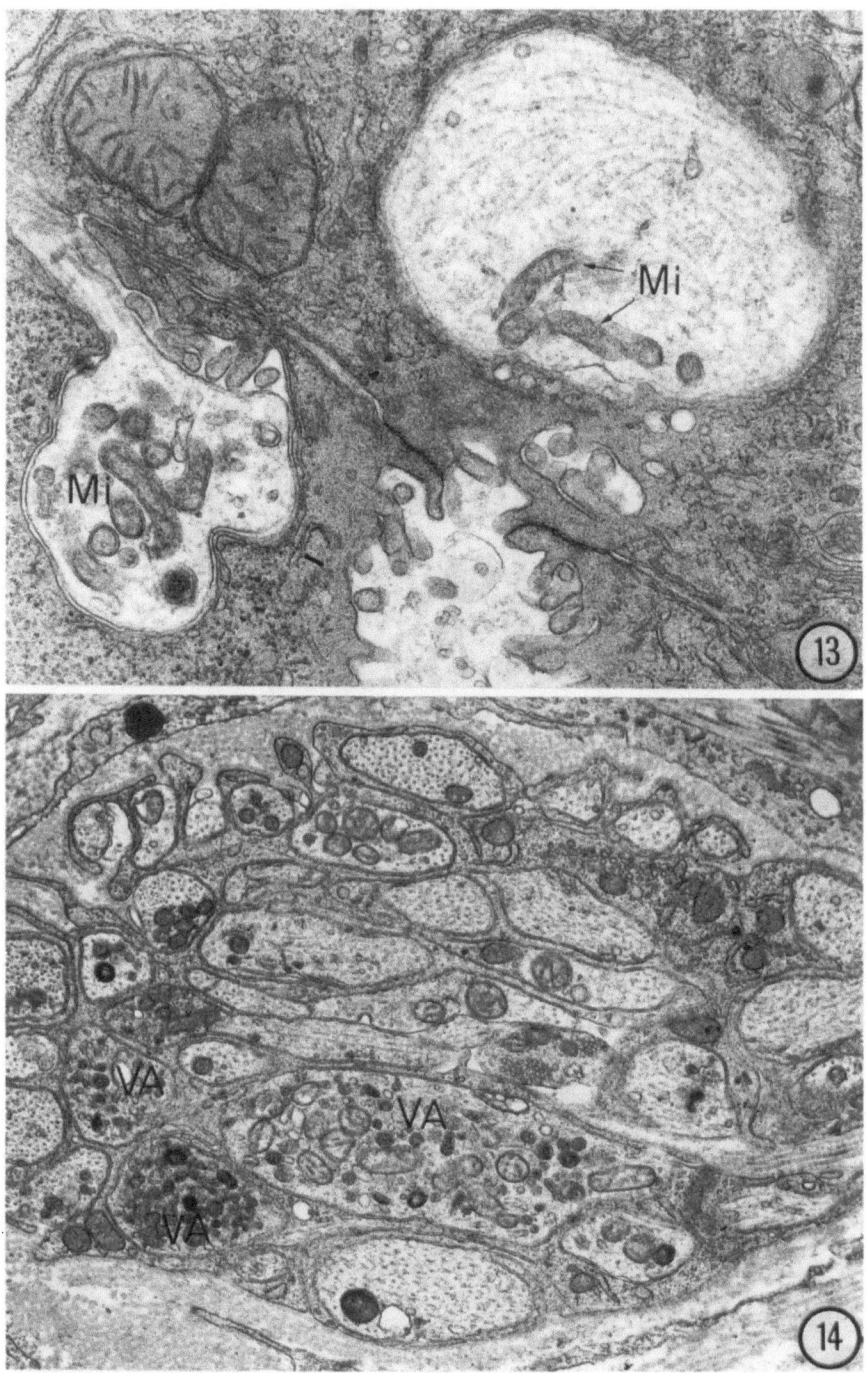

Figures 13–14 Mitochondria containing nerves in the hepatic parenchyma and heteromorphous nerves in the periportal nerve bundles Rarely, as in Figure 13, the intraparenchymatous nerves exhibit agglomerations of mitochondria (Mi) which are seen in this electron micrograph of a monkey (*Tupaia*) liver (× 30 300). In Figure 14, an axon bundle, containing several varicosities (VA) with agglomerations of mitochondria and heteromorphous dense-cored vesicles, is seen in a periportal region of Japanese-dancing-mouse liver (× 17 200)

ened part of the axon; however, the varicosity still exhibits a surface of the axon membrane open to the space Disse. The synapic vesicles are a polymorphic mixture of empty vesicles, small dense-cored vesicles with a distinct halo and some dense-cored vesicles of medium size. Large dense-cored vesicles occur rarely. It must be noted that the vesicle composition is strongly species dependent. With respect to the vesicle composition, the varicosities in one species are very similar in the plexus parenchymatosus.

ULTRASTRUCTURAL HISTOCHEMISTRY AND LIVER DENERVATION AS A TOOL FOR THE CHARACTERIZATION OF THE INTRAHEPATIC NERVES

Few studies on mechanical denervation of the liver are available to date[44-47]. The only success of an ultrastructural characterization of liver nerves was achieved by autoradiography (Figures 15 and 16). From these experiments it is clear that all nerves of the plexus paren-

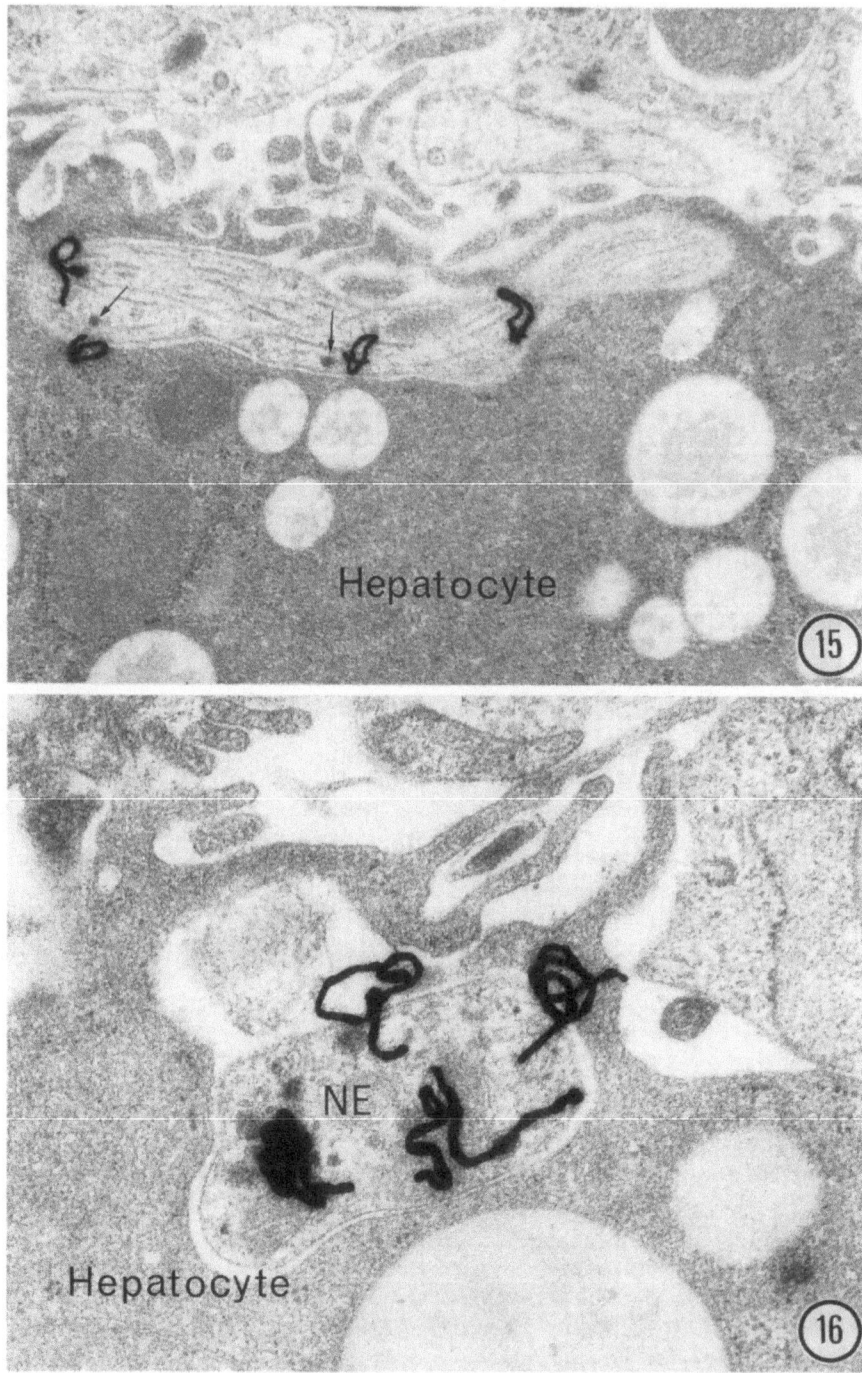

Figures 15–16 Histochemical characterization of liver nerves by high-resolution autoradiography Catecholamine uptake is observed in all intraparenchymatous liver nerves of the monkey (*Tupaia belangeri*); as seen in Figure 15, even in the intervaricose region, where few dense-cored vesicles are seen (arrows) (× 32 200). Figure 16, of the same preparation as above, demonstrates that nerve endings (NE) with the nerve–hepatocyte contact are intensely labelled after *in vivo* application of radioactive, tritiated norepinephrine (× 54 600)

chymatosus are catecholaminergic in nature[29], whereas a considerable population of the axons in the plexus perivasculosus is not related to catecholamine metabolism. This is confirmed by chemical treatment: when 6-OH-dopamine is applied, it is shown that the corresponding nerves undergo degeneration (Figures 17 and 18).

The degeneration of liver nerves has been carried out by both chemical methods and dissection of the visceral nerves, i.e. the vagus and the coeliac ganglion. Chemical denervation with 6-OH-dopamine results in a complete disappearance of the plexus parenchymatosus and a large number of nerve axons in the plexus perivasculosus, showing their adrenergic nature (Figures 17 and 18). This denervation is reversible: within 3 to 6 months, the nerves sprout into the hepatic perivascular and parenchymatosus

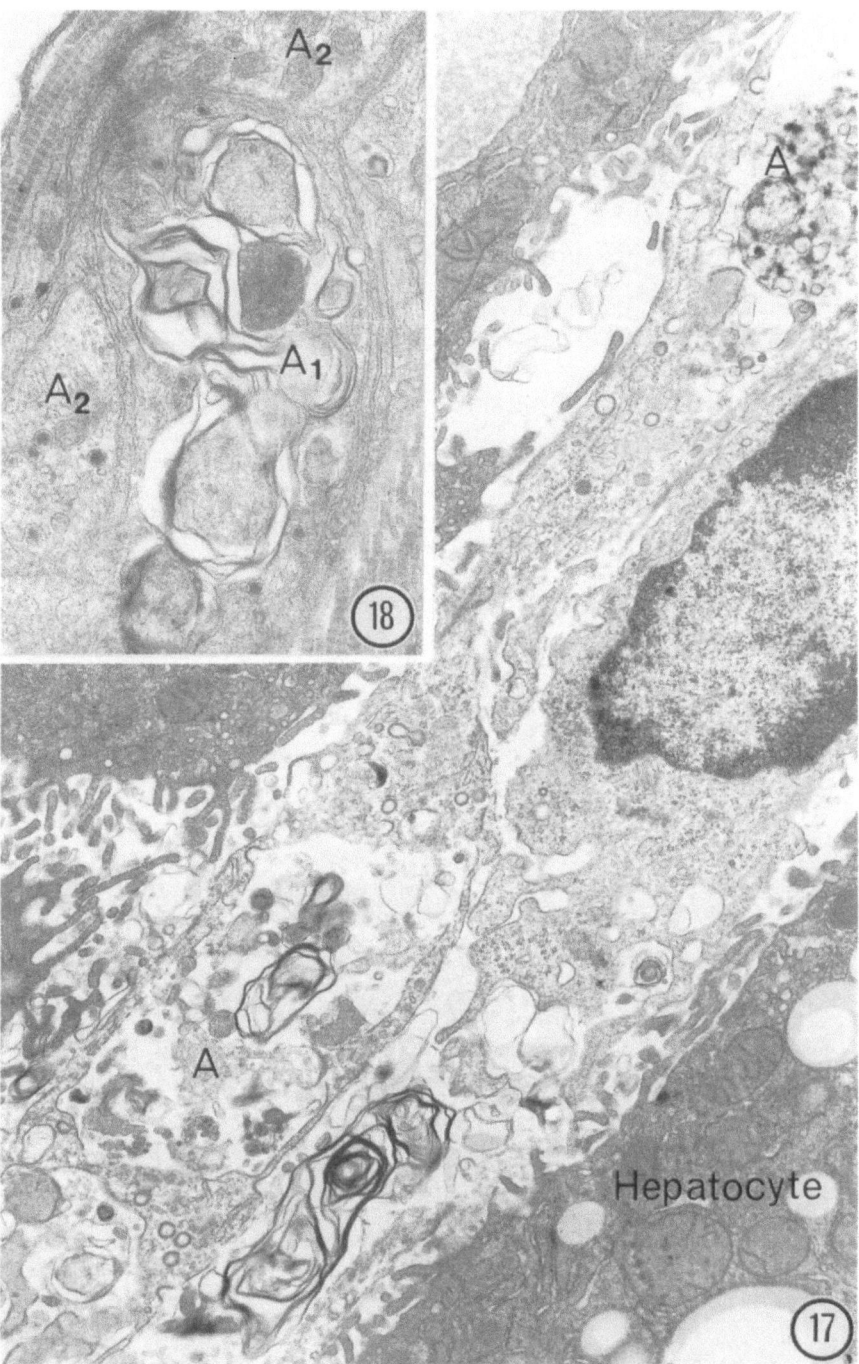

Figures 17–18   Selective chemical denervation of catecholaminergic nerves of the liver   Figure 17 shows that the application of 6-OH-dopamine results in a complete destruction of all intralobular liver nerves in the monkey liver. The degenerating axons (A) are seen 3 to 6 days after application of this substance producing a chemical denervation of sympathetic adrenergic nerves (× 35 900). Similarly, Figure 18 illustrates some of the adrenergic axons (A₁) in the periportal nerves which are destroyed by 6-OH-dopamine. However, some large dense-core vesicle-containing axons (A₂) are still persisting after chemical denervation showing their non-catecholaminergic nature (× 35 000)

plexus resulting in normal innervation. Denervation by cutting the vagal and sympathetic fibres to the liver, i.e. supradiaphragmatic vagotomia combined with the excision of the coeliac ganglion, does not affect the plexus parenchymatosus (Figures 19–22). The axons of the plexus perivasculosus are partially degenerated under the same conditions. Although no conclusive investigations

are available yet, it may be concluded that most of the intrinsic liver nerves are efferent fibres which are axons of the hilus ganglia. A minor proportion of intrinsic liver nerves is afferent or – most questionably – direct efferent nerves from the vagus or the sympathetic fibres of the coeliac ganglion. This structural arrangement is also illustrated in Figure 1.

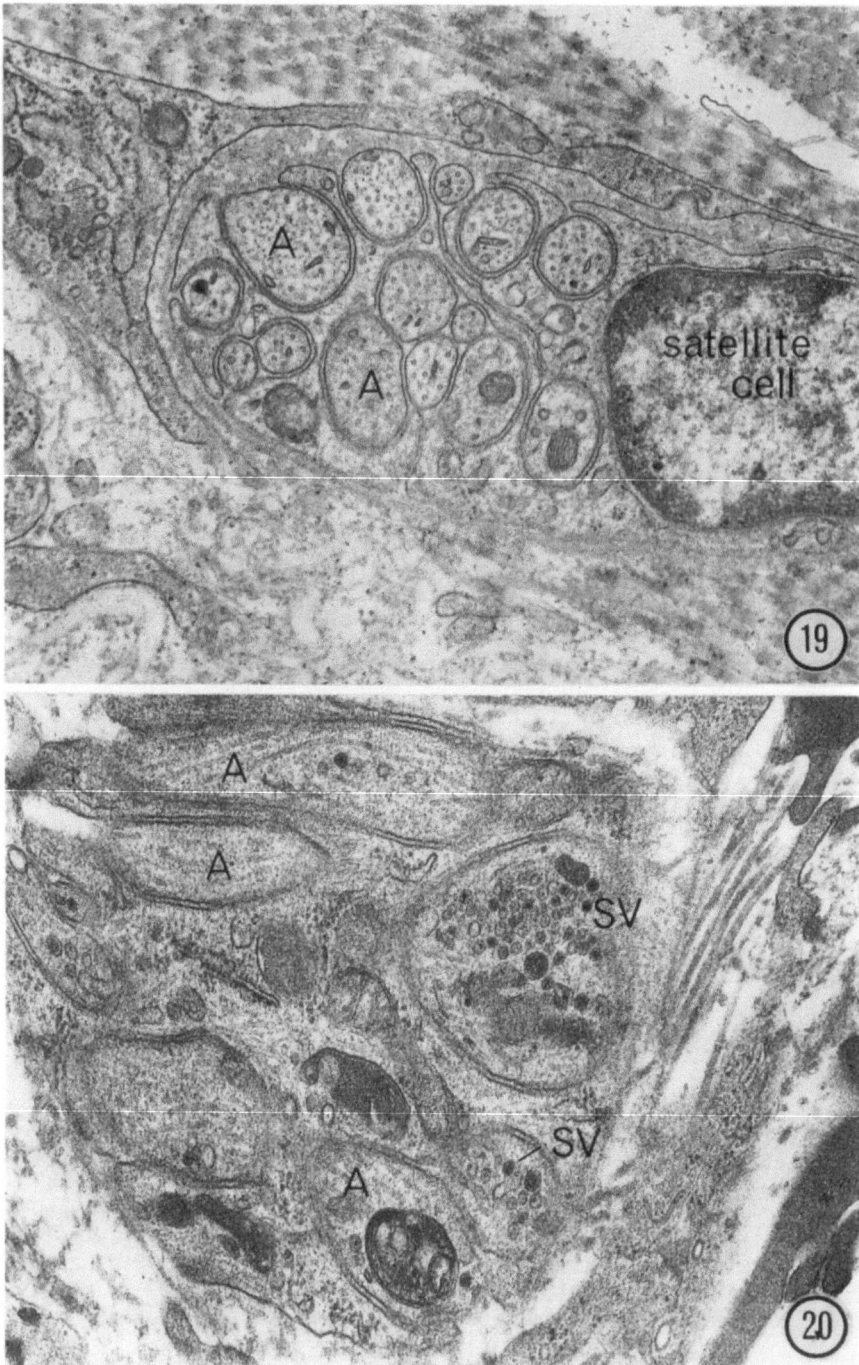

Figures 19–20 Mechanical denervation does not alter the intrinsic liver innervation in dog In Figure 19, the persistence of an intrahepatic nerve after vagotomy (subdiaphragmatic) and sympathectomy (excision of the coeliac ganglion) in dog liver is seen. Note the normal axons (A) surrounded by a satellite cell from a region close to the large intrahepatic branches of liver arteries (× 35 900). Figure 20 shows an intrahepatic nerve of the same specimen as above, but observed in a periportal trias deep in the liver. Note the axons (A) of the intervaricose type containing few or no synaptic vesicles at all; some varicosities which are rich in vesicles (SV) are seen (× 45 000)

FUNCTIONAL ROLE OF LIVER NERVES

In the last few years, the functional role of liver nerves has been studied more extensively than its morphology[9,11,12]. It may be summarized that afferent nerves are involved in: (1) pressure and volume reception, (2) osmoreception, (3) ion composition reception, and (4) reception of the metabolic status of the liver (for review, see Lautt[11]). The

corresponding, functionally well-known nerves have not been analysed by ultrastructural means so far. Efferent liver nerves are involved in (1) the regulation of liver blood flow, and (2) many metabolic functions of the liver, such as glucose metabolism, lipid metabolism, etc[11,14,19,49]. Many of the well-known hepatocyte membrane receptors may be influenced by the transmitters found in the efferent hepatic nerves.

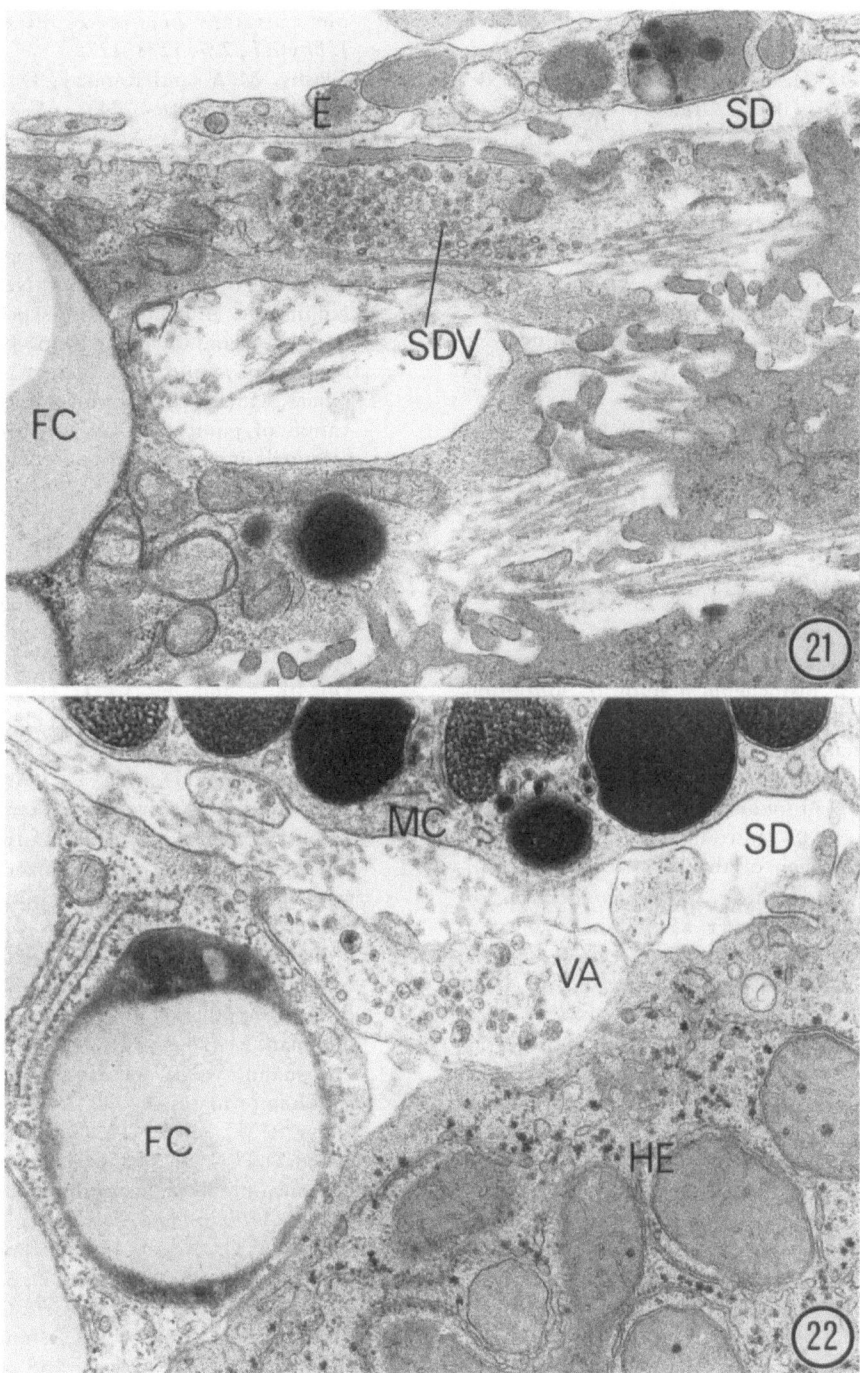

Figures 21–22 Mechanical denervation and intraparenchymatous innervation in dog liver Figure 21 illustrates a liver nerve after complete mechanical denervation (see Figures 19 and 20) of the peripheral region of a liver lobule in the dog. The nerve contains densely packed small dense-cored vesicles (SDV) and runs subjacent to the endothelium (E) in the space of Disse (SD) and in contact with a fat-storing cell (FC) (× 33 800). Figure 22 shows a parenchymatous nerve of the vagotomized and sympathectomized dog liver: a varicosity (VA) containing numerous small dense-cored vesicles innervates a fat-storing cell (FC) and a hepatocyte (HE) at the same time. Note further the space of Disse (SD) bordered by a mast cell (MC) (× 39 000)

CONCLUSIONS

This short survey of the morphological basis of liver innervation reveals many links between ultrastructure and general morphology of liver innervation. However, it must be stressed that there is still a lack of knowledge about the structure of afferent liver nerves and the intrahepatic circuits or the structural organization of the intrinsic hepatic ganglia.

The structural arrangement of the peripheral innervation of the liver is complex and barely understood to date. There exists a local system: the terminal intrinsic innervation is predominantly a part of the intrinsic ganglia. It is questionable whether any efferent vagal or sympathetic fibres directly reach these intrahepatic plexus. Afferent nerves have not yet been identified satisfactorily, in spite of the fact that their existence is evident from many functional studies.

References

1. Forssmann, W. G. (1987). Anatomische Grundlagen der nervalen Regulation der Organe des Gastrointestinaltraktes. *Z. Gastroenterologie*, **25** (Suppl. 1), 1–11
2. Forssmann, W. G. and Reinecke, M. (1984). Organ-specific innervation by autonomic nerve fibres as revealed by electron microscopy and immunohistochemistry. *Front. Horm. Res.*, **12**, 59–73
3. Adachi, A. (1981). Electrophysiological study of hepatic vagal projection to the medulla. *Neurosci. Lett.*, **24**, 19–23
4. Adachi, A. (1984). Projection of the hepatic vagal nerve in the medulla oblongata. *J. Autonom. Nerv. Syst.*, **10**, 287–293
5. Carobi, C. and Magni, F. (1981). The afferent innervation of the liver: a horseradish peroxidase study in the rat. *Neurosci. Lett.*, **23**, 269–274
6. Magni, F. and Carobi, C. (1983). The afferent and preganglionic parasympathetic innervation of the rat liver, demonstrated by the retrograde transport of horseradish peroxidase. *J. Autonom. Nerv. Syst.*, **8**, 237–260
7. Rogers, R. C. and Hermann, G. E. (1983). Central connections of the hepatic branch of the vagus nerve: a horseradish peroxidase histochemical study. *J. Autonom. Nerv. Syst.*, **7**, 165–174
8. Rogers, R. C., Kahrilas, P. J. and Hermann, G. E. (1984). Projection of the hepatic branch of the splanchnic nerve brainstem of the rat. *J. Autonom. Nerv. Syst.*, **11**, 223–225
9. Forssmann, W. G. (1980). Introduction and historical remarks on the innervation of the liver. In Popper, H., Bianchi, L., Gudat, F. and Reutter, W. *Communications of Liver Cells*, pp. 109–114 (Lancaster: MTP Press)
10. Lautt, W. W. (1980). Hepatic nerves: a review of their functions and effects. *Can. J. Physiol. Pharmacol.*, **58**, 105–123
11. Lautt, W. W. (1983). Afferent and efferent neural roles in liver function. *Prog. Neurobiol.*, **21**, 323–348
12. Niijima, A. (1979). Control of liver functions and neuroendocrine regulation of blood glucose levels. In Brooks, Ch. McC., Koizumi, K. and Sato, A. (eds.) *Integrative Functions of the Autonomic Nervous System*, pp. 68–83 (University of Tokyo Press, Tokyo; Elsevier/North Holland Biomedical Press, Amsterdam)
13. Niijima, A. and Fukuda, A. (1973). A reflex effect on glucose release from the liver of the toad. *Jpn. J. Physiol.*, **23**, 559–567
14. Niijima, A. and Fukuda, A. (1973). Release of glucose from perfused liver preparation in response to stimulation of the splanchnic nerves in the toad. *Jpn. J. Physiol.*, **23**, 497–508
15. Lautt, W. W. and Wong, Ch. (1978). Hepatic glucose balance in response to direct stimulation of sympathetic nerves in the intact liver of cats. *Can. J. Physiol. Pharmacol.*, **56**, 1022–1028
16. Hansson, P., Lindfeldt, J., Ekelund, M., Kullendorff, C-M., Holmin, T. and Nilsson-Ehle, P. (1985). Hepatic lipase activity increases after liver denervation in the rat. *Biochim. Biophys. Acta*, **833**, 351–353
17. Andrews, W. H. H. and Orbach, J. (1973). Sensitivity of nerve endings to changes of osmolarity in the perfused rabbit liver. *J. Physiol. (London)*, **231**, 115P–116P
18. Bennett, W. M., Hennes, D., Elliot, D. and Porter, G. A. (1974). In search of a hepatic osmoreceptor in man. *Dig. Dis.*, **19**, 143–148
19. Andrews, W. H. H. and Orbach, J. (1974). Sodium receptors activating some nerves of perfused rabbit livers. *Am. J. Physiol.*, **227**, 1273–1275
20. Glasby, M. A. and Ramsay, D. J. (1974). Hepatic osmoreceptors? *J. Physiol.*, **243**, 765–776
21. Niijima, A. (1977). Afferent discharges from venous pressoreceptors in liver. *Am. J. Physiol.*, **232**, C76–C81
22. Rogers, R. C., Novin, D. and Butcher, L. L. (1979). Electrophysiological and neuroanatomical studies of hepatic portal osmo- and sodium-receptive afferent projections within the brain. *J. Autonom. Nerv. Syst.*, **1**, 183–202
23. Niijima, A. (1983). Glucose-sensitive afferent nerve fibres in the liver and their role in food intake and blood glucose regulation. *J. Autonom. Nerv. Syst.*, **9**, 207–220
24. Ohata, M. (1984). Electron microscope study of the innervation of guinea pig liver – proposal of sensory nerve terminals in the hepatic parenchyme. *Arch. Histol. Jpn.*, **47**, 149–178
25. Prechtl, J. C. and Powley, T. L. (1987). A light and electron microscopic examination of the vagal hepatic branch of the rat. *Anat. Embryol.*, **176**, 115–126
26. Schubert, W., Metz, J. and Forssmann, W. G. (1984). Zur peptidergen Innervation der Leber. *Verh. Anat. Ges.*, **78**, 461–462
27. Donath, T. and Ungvary, G. (1970). Beiträge zur monoaminergischen Innervation der Leber. *Verh. Anat. Ges.*, **68**, 325–328
28. Ungváry, G. and Donáth, T. (1969). On the monoaminergic innervation of the liver. *Acta Anat. (Basel)*, **72**, 446–459
29. Nobin, A., Falck, B., Ingemansson, S., Järhult, J. and Rosengren, E. (1977). Organization and function of the sympathetic innervation of human liver. *Acta Physiol. Scand. Suppl.*, **452**, 103–106
30. Nobin, A., Baumgarten, H. G., Falck, B., Ingemansson, S., Moghimzadeh, E. and Rosengren, E. (1978). Organization of the sympathetic innervation in liver tissue from monkey and man. *Cell. Tiss. Res.*, **195**, 371–380
31. Forssmann, W. G. and Ito, S. (1977). Hepatocyte innervation in primates. *J. Cell. Biol.*, **74**, 299–313
32. Fuller, R. W., Felten, S. Y., Perry, K. W., Snoddy, H. D. and Felten, D. L. (1981). Sympathetic noradrenergic innervation of guinea-pig liver: histofluorescence and pharmacological studies. *J. Pharmacol. Exp. Ther.*, **218**, 282–288
33. Allman, F. D., Rogers, E. L., Caniano, D. C., Jacobowitz, D. M. and Rogers, M. C. (1982). Selective chemical hepatic sympathectomy in the dog. *Crit. Care Med.*, **10**, 100–103
34. Moghimzadeh, E., Nobin, A. and Rosengren, E. (1983). Fluorescence microscopical and chemical characterization of the adrenergic innervation in mammalian liver tissue. *Cell. Tiss. Res.*, **230**, 605–613
35. Metz, W. and Forssmann, W. G. (1980). Innervation of the liver in guinea pig and rat. *Anat. Embryol.*, **160**, 239–252
36. Yamada, E. (1965). Some observations on the nerve terminal on the liver parenchyma cell of the mouse as revealed by electron microscopy. *Okajimas Fol. Anat. Jpn.*, **40**, 663–677
37. Ito, T. and Shibasaki, S. (1968). Electron microscopic study on the hepatic sinusoidal wall and the fat-storing cells in the normal human liver. *Arch. Histol. Jpn.*, **29**, 137–192
38. Blouin, A. and Coté, M. G. (1973). Cartographie de l'innervation sympathique de lobes gauche et médians du foie du rat. *Rev. Can. Biol.*, **32**, 187–211
39. Forssmann, W. G. and Ito, S. (1975). Innervation of hepatocytes in the tree shrew. In *10th International Congress of Anatomy, Tokyo*, p. 540

40. Skaaring, P. and Bierring, F. (1976). On the intrinsic inner-vation of normal rat liver. *Cell. Tiss. Res.*, **171**, 141–155

41. Reilly, F. D., McCuskey, P. A. and McCuskey, R. S. (1978). Intrahepatic distribution of nerves in the rat. *Anat. Rec.*, **191**, 55–68

42. Tsuneki, K. and Ichihara, K. (1981). Electron microscope study of vertebrate liver innervation. *Arch. Histol. Jpn.*, **44**, 1–13

43. Metz, J. and Forssmann, W. G. (1979). Comparative mor-phology of liver innervation. In Popper, H., Bianchi, L., Gudat, F. and Reutter, W. *Communications of Liver Cells*, pp. 121–127. (Lancaster: MTP Press)

44. Ungváry, G. and Donáth, T. (1975). Neurohistochemical changes in the liver of guinea pigs following ligation of the common bile duct. *Exp. Mol. Pathol.*, **22**, 29–34

45. Mathie, R. T., Lam, P. H. M., Harper, A. M. and Blumgart, L. H. 1980). The hepatic arterial blood flow response to portal vein occlusion in the dog. *Pflügers Arch.*, **386**, 77–83

46. McKelvey, S. T. D., Toner, D., Connell, A. M. and Kennedy, T. L. (1976). Coeliac and hepatic nerve function following selective vagotomy. *Br. J. Surg.*, **60**, 219–221

47. Lautt, W. W. (1981). Evaluation of surgical denervation of the liver in cats. *Can. J. Physiol. Pharmacol.*, **59**, 1013–1016

48. Jungermann, K. (1987). Regulation von Stoffwechsel und Hämodynamik der Leber durch die hepatischen Nerven. *Z. Gastroenterelogie,* **25** (Suppl. 1), 44–54

49. Hartmann, H., Beckh, K. and Jungermann, K. (1982). Direct control of glycogen metabolism in the perfused rat liver by the sympathetic innervation. *Eur. J. Biochem.*, **123**, 521–526

7

The microvascularization of the liver, the bile duct and the gallbladder

O. OHTANI

INTRODUCTION

The combination of Murakami's technique[1] for obtaining vascular corrosion casts and scanning electron microscopy has been widely used to visualize fine blood vessels and has revolutionized current knowledge of the three-dimensional organization of the microvasculature of a variety of tissues and organs, including the liver. More recently, methods have been developed for making corrosion casts of the biliary system, including the bile canaliculi[2], and of lymphatic microvessels[3–7].

This chapter briefly describes these methods and reviews liver, bile ducts and gallbladder findings in humans and in laboratory animals.

MATERIALS AND METHODS

The human liver was obtained by necropsy from a Japanese individual who had suffered from chronic renal failure and had been treated with artificial dialysis. Light microscopy of the tissues stained with haematoxylin and eosin showed no pathological changes. Experimental animals used were normal adult Wistar rats, Japanese rabbits and cats. Bullfrogs, *Rana catesbiana*, were also used.

Thorough casting of blood vessels

In the human liver, cannulae were inserted into the hepatic artery and the portal vein, through which Ringer's solution or physiological saline was perfused in order to remove as much blood as possible from the vascular bed. The experimental animals were anaesthetized by inhalation of diethyl ether or intravenous administration of pentobarbital sodium (Nembutal, Abbot Lab., North Chicago). A cannula was inserted either into the thoracic aorta or the coeliac artery, and physiological saline was perfused through the cannulated vessel.

Following this procedure, the casting medium was prepared according to the method described by Murakami (1971)[1] or a commercially available one (Mercox, Oken Shoji, Tokyo, Japan) whose viscosity was adjusted to 3–4 centistokes by supplementing with methyl methacrylate monomer (Katayama Chemicals, Osaka, Japan). This was injected through the cannulated vessels until the draining vessels of the liver (and the gallbladder) were filled with injected resin. Injection was performed by syringe with applied hand pressure, while observing the casting medium filling the vascular bed of the liver. The injected organs were placed for several hours in a warm water bath (60° C), corroded overnight in a warm 10–20% NaOH solution, and washed in warm (60° C) running water.

Partial casting of blood vessels

Partial casting of blood vessels is useful in studying the distribution pattern of the arterial and/or venous systems.

Partial casting of the hepatic venous system

Either the hepatic vein or the inferior vena cava in the rat was cannulated. The inferior vena cava was ligated just cranial to the renal veins, and the portal vein was cut open just before the point at which it enters the liver. Through the cannula, physiological saline was perfused, after which 10% formalin in $0.1 \, mol \, L^{-1}$ phosphate buffer was perfused. About 10 ml of resin was infused through the cannulated vessel until the hepatic sinusoids were partially filled. The resin-infused organ was treated in the same way as in the thorough casting of blood vessels.

Partial casting of the portal vein and hepatic artery

The thoracic aorta was cannulated and the inferior vena cava was cut open just cranial to the diaphragm. Physiological saline was perfused through the cannulated vessel, after which 10% formalin in $0.1 \, mol \, L^{-1}$ phosphate buffer was perfused. About 10 ml of resin was infused through the cannulated vessel until the colour of the liver surface around the portal tracts changed to the colour of the resin injected. The resin-infused organ was treated in the same way as in the partial casting of the hepatic venous system.

Corrosion casting of lymphatic vessels

Recently, methods have been developed for making lymphatic corrosion casts. Retrograde injection of partially polymerized methacrylate (Mercox) into the bile duct may fill the lymphatic system located in the portal canal of the liver[7]. The lymphatic system of the lymph node can be replicated by injection of resin into the afferent lymphatics of the lymph node[8,9]. In order to make corrosion casts of the lymphatic capillaries of the gastrointestinal tract, a small volume of low-viscosity resin (Mercox supplemented with methyl methacrylate monomer to give a viscosity of 1.5–2.0 centistokes) was injected intraparenchymally into the submucosa and deep mucosa by needle punctures (Figure 1)[4–6]. The intraparenchymal injection of resin can replicate the lymphatics of the thyroid gland[3] as well as the tongue[10]. In newborn animals, the intra-arterial injection of low-viscosity resin (see above) filled lymphatic vessels as well as blood vessels in some organs, such as the stomach[11].

Simultaneous casting of blood and lymphatic vessels

Scanning electron microscopic observations of the simultaneously cast blood and lymphatic vessels clearly show the three-dimensional relationships between the two vascular systems. However, this method has not yet been employed for the study of the microcirculation of the liver, but only for that of the small intestine in the rat and rabbit (Figure 2)[6].

Under anaesthesia, a cannula was inserted into the main feeding artery of the organ. The blood vascular bed was perfused with physiological saline or Ringer's solution through the cannula. A small volume of low-viscosity casting medium (Mercox diluted with methyl methacrylate monomer, see above) was injected intraparenchymally by needle punctures, as in the lymphatic corrosion casting, following the infusion of Mercox into the blood vascular system. The injected organ was treated in the same way as in lymphatic or blood vascular corrosion casting.

Corrosion casting of bile canaliculi

Casting medium

Methyl methacrylate monomer (Katayama Chemicals) and 2-hydroxypropyl methacrylate monomer (Nakarai Chemical, Kyoto, Japan) was mixed in the volume ratio of 5:4 to 6:5. This mixture was supplemented with N,N-dimethylanilin (Katayama Chemicals) to give a concentration of 1.5% shortly before injection.

Injection into bile canaliculi

Under anaesthesia with pentobarbital sodium (Nembutal, Abbot Lab.), the thoracic aorta and the common bile duct were cannulated. The animals were perfused with physiological saline through the cannulated aorta, followed by perfusion with 2% glutaraldehyde in 0.1 mol L^{-1} phosphate buffer. Immediately after this procedure, the casting medium was injected into the cannulated duct by a syringe with applied force at a pressure of about 70–80 mmHg. The injection was continued until the casting medium in the syringe hardened. Injected organs were treated in the same way as in blood vascular corrosion casting except that the corrosion casts of the bile canaliculi were freeze-dried in a Model 2FS5 freeze-dryer (Hull, PA, USA).

Scanning electron microscopic observation

The corrosion casts were frozen in water, cut into blocks of a suitable size for scanning electron microscopic observation, and air-dried. The corrosion casts of the bile canaliculi were freeze-dried in a Model 2FS5 freeze-dryer (Hull, PA, USA). Blocks were mounted on metal stubs with silver paste (Dotite Type 550, Fujikura Kasei, Sano, Japan), coated with a thin layer of gold in an Eiko IB-3 ion coater (Eiko Engineering, Tokyo, Japan), and observed in a JSM U3 scanning electron microscope (JEOL, Tokyo, Japan) with an accelerating voltage of 5 kV. Prior to scanning electron microscopic observation, some casts were microdissected with fine tweezers and sharpened needles under a binocular microscope to expose deeper structures. Scanning electron microscopic observation and the following microdissection was repeated until the microvascular organization was satisfactorily revealed. Stereo pairs of scanning electron micrographs were frequently taken with tilt separation of 6–10° to assess the connections of fine structures.

MICROVASCULARIZATION OF THE LIVER

General

The liver is made up of innumerable small lobules which are considered the anatomical units of liver. This concept of 'classical' hepatic lobule was initially proposed by Kiernan[12] more than a century ago. Histologically, the hepatic lobule consists of an epithelial parenchyma and a system of extensively interconnecting sinusoids. The parenchyma is made up of hepatic cells aligned in broad plates or sheets which form partitions between blood sinusoids[13,14].

The liver has a dual blood supply. It is generally accepted that approximately 80% of the blood entering the liver is poorly oxygenated but nutrient-rich venous blood supplied by the portal vein, while the remainder is well oxygenated and supplied by the hepatic artery.

In general, the interlobular (or hepatic) artery runs with the much thicker interlobular portal vein, intrahepatic bile duct, lymphatics and nerves in the stroma of the portal tract (Figures 3 and 4).

The portal veins branch out into the hepatic sinusoids (Figures 3–8) and the hepatic arterial branches also drain into the sinusoids either directly, via the peribiliary plexus or through the portal venules (i.e. through the arterioportal anastomoses) (see below). The sinusoids converge into the central veins which, in turn, drain into the sublobular veins and ultimately lead into the hepatic vein (Figures 3 and 4).

The hepatic artery

The interlobular (hepatic) arteries largely contribute to formation of the peribiliary (or periductal) plexus circumscribing the intrahepatic bile ducts[15–18] (Figure 3). Other arterial branches bypass the peribiliary plexus and break up into the sinusoids[19] (Figure 7). The arteriolar capillaries connect with the sinusoids only at the periphery of the lobule (Figures 5 and 9). The interlobular arterioles occasionally anastomose with the accompanying interlobular (portal) venules (arterioportal anas-

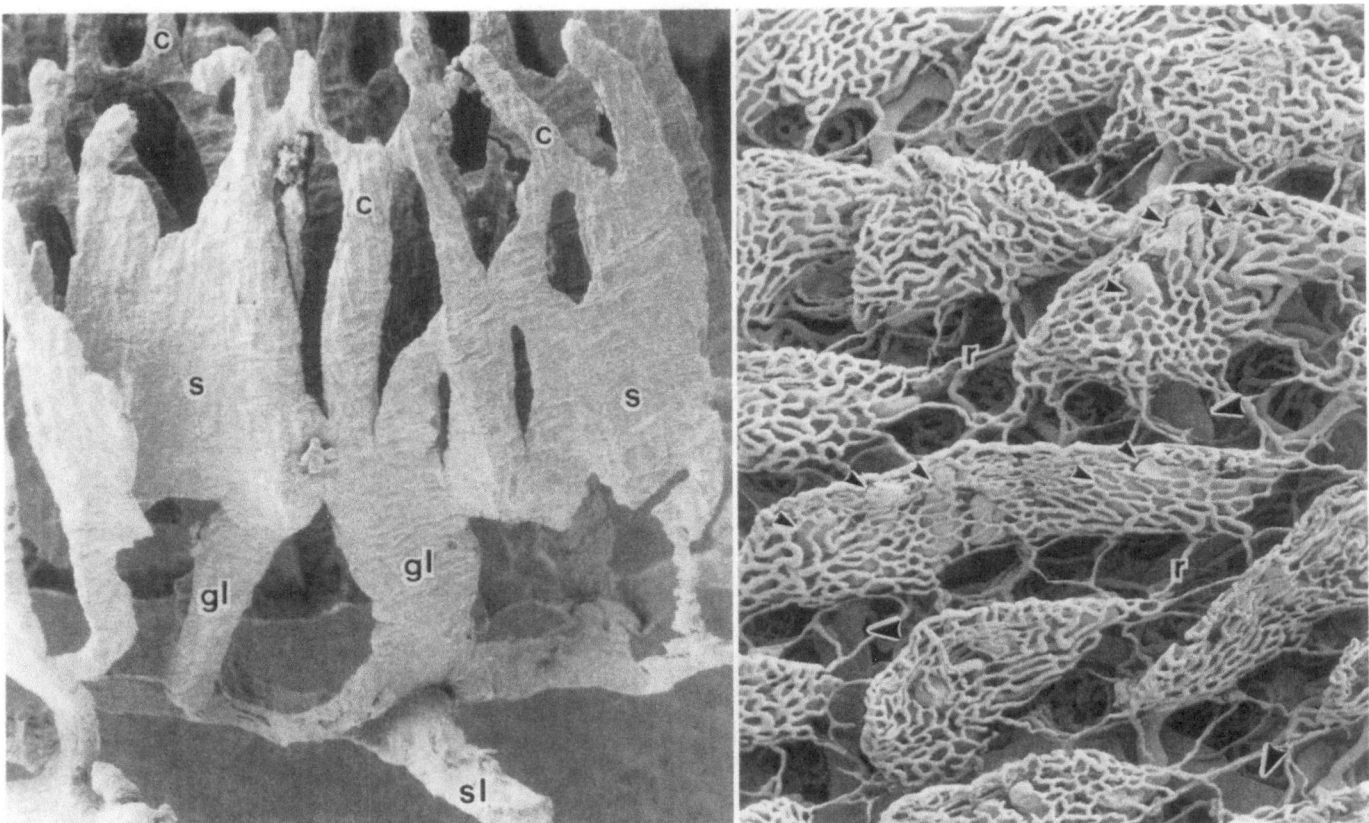

Figure 1 A scanning electron micrograph of a lymphatic corrosion cast of the upper small intestine in the rat (lateral view). The central lacteals (c) in each villus have many transverse connections, and, at the villous base, the lacteals fuse to form a flat but broad sinus (s). From the bottom of the sinus, two or three perpendicularly oriented lymphatics (gl) descend through the glandular layer and lead into the submucosal lymphatic network (sl). × 180

Figure 2 A scanning electron micrograph of a lymphatic/blood vascular corrosion cast of the lower small intestine in the rat. There are many close-meshed networks of the villous subepithelial capillaries. Each network shows the shape of a villus and completely surrounds the central lacteals, some of which are indicated by small arrow-heads. Between the villous capillary networks, there are many capillary rings (r) surrounding the intestinal glands. The submucosal lymphatics (large arrow-heads) are also seen, deeper than the glandular capillaries. × 95

tomoses)[16,20–25] (Figure 6). Such arterioportal anastomoses are frequently seen in the rat[16] but rarely in the rabbit[17]. However, to date, it is unknown how much of the arterial blood flows through the peribiliary plexus and how much drains directly into the sinusoids or into the portal venules.

Neither arteriohepatic venous anastomoses[26] nor intralobular arterioles which travel deep into the hepatic lobule to connect with the sinusoids[27] have been confirmed by scanning electron microscopy of vascular corrosion casts[16–18].

The hepatic sinusoids

The hepatic sinusoids are the principal sites for transvascular exchange between the blood and the hepatocytes. The sinusoid is composed of endothelial cells, Kupffer cells with many pseudopodia[28] and Ito cells (or perisinusoidal cells) located within the perisinusoidal space of Disse[29]. The endothelial cell possesses an attenuated cytoplasm with numerous fenestrae, none of which has a diaphragm. The majority of fenestrae are 100–150 nm in diameter and tend to be clustered together

to form sieve plates, while there are occasionally large fenestrae where Kupffer cells frequently attach[30]. The Kupffer cell is a macrophage which is a source of a variety of toxic and vasoactive substances and a principal source of beneficial mediators which contribute toward the non-specific host defence mechanism[31]. Ito cells possess thin, multiple cytoplasmic processes which embrace the abluminal surfaces of the endothelium of the sinusoids[32]. Ito cells (or perisinusoidal cells) contain fat droplets and are a storage site for vitamin A[33–37].

In many places, the interlobular veins give off short side branches or inlet venules which rather abruptly diverge into the sinusoids at the margin of the lobule (Figure 3 and 4). The terminal divisions of the distributing portal veins also branch out into the sinusoids (Figure 4). In general, the sinusoids are organized into dense, extensively interconnecting capillary masses. There are some regional differences in the organization of the sinusoids. Near their origins from the portal veins, the sinusoids are slightly narrower, more tortuous and more extensively interconnected than their terminations in central venules (or veins) (Figures 3, 4, 9 and 10).

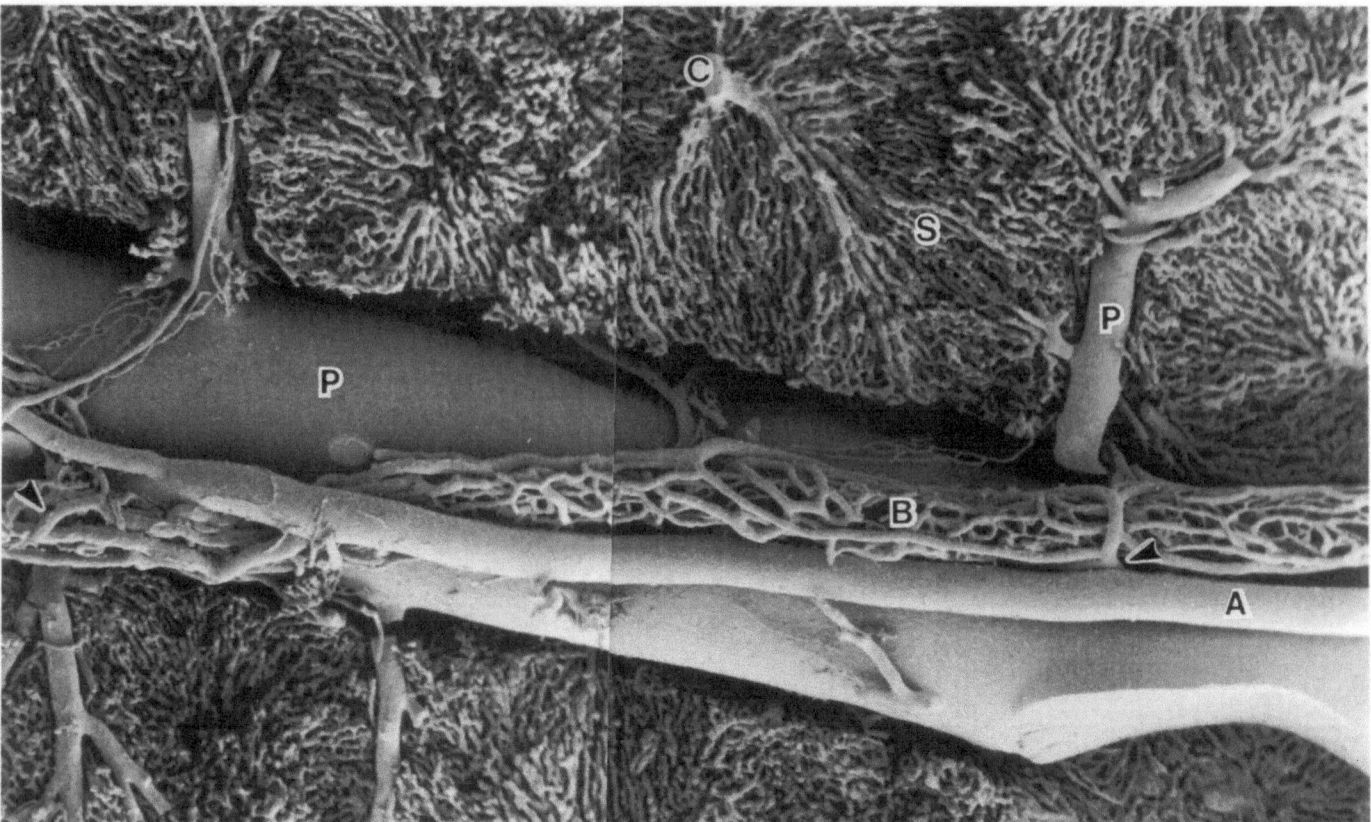

Figure 3   A scanning electron micrograph of a vascular corrosion cast of the rat liver. The portal vein branch (P) runs together with the hepatic arterial branch (A) and the peribiliary plexus (B) in the portal canal. The portal veins branch out into the hepatic sinusoids (S) which, in turn, converge into the central vein (C). The hepatic arterial branches (arrow-heads) supply the peribiliary plexus. × 70. (Micrograph from Ohtani *et al.*[16])

The liver lobule and functional unit of the liver

The liver lobule, as seen in vascular corrosion casts, is represented by a dense network of extensively interconnected sinusoids which converge into the central vein (Figures 3, 4 and 9). The vascular corrosion casts of the liver surface show a hexagonal pattern consisting of the tapered origins of the central veins (or collecting veins) into which sinusoids converge (Figure 10). The sinusoids on the periphery of the hexagon are slender, tortuous and extensively interconnected, but they become thicker, less interconnected and straighter as they run towards the central venules (Figure 10). The terminal hepatic arterioles and portal venules connecting with the hepatic sinusoids also appear on the surface of the liver in the monkey[15] and human[18]. In the rat, rabbit and cat, however, the hepatic arterioles and portal venules are not usually seen on the liver surface[16,17].

In most mammals, the peripheral boundaries of the lobules are not well defined, except in pigs where a definitive layer of connective tissue circumscribes the lobule. Thus, in most mammals, considerable numbers of sinusoids interconnect the adjacent lobules (Figures 3, 4 and 10). Because of this and the intralobular regional differences in oxygenation, metabolic functions and response to disease, the concept of 'acinus' has been proposed to define the hepatic functional unit[38,39]. The axis of the acinus is a portal tract containing terminal portal venules

and hepatic arterioles. Its peripheral boundary is, however, circumscribed only by an imaginary line connecting the neighbouring central venules (or so-called terminal hepatic venules). Each acinus has been proposed to contain three zones, each having different levels of oxygenation and metabolic function, though no-one can draw a definite line separating one zone from another.

Partial injection of resin into the portal venous and hepatic arterial systems reproduces the hepatic sinusoids only around the portal tract (Figure 11). This would indicate that the periphery of the polyhedral lobule is not evenly supplied by portal venules and hepatic arterioles, although the hepatic sinusoids around the portal tracts are sites where oxygen- and nutrient-rich blood flows first. In some areas of the partially injected liver casts, the replicated hepatic sinusoids reach as far as the central venules (Figure 11), which may support the acinar concept proposed by Rappaport.

Morphological sites regulating the hepatic microcirculation

Hepatic arterioles are invested with smooth muscle and are probably responsible for regulating the hepatic microcirculation. Since portal venules and central venules contain smooth muscle, though less than arterioles, they too may participate in regulating the hepatic microcirculation. According to McCuskey, the endothelial cells

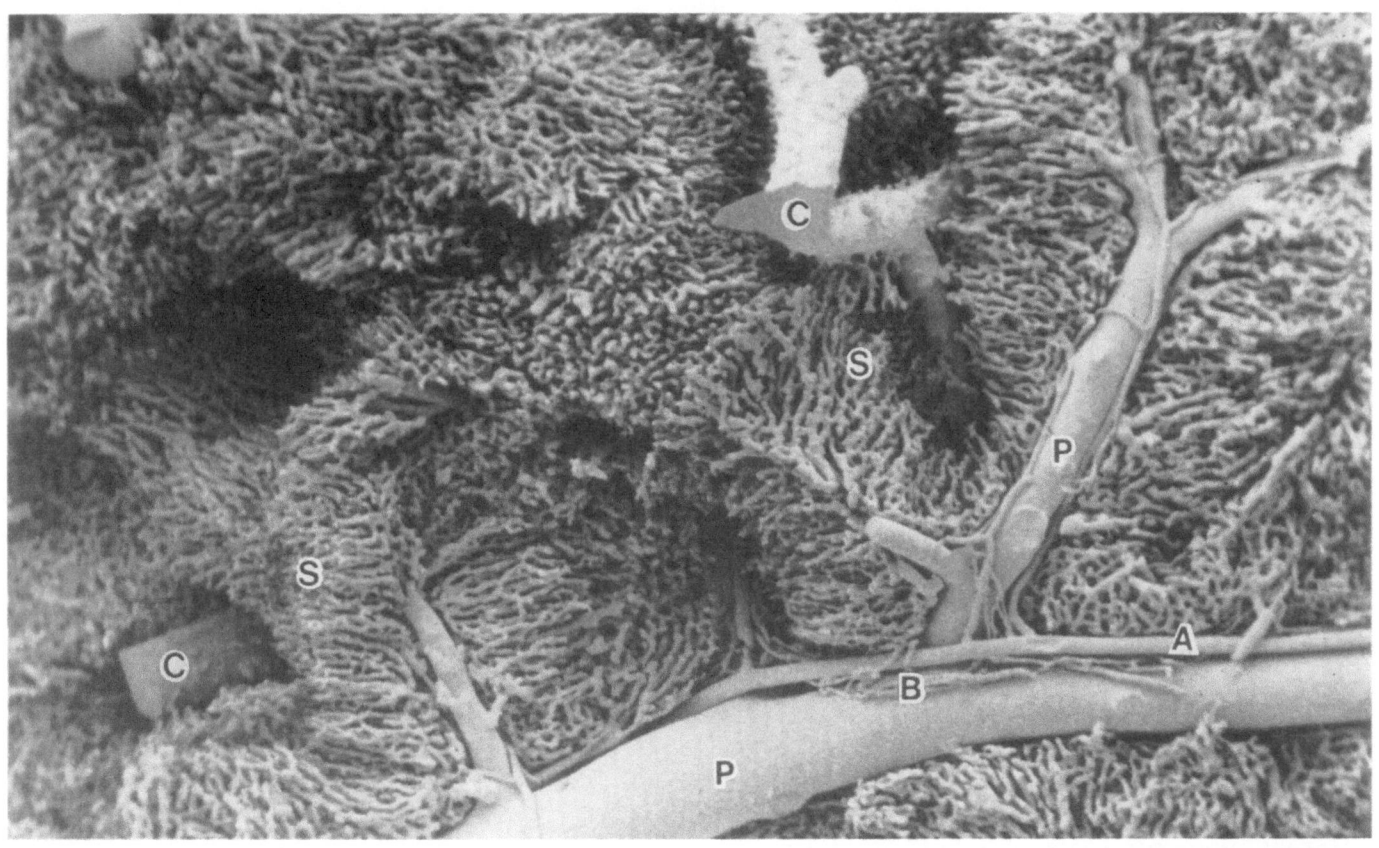

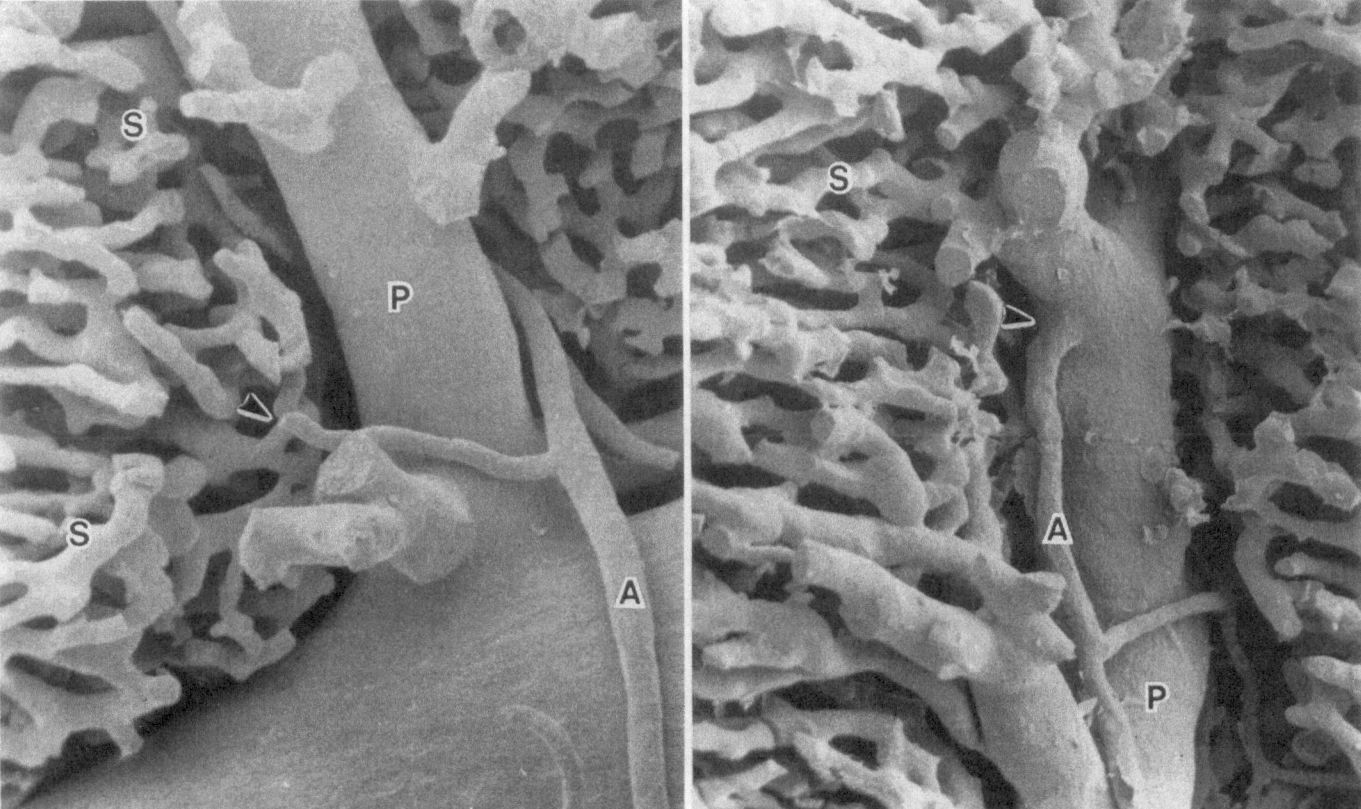

Figure 4 A scanning electron micrograph of a microdissected vascular corrosion cast of the rat liver. The interlobular (portal) vein branch (P), hepatic artery branch (A) and peribiliary plexus (B) run together in the portal tract. The interlobular veins branch out into the extensively interconnecting hepatic sinusoids (S) which converge into the central veins (C). × 95 (Micrograph from Ohtani et al.[18])

Figure 5 A closer view of part of Figure 4. A twig (capillary in size) of the hepatic arterial branch (A) is seen leading into the hepatic sinusoids (S) as indicated by an arrow-head. P: interlobular (portal) vein. × 495

Figure 6 A closer view of part of Figure 4 showing an anastomosis (arrow-head) between the terminal branch of the hepatic artery (A) and the interlobular portal venule (P) (i.e. arterioportal anastomosis). S: hepatic sinusoids. × 535

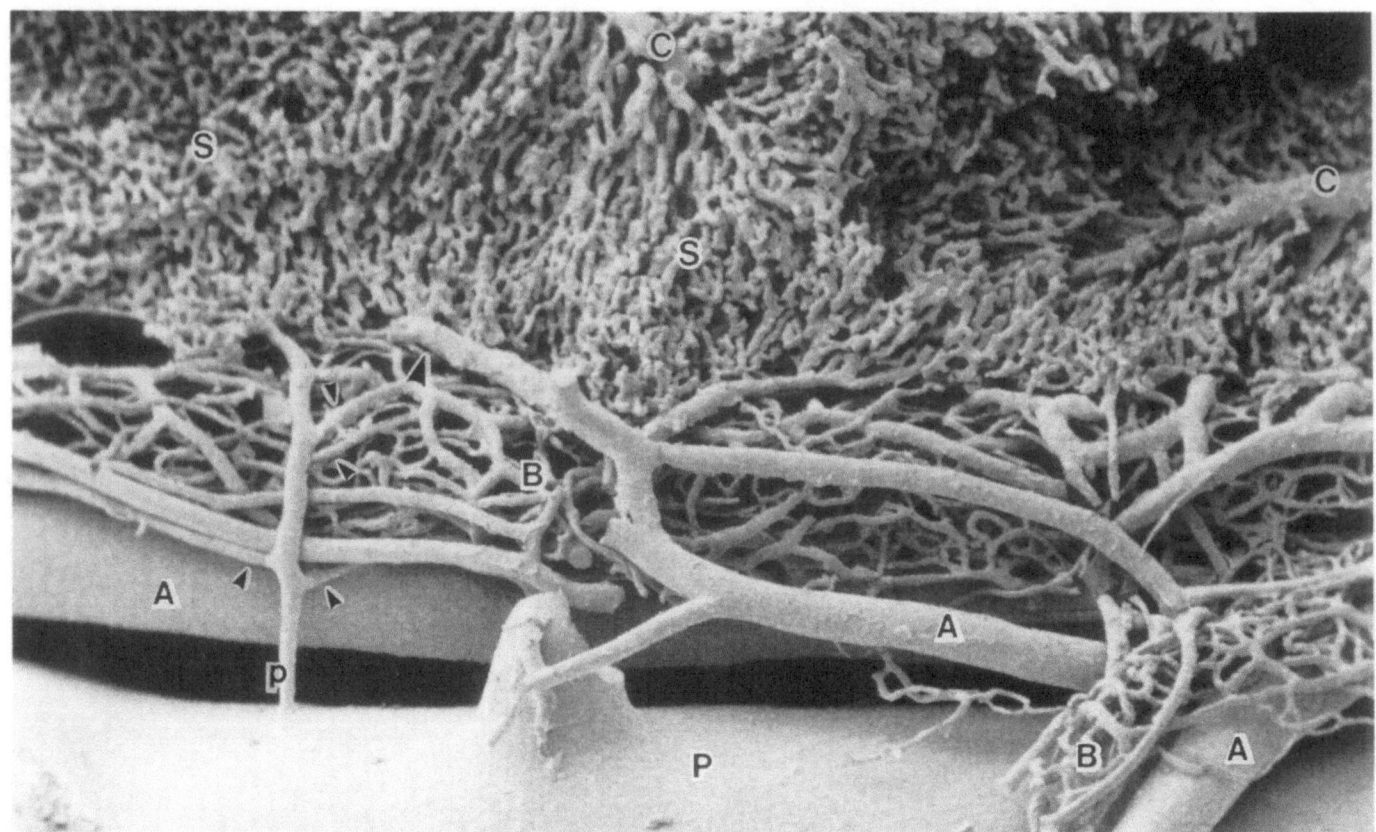

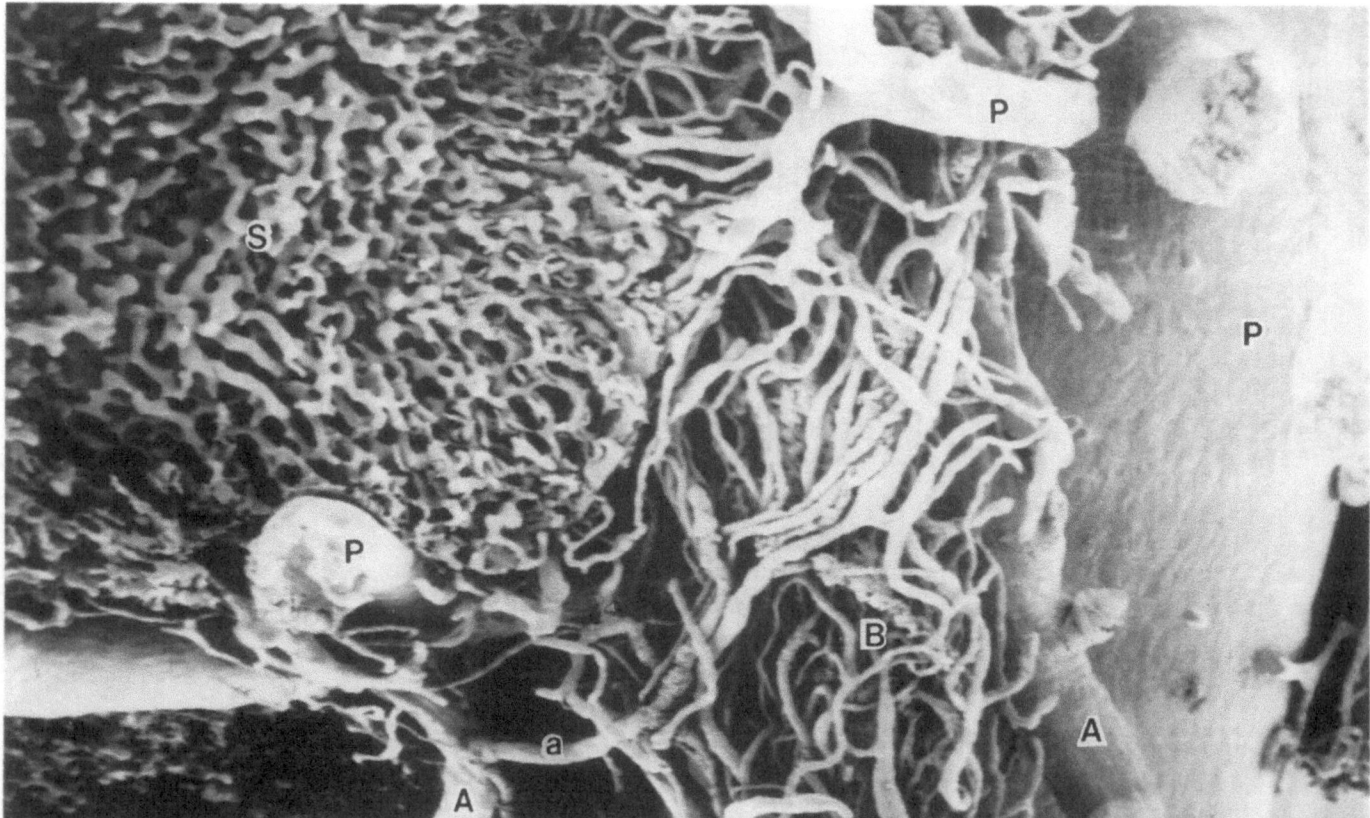

Figure 7 A scanning electron micrograph of a vascular corrosion cast of the rat liver. The branches of the hepatic artery (A) supply the hepatic sinusoids (S) (indicated by a large arrow-head) as well as the peribiliary plexus (B). Note that a small branch (p) of the interlobular (portal) vein (P) collects the efferent vessels (small arrow-heads) of the peribiliary plexus and branches out into the hepatic sinusoids. × 95

Figure 8 A scanning electron micrograph of a vascular corrosion cast of the human liver. The portal vein branch (P), the hepatic arterial branch (A) and the peribiliary plexus (B) run in the portal canal. The hepatic arterial branch (a) can be seen supplying the peribiliary plexus. The portal vein branches break up into the extensively interconnected hepatic sinusoids (S). × 120

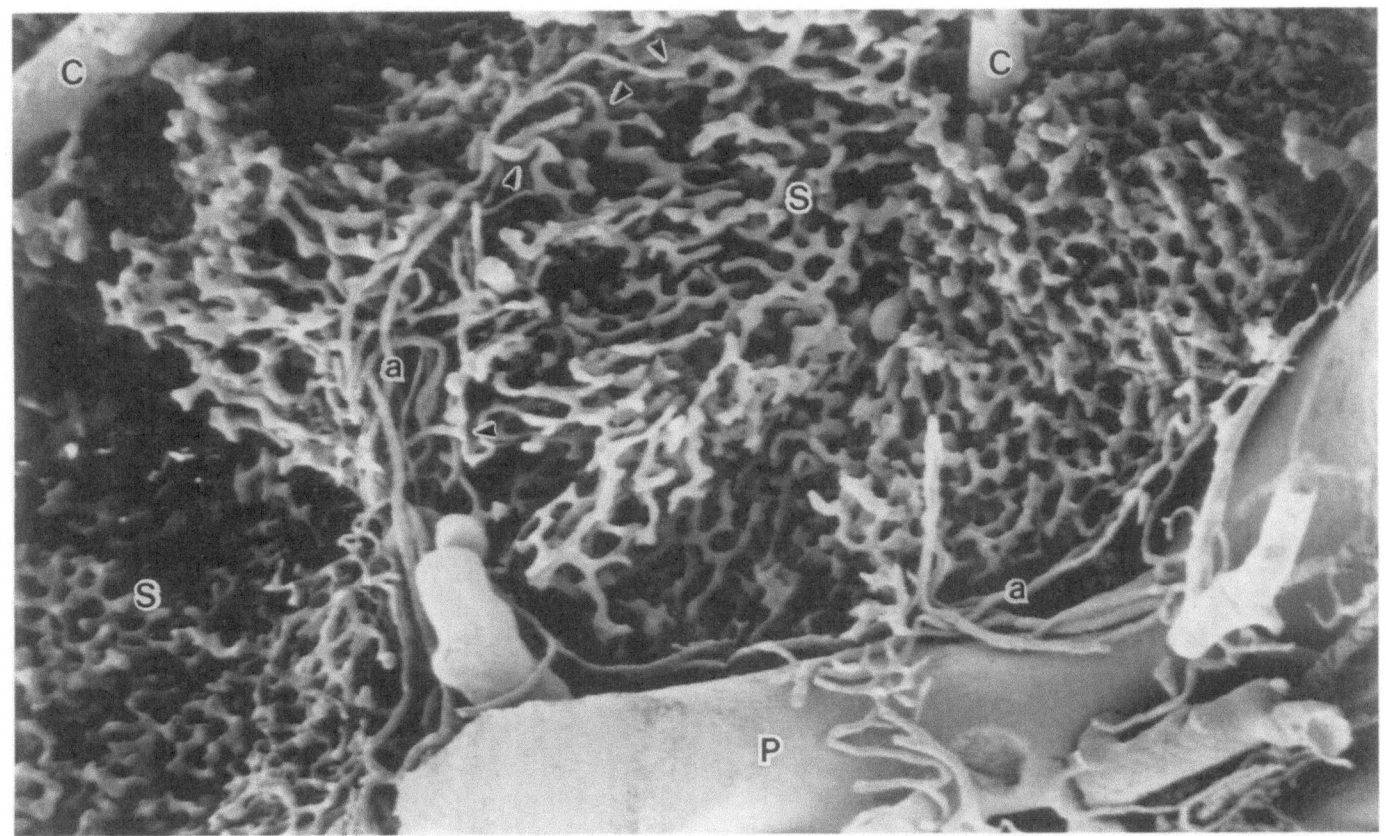

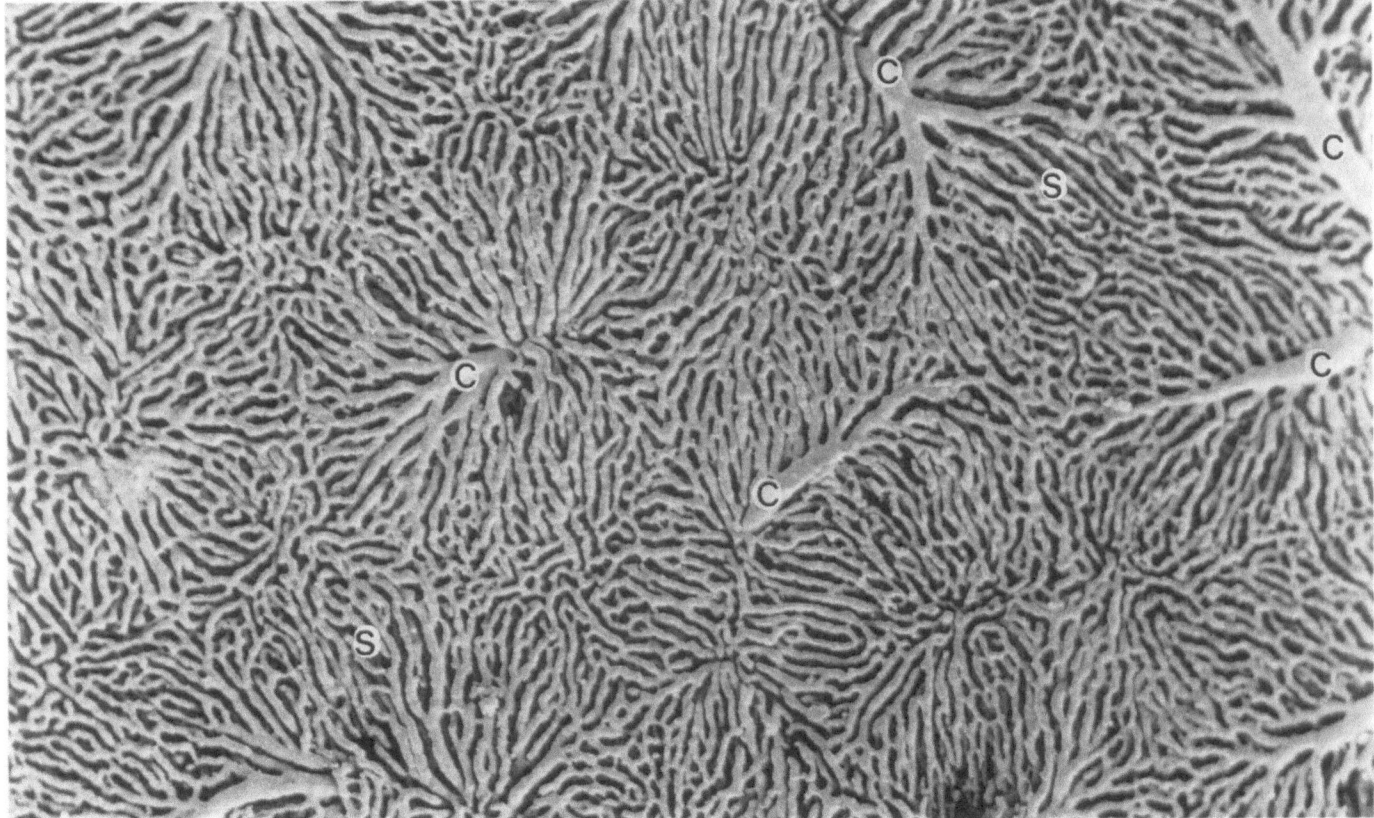

Figure 9 A scanning electron micrograph of a vascular corrosion cast of the human liver. Terminals of the hepatic arterioles (a) lead into the hepatic sinusoids (S) as indicated by arrow-heads. P: portal vein branch, C: central vein. × 120

Figure 10 A scanning electron micrograph of a vascular corrosion cast of the rat liver surface. There are tapered origins of the central venules (C) into which converge numerous hepatic sinusoids (S). The sinusoids at the periphery of the lobule are somewhat slender and tortuous, and become thicker and straighter as they run towards the central venules. × 95 (Micrograph from Ohtani *et al.*[18])

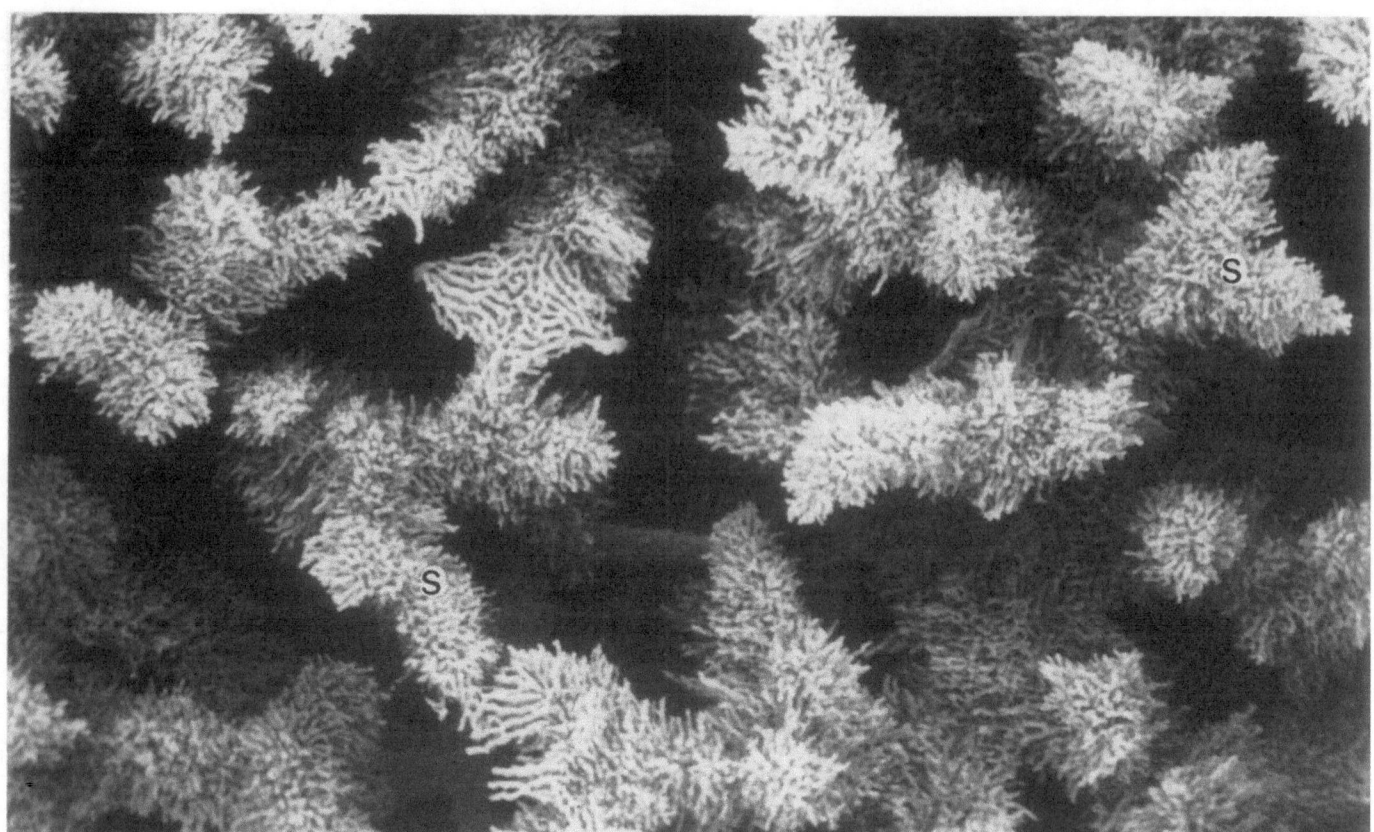

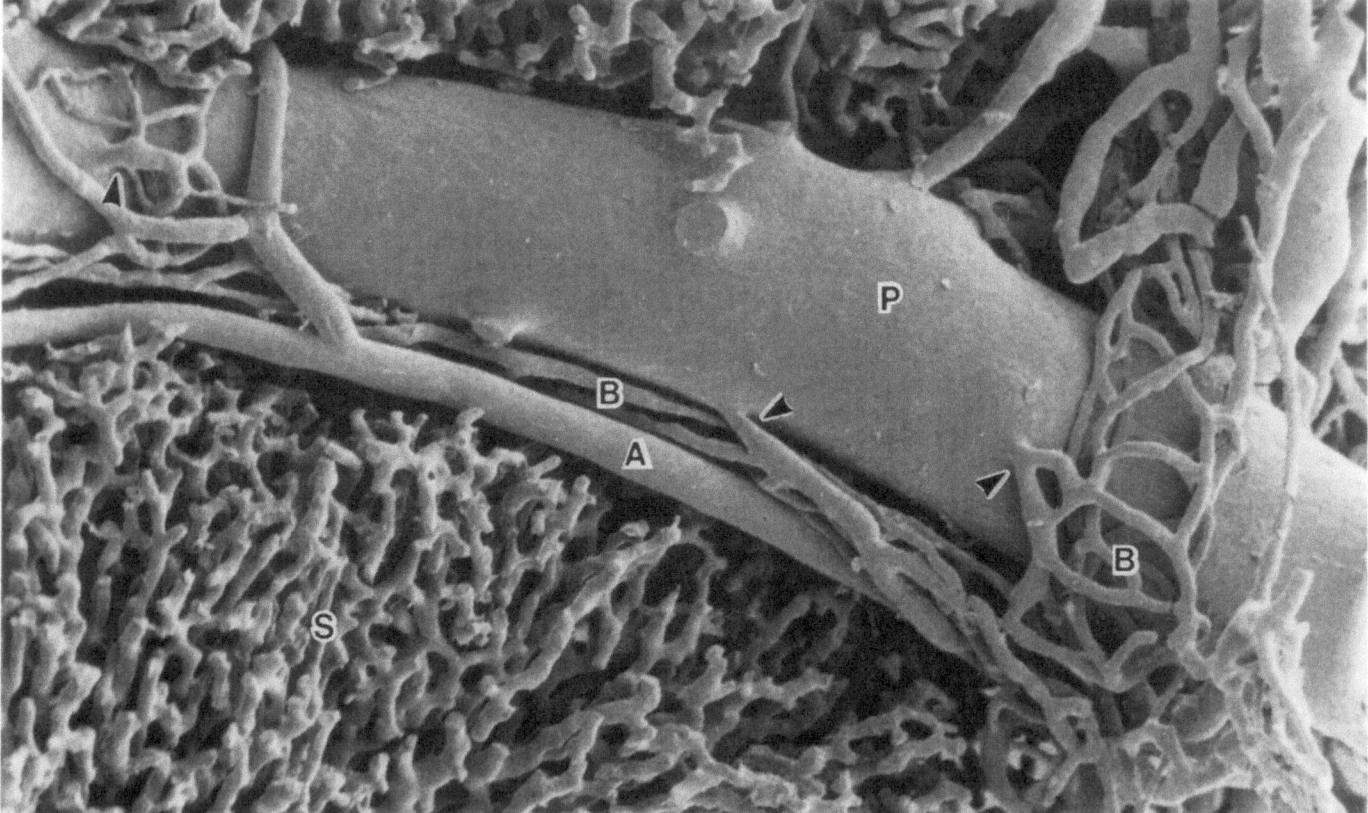

Figure 11   A scanning electron micrograph of a partial cast of the portal venous and hepatic arterial systems of the rat liver (viewed from the liver surface). The hepatic sinusoids (S) are replicated only around the portal tracts, and incompletely surround the periphery of the hepatic lobules. × 70

Figure 12   A scanning electron micrograph of a corrosion cast of the rat liver. The efferent vessels (arrow-heads) of the peribiliary plexus (B) lead into the interlobular (or portal) vein (P). A: hepatic artery, S: hepatic sinusoids. × 280

of the sinusoids and Kupffer cells are responsive to a wide variety of pharmacodynamic substances, and by contracting or swelling, these cells regulate the rate and distribution of blood through the sinusoids[31,40]. Although the participation of Ito cells remains to be clarified, their multiple cytoplasmic processes embracing the sinusoids[32] suggest a pericyte-like contractile activity. It should also be noted that endothelial cells, Kupffer cells and Ito cells contain filaments and tubules possibly related to contractile activity[31].

THE INTRAHEPATIC BILIARY SYSTEM AND THE PERIBILIARY PORTAL SYSTEM

The organization of the intrahepatic biliary system

The duct system of the liver serves to transport the bile to the duodenum. This system starts with intralobular bile canaliculi of approximately 0.5 to a little over 1.0 μm in diameter[41]. The bile canaliculi form a ramifying network of channels between the parenchymal cells of the hepatic lobule[42,43]. In many places, the bile canaliculi possess branches ending blindly very close to the sinusoidal surface of the hepatocyte[44-46]. The canaliculi drain through terminal ductules (or canals of Hering, or intercalated ducts) into small interlobular bile ducts located at the periphery of a lobule. At the canaliculo-ductular junctions, ampullary dilatations were frequently observed[46,47]. The bile ductules are lined by cuboidal cells, each of which has a cilium. Many of the bile ductules run for long distances and repeatedly branch and anastomose each other to form a coarse network in the portal tract, and become progressively larger ducts lined by cuboidal or columnar epithelium.

Scanning electron microscopic observation of corrosion casts of the biliary system clearly shows three-dimensional organization of the system, including the bile canaliculi[2].

The peribiliary portal system

As noted by Mall (1906)[48] and confirmed later by injection studies[49], most branches of the interlobular arteries contribute to formation of the dense capillary network termed 'peribiliary plexus' which supplies the intrahepatic bile ducts and ductules (Figures 3, 7, 8 and 12). The peribiliary plexus starts with one or two capillaries with interconnections or a rope ladder-like capillary mesh running along the bile ductules or ducts (Figures 3 and 12). As the ducts become larger, the plexus becomes two vascular layers: an inner network of subepithelial capillaries, and an outer layer of venules and arterioles (Figures 3, 7, 8, 13 and 14).

The peribiliary plexus is collected into fairly independent vessels, leading either into the hepatic sinusoids (Figure 13) or into the interlobular veins (Figures 7 and 12). The former route, which drains into the hepatic sinusoids, is designated the 'lobular branch', while the latter, ending in the interlobular vein, is designated the 'prelobular branch'[17].

The occurrence of the 'lobular' and 'prelobular branches' of the peribiliary efferent vessels shows species differences. In the rabbit and human, both branches occur at almost the same frequency[17,18]. In the rat, the 'pre-lobular branches' are seen more frequently than the 'lobular branches'[16], whereas, in the monkey, the 'lobular branches' occur almost exclusively with few 'prelobular branches'[15]. In lower vertebrates, e.g. the bullfrog, *Rana catesbeiana*, a similarly arranged peribiliary plexus exists, the efferent vessels of which more frequently tend to drain directly into the hepatic sinusoids (i.e. through the 'lobular branches')[50] (Figure 15).

Functional significance of the peribiliary portal system

Since the peribiliary plexus has an elaborate network of capillaries with efferent vessels re-entering the hepatic sinusoids, the vascular route from the peribiliary capillary plexus through the efferent vessels to the hepatic sinusoids qualifies for the term 'portal' system, and should be referred to as the 'peribiliary portal system'[15]. However, to date, it is unknown whether the efferent vessels of the peribiliary plexus possess a wall structure similar to that of veins, though some of the efferent vessels are quite large in calibre and appear to be veins.

The possible function of the peribiliary portal system has been considered in terms of a countercurrent mechanism which could facilitate the reabsorption of substances from bile[51]. It has also been suggested that hormones released from the endocrine cells in the bile ducts in response to chemical information in the bile, might be transported by this portal system back to the interlobular portal veins, venules and the hepatic lobule, where they would exert their actions[52].

THE MICROVASCULARIZATION OF THE EXTRAHEPATIC BILE DUCTS

The extrahepatic bile duct consists of three parts: the cystic duct, the hepatic duct and the common bile duct. The rat, however, possesses neither a cystic duct nor a gallbladder. The hepatic duct conducts bile from the liver to a point where the cystic duct from the gallbladder meets the common bile duct leading into the duodenum. The extrahepatic bile ducts are lined with a columnar epithelium similar to that of the gallbladder.

On reaching the extrahepatic bile duct, the arterial branches ramify into many arterioles which, giving off capillaries in the adventitia *en route*, enter the lamina propria of the duct (Figure 16). There, these arterioles break up into capillaries to form a close-meshed network immediately below the epithelium[53] (Figure 17). The subepithelial capillary network resembles that of the intrahepatic bile duct.

The luminal view of the corrosion casts of the extrahepatic bile duct frequently shows oval pits surrounded by a dense capillary network[53] (Figure 17). These pits accommodate outpouchings simulating irregularly distributed glands. It is believed that mitoses of epithelial cells occur mainly in these outpouchings, and that the cells move upward to replace worn cells of the luminal surface.

The capillaries in the lamina propria and in the adventitia are collected into venules which repeatedly anastomose and branch to form a venular plexus in the adventitia, similar to that seen in the intrahepatic bile duct (Figure 16). The venular plexus drains into thicker

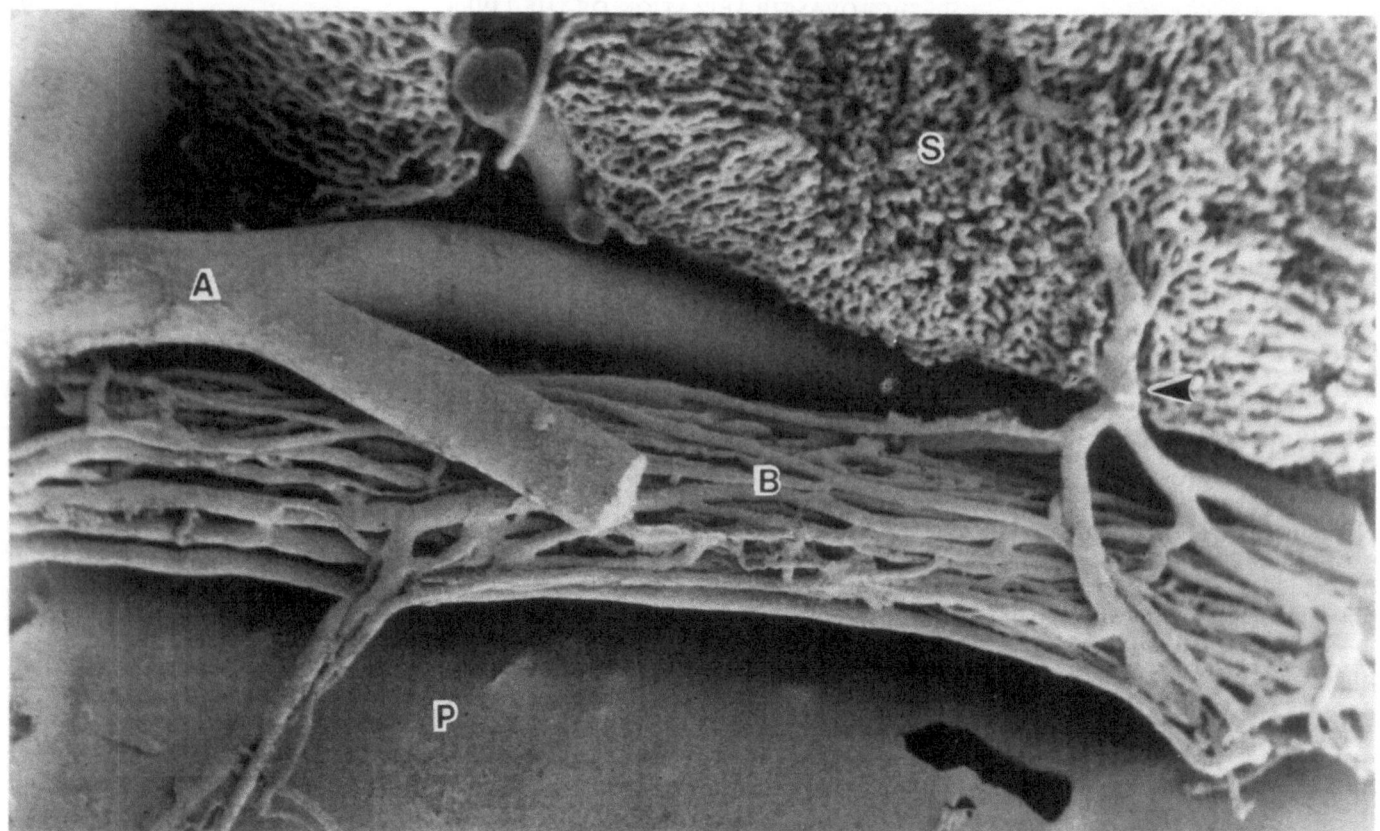

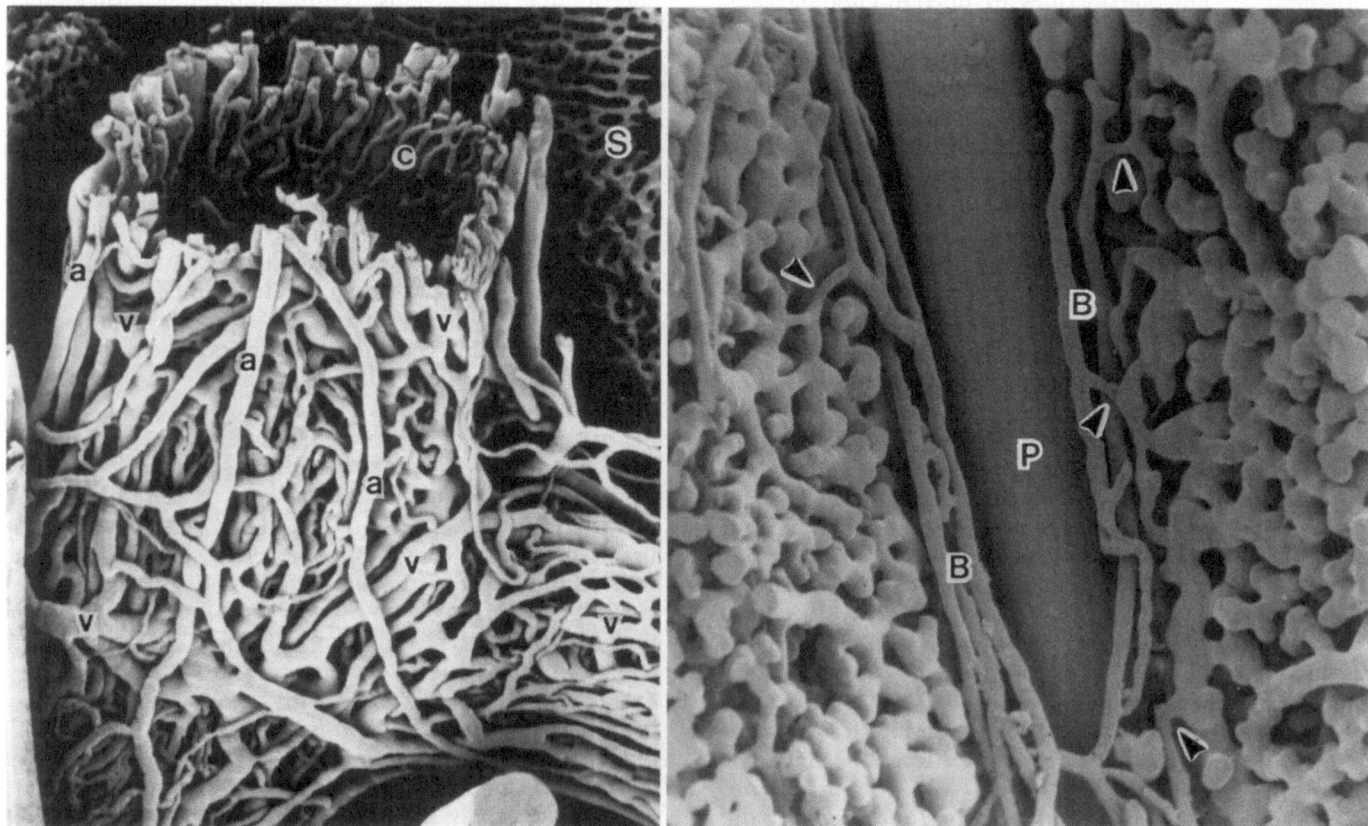

Figure 13 A scanning electron micrograph of a vascular corrosion cast of the rabbit liver. The efferent vessel (arrow-head) of the peribiliary plexus (B) branches out into the hepatic sinusoids (S). A: hepatic artery, P: portal vein branch. × 110.

Figure 14 A scanning electron micrograph of a vascular corrosion cast of the rabbit liver showing the peribiliary plexus circumscribing the larger intrahepatic bile duct. The plexus consists of two vascular layers: an inner capillary (c) network and an outer venous (v) and arterial (a) network. S: hepatic sinusoids. × 110. (Micrograph from Ohtani[17])

Figure 15 A scanning electron micrograph of a vascular corrosion cast of the liver in the bullfrog, *Rana catesbeiana*. The efferent vessels (arrow-heads) of the peribiliary plexus (B) drain into the hepatic sinusoids (S). P: portal vein. × 120. (Micrograph from Ohtani et al.[50])

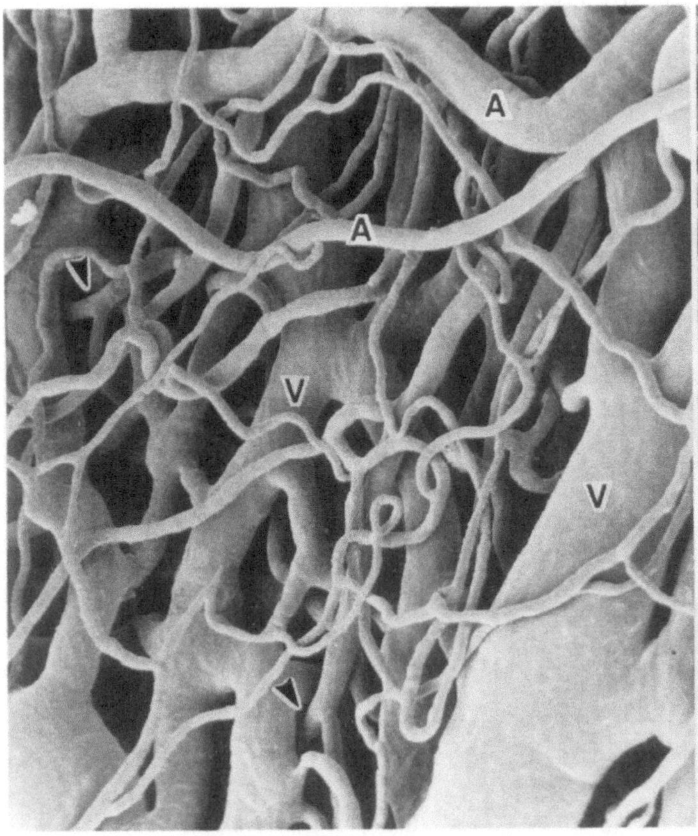

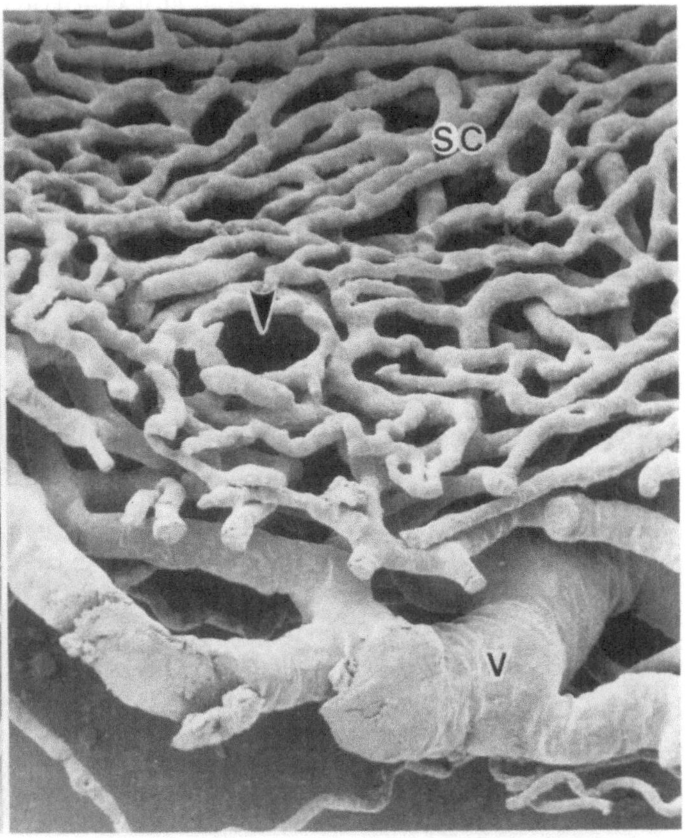

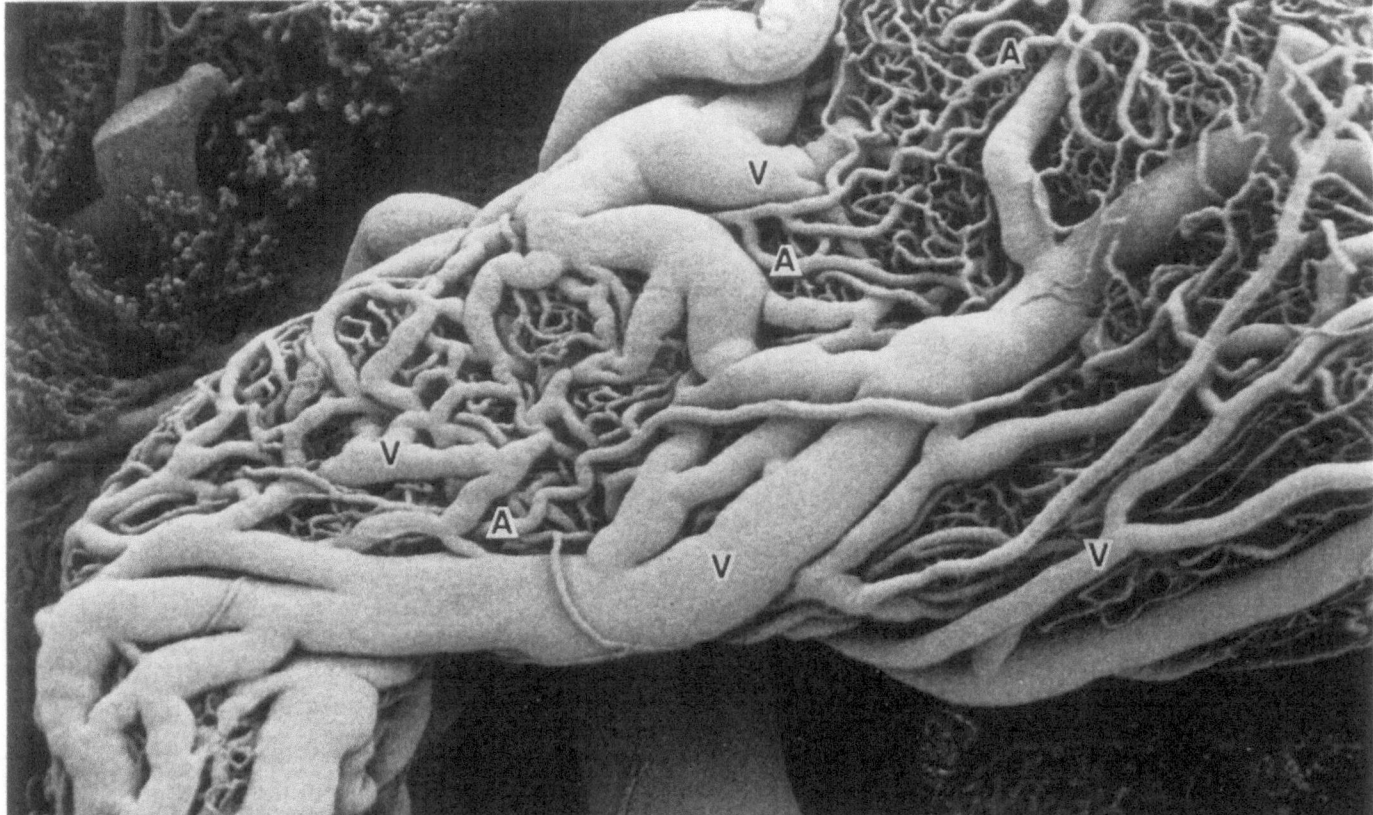

Figure 16 A scanning electron micrograph of a vascular corrosion cast of the extrahepatic bile duct in the rat (viewed from the outer surface). The arterioles (A), giving off capillaries in the superficial layer *en route*, enter deep to supply the subepithelial capillaries (indicated by arrow-heads). Deeper than the superficial vascular network, there is a network of venules (V) gathering the subepithelial capillaries. × 180

Figure 17 A scanning electron micrograph of a vascular corrosion cast of the extrahepatic bile duct in the rat. There is a close-meshed network of subepithelial capillaries (SC) which are gathered into the venules (V) located in the adventitia. There is also a pit surrounded by capillaries (arrow-head). × 240

Figure 18 A scanning electron micrograph of a corrosion cast of the rabbit gallbladder (surface view). Slender arterioles (A) give off some capillaries in the adventitia *en route*, and penetrate deeply to supply the subepithelial capillary network. This network is collected into venules which, in turn, form a venular network (V) in the adventitia. × 75

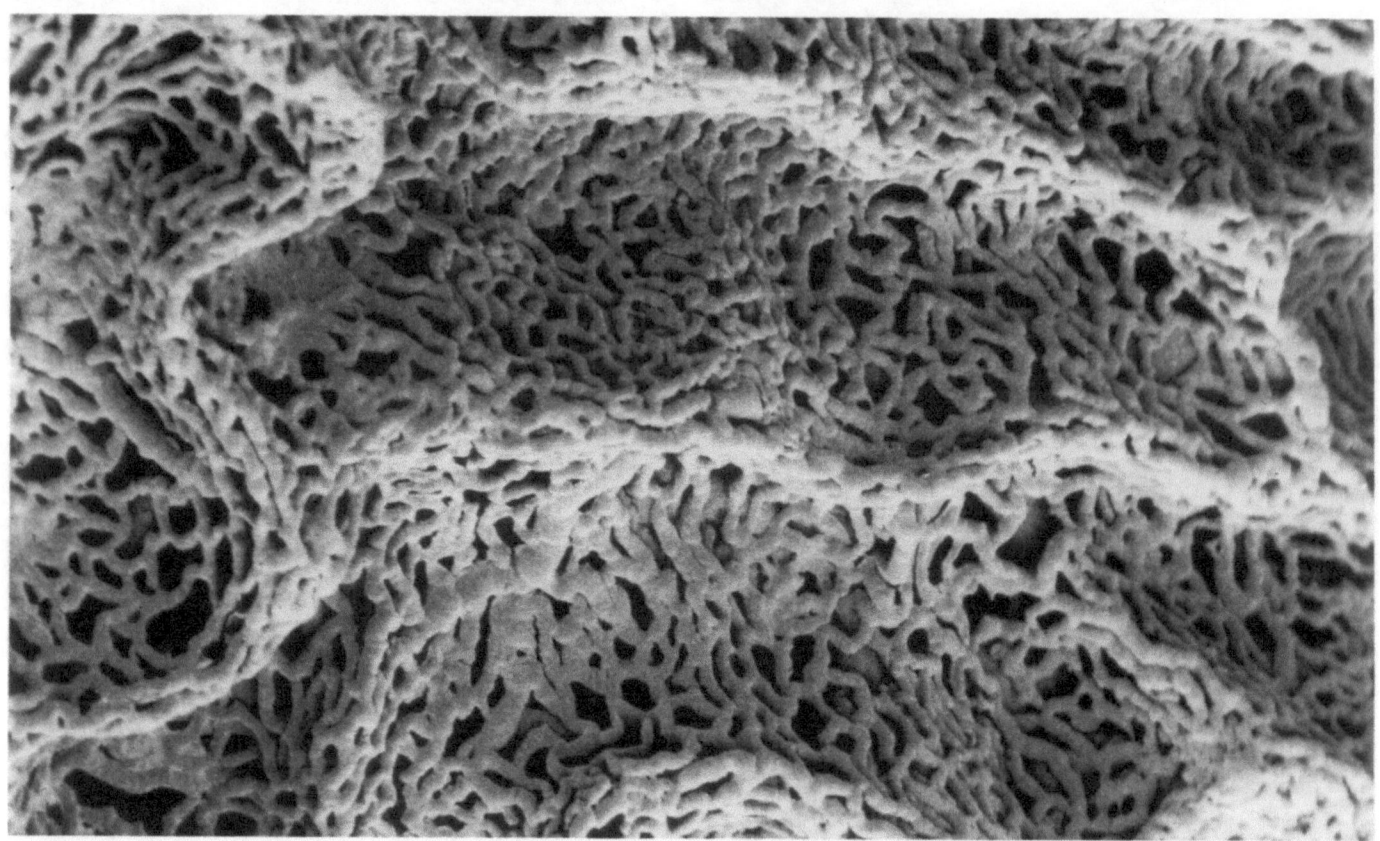

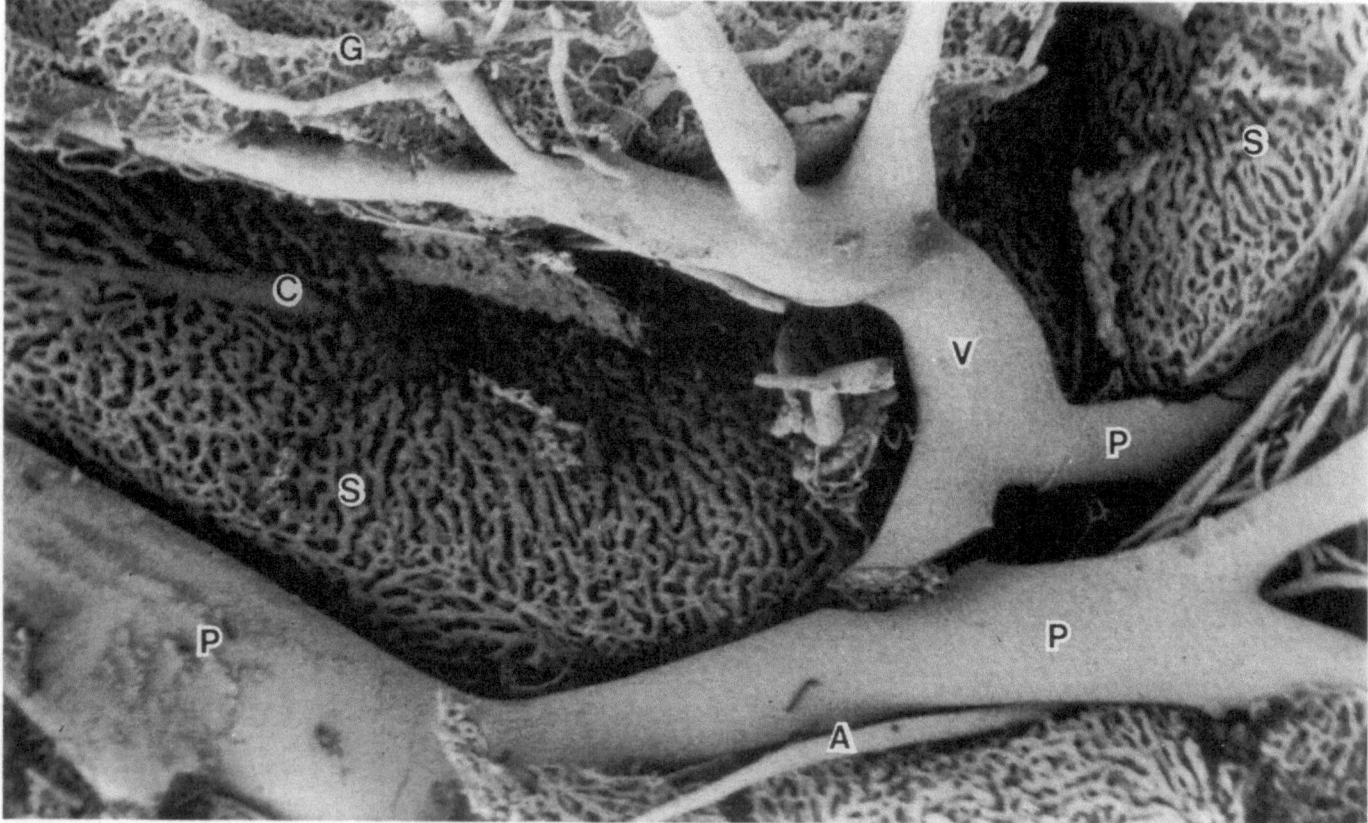

Figure 19 A scanning electron micrograph of a vascular corrosion cast showing an extremely dense network of subepithelial capillaries of the rabbit gallbladder. Note the folds of the network which correspond with the muscosal folds of the organ. × 285

Figure 20 A scanning electron micrograph of a vascular corrosion cast of the gallbladder (G) and the liver in the rabbit. A vein (V) draining the gallbladder leads into the branch of the hepatic portal vein (P). S: hepatic sinusoids. C: central vein, A: hepatic artery branch. × 90

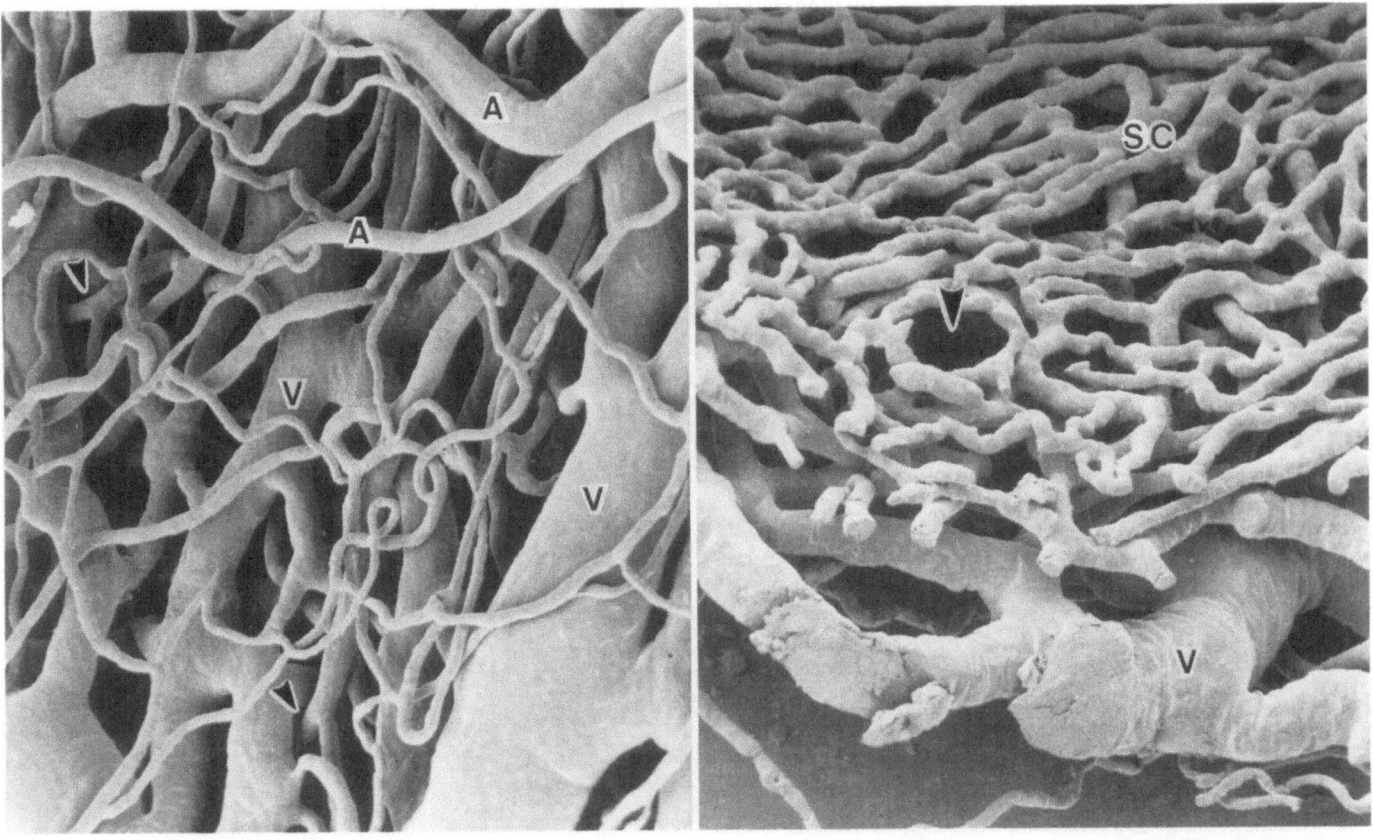

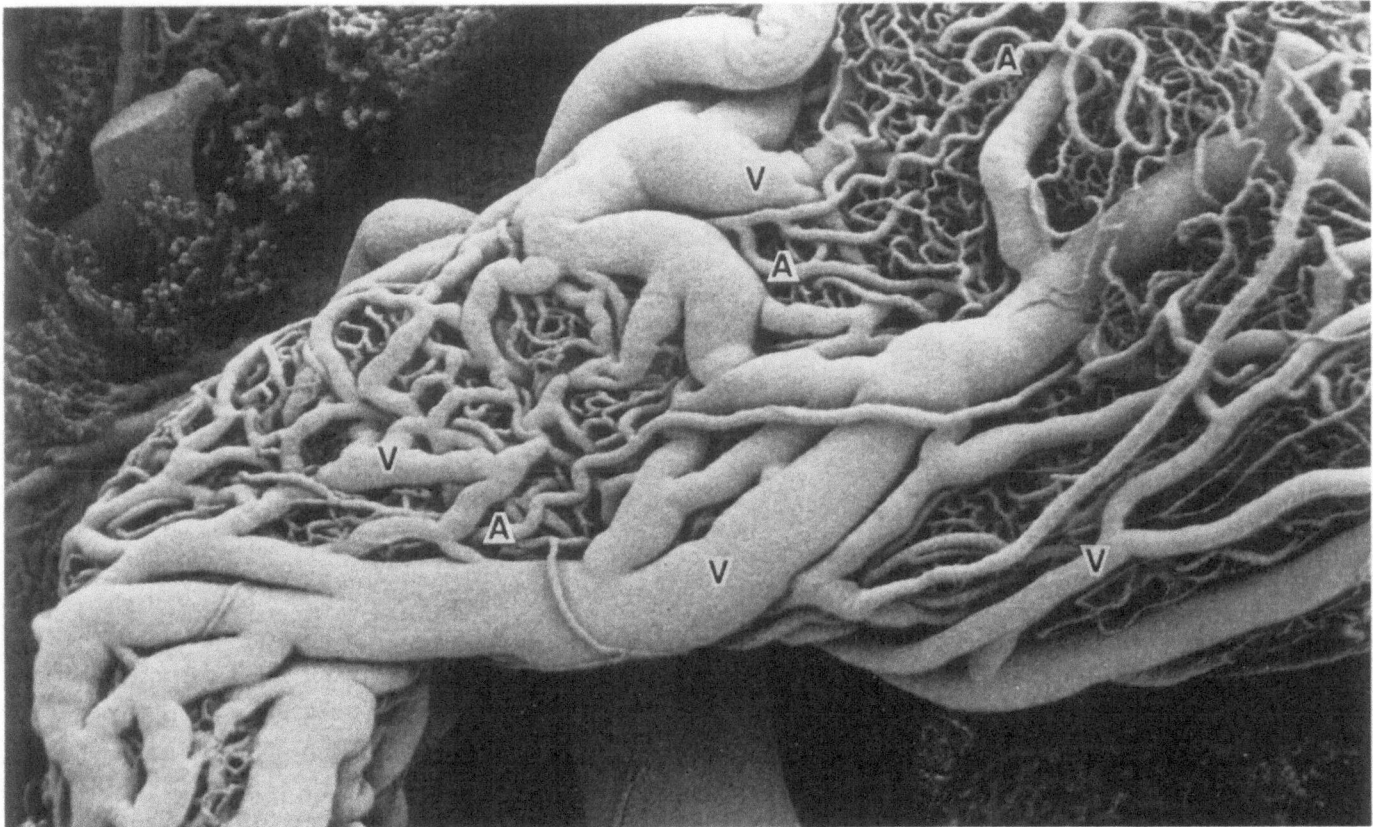

Figure 16 A scanning electron micrograph of a vascular corrosion cast of the extrahepatic bile duct in the rat (viewed from the outer surface). The arterioles (A), giving off capillaries in the superficial layer *en route*, enter deep to supply the subepithelial capillaries (indicated by arrow-heads). Deeper than the superficial vascular network, there is a network of venules (V) gathering the subepithelial capillaries. × 180

Figure 17 A scanning electron micrograph of a vascular corrosion cast of the extrahepatic bile duct in the rat. There is a close-meshed network of subepithelial capillaries (SC) which are gathered into the venules (V) located in the adventitia. There is also a pit surrounded by capillaries (arrow-head). × 240

Figure 18 A scanning electron micrograph of a corrosion cast of the rabbit gallbladder (surface view). Slender arterioles (A) give off some capillaries in the adventitia *en route*, and penetrate deeply to supply the subepithelial capillary network. This network is collected into venules which, in turn, form a venular network (V) in the adventitia. × 75

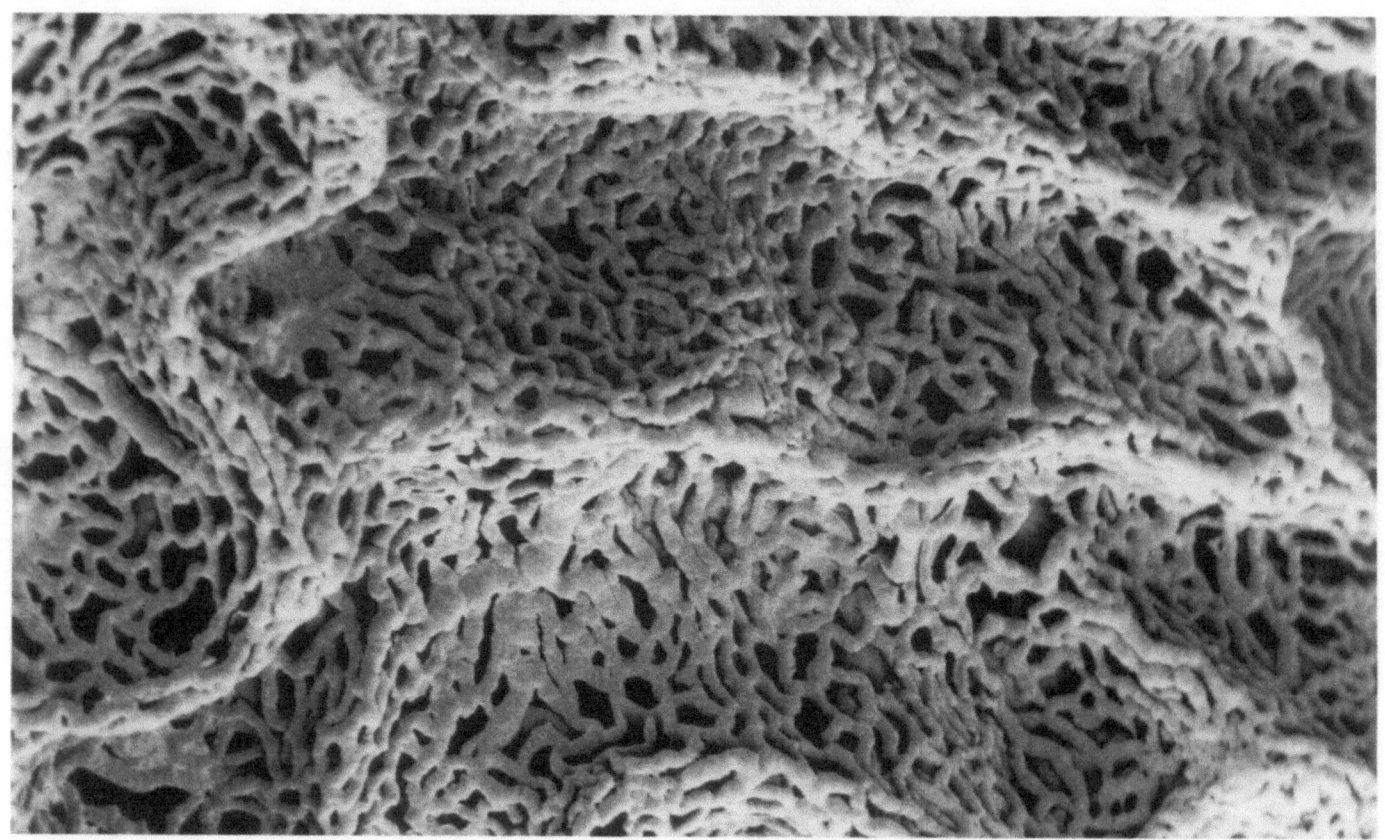

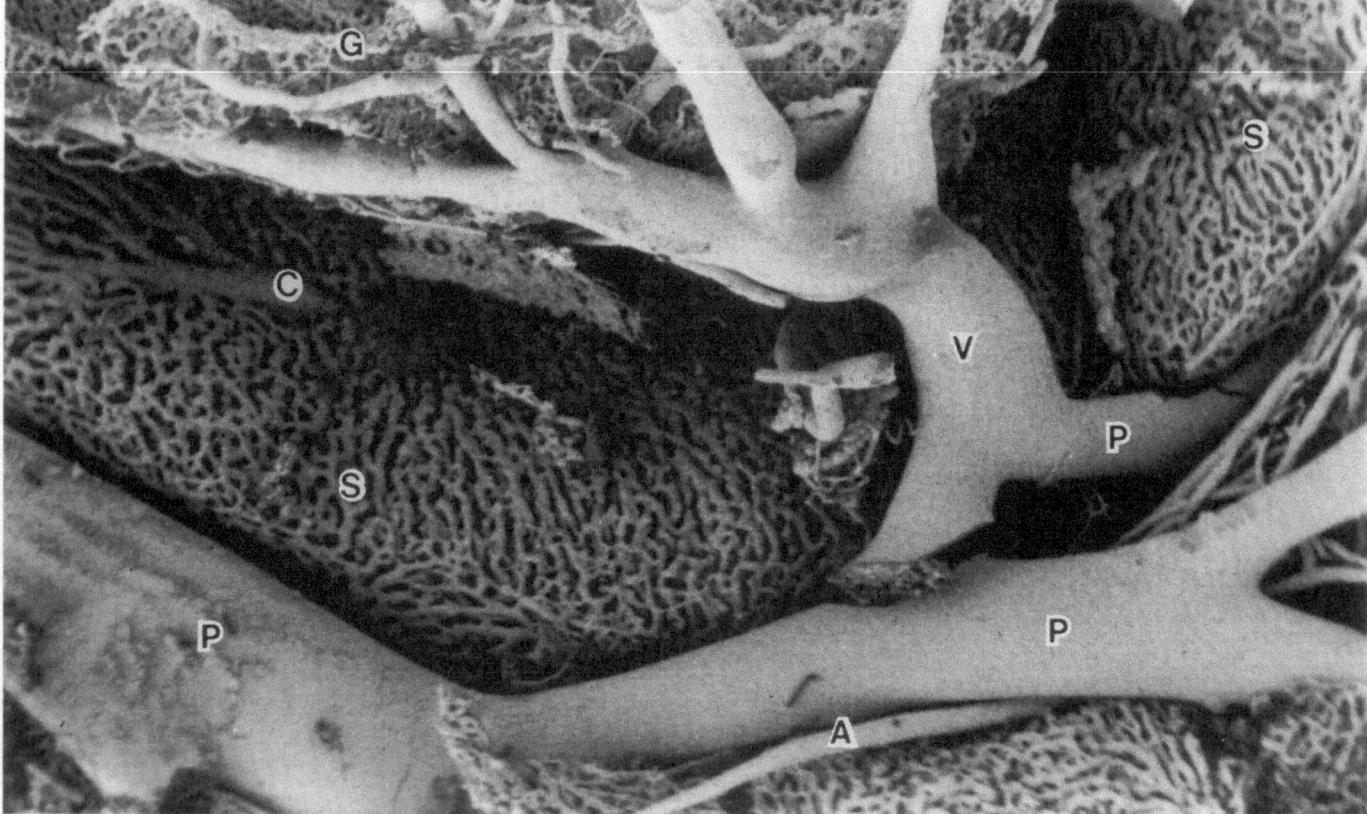

Figure 19   A scanning electron micrograph of a vascular corrosion cast showing an extremely dense network of subepithelial capillaries of the rabbit gallbladder. Note the folds of the network which correspond with the muscosal folds of the organ. × 285

Figure 20   A scanning electron micrograph of a vascular corrosion cast of the gallblader (G) and the liver in the rabbit. A vein (V) draining the gallbladder leads into the branch of the hepatic portal vein (P). S: hepatic sinusoids. C: central vein, A: hepatic artery branch. × 90

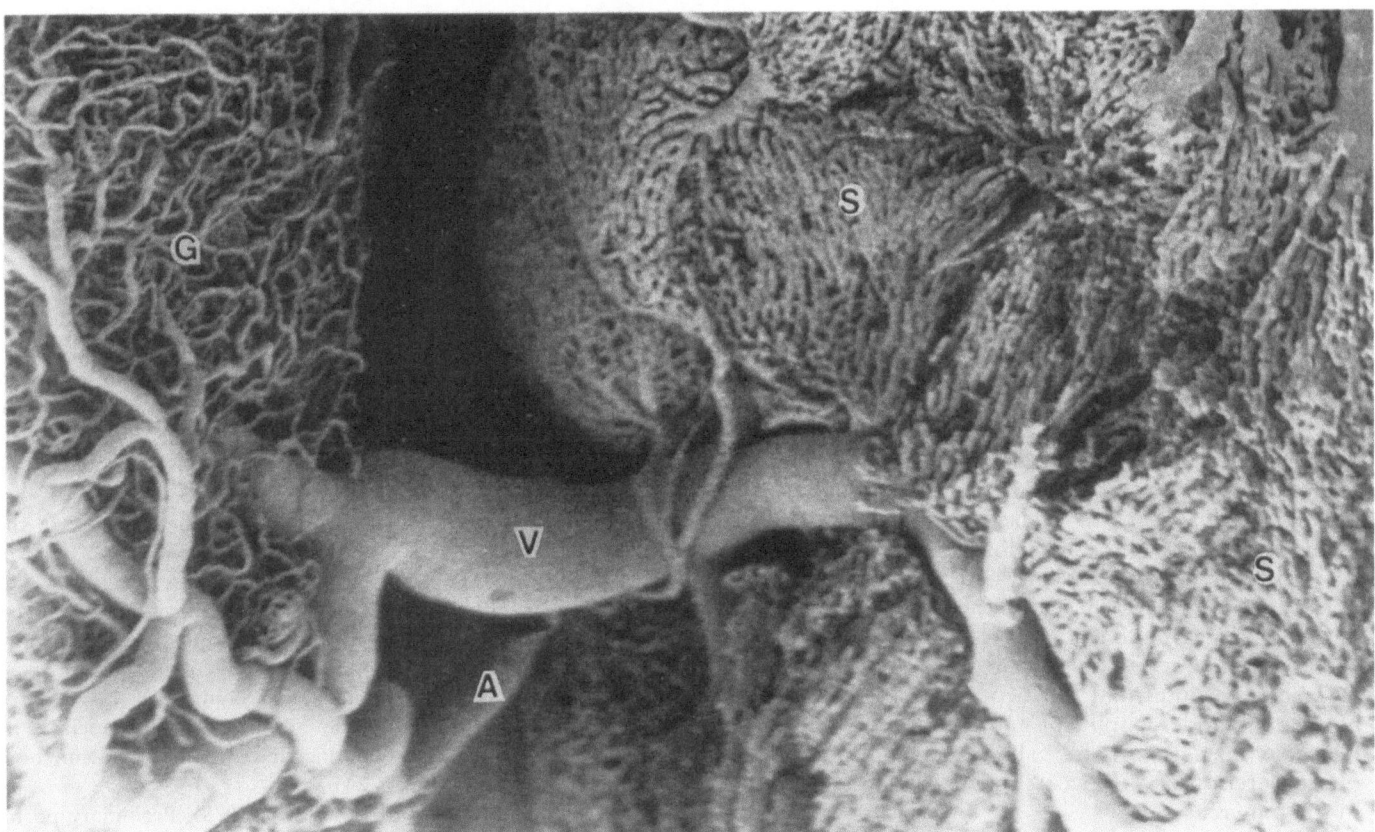

Figure 21 A scanning electron micrograph of a vascular corrosion cast of the gallbladder and the liver in the rabbit. A vein (V) draining the gallbladder (G) directly branches out into the hepatic sinusoids (S). This vein qualifies for the term 'portal' vessel. A: arterial branch coming off the hepatic arterial branch. × 80

venules and veins which ultimately lead into the hepatic portal vein.

The extensive dense network of capillaries in the lamina propria (or subepithelial capillary network) suggests its involvement in reabsorbing some substances in the bile, and in taking up any hormonal substances released by endocrine cells and transporting them to the portal venules and the sinusoids to regulate the microcirculation of the liver lobule and/or to exert their actions on the liver parenchyma.

THE MICROVASCULARIZATION OF THE GALLBLADDER

The gallbladder is a pear- or eggplant-shaped sac positioned in the gallbladder fossa of the caudal surface of the liver, and is connected with the common bile duct and the hepatic duct by way of the cystic duct. The gallbladder is a modified bile duct for concentrating and storing bile. Its wall is made up of mucosa, lamina propria, interlacing sheets of smooth muscles, and an adventitial layer. The luminal aspect shows folded mucosa which consists of a sheet of columnar epithelial cells anchored by a basement membrane to an underlying connective tissue layer. The extensive folding of the mucosa, together with numerous microvilli of the epithelium, perhaps functions to increase the absorptive surface in contact with bile.

The gallbladder is supplied by the cystic artery which

usually arises from the proper hepatic artery, and by some additional slender arteries which come from a branch of the proper hepatic artery during its passage between the gallbladder and the liver. In the adventitia of the gallbladder, these arteries give off many branches. Some of them break up into capillaries in the adventitia and in the layers of smooth muscle, but most of them enter the lamina propria where the arterial branches break up into capillaries to form a close-meshed reticular network immediately below the epithelium (Figures 18 and 19).

The subepithelial capillary network would be appropriate for the absorptive functions of the gallbladder as well as supplying vital nutrients and oxygen to the overlying epithelium.

In the subepithelial capillary network, there are tapered origins of collecting venules (Figure 19). These venules lead into veins that repeatedly branch and anastomose to form a meshwork in the adventitial layer (Figure 18). The efferent veins of the gallbladder lead either into the hepatic portal vein (Figure 20) or directly break up into the sinusoids in the hepatic lobules surrounding the gallbladder[54] (Figure 21). In the rabbit, the latter veins seem to be the main venous drainage of the gallbladder and the former veins drain only the neck region or part of the caudal surface of the gallbladder. In human, two types of veins of the gallbladder have been described by the famous French anatomist, Sappey[55]: the veins which originate in the superior surface of the gallbladder usually give rise to two trunks and empty into the right branch of the hepatic portal vein; and those, twelve to fifteen in number, originating from the inferior surface of the organ leave the gallbladder to ramify in the liver lobules which surround the gallbladder fossa. Sappey's description has later been supported[56]. However, scanning electron microscopy of the human gallbladder has not been reported yet.

The vascular route from the subepithelial capillaries in the gallbladder to the liver qualifies for the term 'portal system' similar to the peribiliary portal system. Thus, we propose that the term 'peribiliary portal system' should be applied to the portal system associated with the extrahepatic bile ducts and the gallbladder as well as the intrahepatic biliary ducts.

The portal system could play an important role in concentrating bile and in transporting reabsorbed substances and any hormonal substances produced by the gallbladder wall back to the hepatic sinusoids to control microcirculation of the liver lobule and to the hepatocytes, presumably to act on them as postulated in the peribiliary portal system within the liver. Recently, motilin-, substance P- and somatostatin-containing cells have been demonstrated in the extrahepatic biliary system[57–59]. A vasoactive intestinal polypeptide (VIP) nerve supply of the gallbladder, papilla of Vater, and sphincter of Oddi has also been reported[60,61]. It has been proposed that neurosecretion of VIP occurs in the islets of Langerhans in the pancreas[62].

The portal veins directly linking the gallbladder and the hepatic sinusoids may be particularly important clinically, since they may provide a short vascular route by which some kinds of disease of the gallbladder spread rapidly into the liver.

References

1. Murakami, T. (1971). Application of the scanning electron microscope to the study of the fine distribution of blood vessels. *Arch. Histol. Jpn.*, **32**, 445–54

2. Murakami, T., Itoshima, T., Hitomi, K., Ohtsuka, A. and Jones, A. L. (1984). A monomeric methyl and hydroxypropyl methacrylate injection medium and its utility in casting blood capillaries and liver bile canaliculi for scanning electron microscopy. *Arch. Histol. Jpn.*, **47**, 223–37

3. Kobayashi, S., Osatake, H. and Kashima, Y. (1976). Corrosion casts of lymphatics. *Arch. Histol. Jpn.*, **39**, 177–81

4. Ohtani, O. and Ohtsuka, A. (1985). Three-dimensional organization of lymphatics and their relationship to blood vessels in rabbit small intestine. A scanning electron microscopic study of corrosion casts. *Arch. Histol. Jpn.*, **48**, 255–68

5. Ohtani, O., Ohtsuka, A. and Owen, R. L. (1986). Three-dimensional organization of the lymphatics in the rabbit appendix. A scanning electron microscopic study. *Gastroenterology*, **91**, 947–55

6. Ohtani, O. (1987). Three-dimensional organization of lymphatics and its relationship to blood vessels in rat small intestine. *Cell Tiss. Res*, **248**, 365–374

7. Yamamoto, K. and Phillips, M. J. (1986). Three-dimensional observation of the intrahepatic lymphatics by scanning electron microscopy of corrosion casts. *Anat. Rec.*, **214**, 67–70

8. Irino, S., Ono, T., Hiraki, K. and Murakami, T. (1974). A study of the lymphatics and lymph nodes by injection

9. Kurokawa, T. and Ogata, T. (1980). A scanning electron microscopic study on the lymphatic microcirculation of the rabbit mesenteric lymph node. A corrosion casts study. *Acta Anat. (Basel)*, **107**, 439–66

10. Castenholz, A. (1984). Morphological characteristics of initial lymphatics in the tongue as shown by scanning electron microscopy. *Scanning Electron Microsc.*, III, 1343–52

11. Ohtani, O. and Murakami, T. (1987). Lymphatics and myenteric plexus in the muscular coat in the rat stomach: A scanning electron microscopic study of corrosion casts made by intra-arterial injection. *Arch. Histol. Jpn.*, **50**, (In press)

12. Kiernan, F. (1833). The anatomy and physiology of the liver. *Philos. Trans. R. Soc. London*, **123**, 711–70

13. Elias, H. (1949). A re-examination of the structure of the mammalian liver: I. Parenchymal architecture. *Am. J. Anat.*, **84**, 311–34

14. Elias, H. (1949). A re-examination of the mammalian liver: II. The hepatic lobule and its relation to the vascular and biliary system. *Am. J. Anat.*, **85**, 379–465

15. Murakamai, T., Itoshima, T. and Shimada, Y. (1974). Peribiliary portal system in the monkey liver as evidenced by the injection replica scanning electron microscope method. *Arch. Histol. Jpn.*, **37**, 245–60

16. Ohtani, O. and Murakamai, T. (1978). Peribiliary portal system in the rat liver as studied by the injection replica scanning electron microscopic method. *Scanning Electron Microsc.*, II, 241–4

17. Ohtani, O. (1979). The peribiliary portal system in the rabbit liver. *Arch. Histol. Jpn.*, **42**, 153–67

18. Ohtani, O., Murakamai, T. and Jones, A. L. (1982). Scanning electron microscopy of replicated liver blood vessels in man and some other animals with special reference to the peribiliary portal system. In Motta, P. M. and DiDio, L. J. A. (eds.) *Basic and Clinical Hepatology*, pp. 85–96. (The Hague: Martinus Nijhoff)

19. Ohtani, O. (1983). Microvascular organization of the liver as visualized by scanning electron microscopy of vascular corrosion casts. In Koo, A., Lam, S. K. and Smaje, L. H. (eds.) *Microcirculation of the Alimentary Tract*, pp. 69–74. (Singapore: World Scientific)

20. Wakim, K. G. (1941). The intrahepatic circulation of blood in the intact animal: preliminary report. *Proc. Staff Mayo Clin.*, **16**, 198

21. Wakim, K. G. and Mann, F. C. (1942). The intrahepatic circulation of blood. *Anat. Rec.*, **82**, 233–53

22. Knisley, M. H., Bloch, E. H. and Warner, L. (1948). Selective phagocytosis. I. Microscopic observations concerning the regulation of the blood flow through the liver and other organs and the mechanism and rate of phagocytic removal of particles from the blood. *Biol. Str.*, **4**, 1–93

23. Block, E. H. (1955). The in vivo microscopic vascular anatomy and physiology of the liver as demonstrated with the quartz rod method of transillumination. *Angiology*, **6**, 340–9

24. Mitra, S. K. (1966). The terminal distribution of the hepatic artery with special reference to arterioportal anastomosis. *J. Anat.*, **100**, 651–63

25. Del Rio Lozano, I. and Andrews, W. H. H. (1966). A study by means of vascular casts of small vessels related to the mammalian portal vein. *J. Anat.*, **100**, 665–73

26. Andrews, W. H. H. and Maegraith, B. G. (1953). Anatomical and physiological evidence of the hepatic artery and hepatic vein within the mammalian liver. *Nature (London)*, **171**, 222–3

27. Elias, H. and Petty, D. (1953). Terminal distribution of the hepatic artery. *Anat. Rec.*, **116**, 9–18

28. Kupffer, C. von (1876). Über Sternzellen der Leber Briefliche Mittheilung an Prof. Waldeyer. *Arch. Mikrosk. Anat.*, **12**, 353–8

29. Ito, T. (1951). Cytological studies on stellate cells of Kupffer and fat storing cells in the capillary wall of the human liver. (Japanese abstr.) *Acta Anat. Nippon.*, **26**, 42

30. Muto, M. (1975). A scanning electron microscopic study on endothelial cells and Kupffer cells in rat liver sinusoids. *Arch. Histol. Jpn.*, **37**, 369–86

31. McCuskey, R. S. (1983). The hepatic microvascular system. In Koo, A., Lam, S. K. and Smaje, L. H. (eds.) *Microcirculation of the Alimentary Tract*, pp. 57–68. (Singapore: World Scientific)

32. Takahashi-Iwanaga, H. and Fujita, T. (1986). Application of an NaOH maceration method to a scanning electron microscopic observation of Ito cells in the rat liver. *Arch. Histol. Jpn.*, **49**, 349–57

33. Ito, T. and Nemoto, M. (1952). Über die Kupfferschen Sternzellen und die 'Fettspeicherungszellen' ('fat-storing cells') in der Blutkapillarenwand der menschlichen Leber. *Okajima's Fol. Anat. Jpn.*, **24**, 243–58

34. Nakane, P. K. (1963). Ito's 'fat-storing cell' of the mouse liver. *Anat. Rec.*, **145**, 265–6

35. Ito, T. and Shibasaki, S. (1968). Electron microscopic study on the hepatic sinusoidal wall and the fat-storing cells in the normal human liver. *Arch. Histol. Jpn.*, **29**, 137–92

36. Wake, K. (1971). 'Sternzellen' in the liver: Perisinusoidal cells with special reference to storage of vitamin A. *Am. J. Anat.*, **133**, 429–62

37. Muto, M., Nishi, M. and Fujita, T. (1977). Scanning electron microscopy of human liver sinusoids. *Arch. Histol. Jpn.*, **40**, 137–51

38. Rappaport, A. M. (1973). The microcirculatory hepatic unit. *Microvasc. Res.*, **6**, 212–28

39. Rappaport, A. M., Borowy, Z. J., Lougheed, W. M. and Lotto, W. N. (1954). Subdivision of hexagonal liver lobules into a structural and functional unit: role in hepatic physiology and pathology. *Anat. Rec.*, **119**, 11–34

40. McCuskey, R. S. (1966). A dynamic and static study of hepatic arterioles and hepatic sphincters. *Am. J. Anat.*, **119**, 455–78

41. Grisham, J. W., Nopanitaya, W., Compagno, J. and Nagel, A. E. H. (1975). Scanning electron microscopy of normal rat liver. The surface structure of its cells and tissue components. *Am. J. Anat.*, **144**, 295–322

42. Andrejevic, J. (1861). Über den feineren Bau der Leber. *Sitzber. Akad. Wiss. Math.-Naturwiss. Kl.*, **34**, 642–57

43. Hering, E. (1866). Über den Bau der Birbeltierleber. *Sitzber. Akad. Wiss. Wien, Math.-Naturwiss. Kl.*, **54**, 496–515

44. Motta, P. and Fumagalli, G. (1975). Structure of rat bile canaliculi as revealed by scanning electron microscopy. *Anat. Rec.*, **182**, 499–514

45. Nopanitaya, W. and Grisham, J. W. (1975). Scanning electron microscopy of mouse intrahepatic structures. *Exp. Molec. Pathol.*, **23**, 441–58

46. Motta, P., Muto, M. and Fujita, T. (1978). *The Liver. An Atlas of Scanning Electron Microscopy*. (Tokyo: Igakushoin)

47. Clara, M. (1930). Untersuchungen an der menschlichen Leber. I. Über den Übergang der Gallenkapillaren in die Gallengange. *Z. Mikr.-Anat. Forsch.*, **20**, 584–607

48. Mall, F. P. (1906). A study of the structural unit of the liver. *Am. J. Anat.*, **5**, 227–308

49. Andrews, W. H. H., Maegraith, B. G. and Wenyon, C. E. (1949). Studies on the liver circulation. II. The microanatomy of the hepatic circulation. *Ann. Trop. Merd. Parasit.*, **43**, 229–37

50. Ohtani, O., Kikuta, A., Ohtsuka, A., Taguchi, T. and Murakami, T. (1983). Microvasculature as studied by the microvascular corrosion casting/scanning electron microscope method. I. Endocrine and digestive system. *Arch. Histol. Jpn.*, **46**, 1–42

51. Henderson, J. R. and Daniel, P. M. (1978). Portal circulations and their relation to countercurrent systems. *Q. J. Exp. Physiol.*, **63**, 355–69

52. Fujita, T. (1977). Concept of paraneuron. *Arch. Histol. Jpn.*, **40**, (Suppl.), 1–12

53. Northover, J. M. A. and Terblanche, J. (1979). A new look at the arterial supply of the bile duct in man and its surgical implications. *Br. J. Surg.*, **66**, 79–84

54. Ohtani, O. (1981). Microcirculation studies by the injection-replica method with special reference to the portal circulation. In Allen, D. J., Motta, P. M. and DiDio, L. J. A. (eds.) *Three Dimensional Microanatomy of Cells and Tissue Surfaces*, pp. 51–70. (New York: Elsevier North-Holland)

55. Sappey, Ph. C. (1889). *Traite D'anatomie Descriptive*, Vol. 4. (Paris)

56. Kreider, P. G. (1933). The anatomy of the veins of the gall bladder. *Surg. Gynec. Obstet.*, **57**, 475–82

57. Judge, O. M., Dickman, P. S. and Trapukdi, S. (1976). Nonfunctioning argyrophilic tumor (APUDoma) of the hepatic duct. Simplified methods for detecting biogenic amines in tissue. *Am. J. Clin. Pathol.*, **66**, 40–5

58. Heitz, P., Polak, J. M., Kasper, M., Timson, C. M. and Pearse, A. G. E. (1977). Immunoelectron cytochemical localization of motilin and substance P in rabbit bile duct enterochromaffine (EC) cells. *Histochemistry*, **50**, 319–25

59. Dancygier, H., Klein, U., Leuschner, U., Hubner, K. and Classen, M. (1984), Somatostatin-containing cells in the extrahepatic biliary tract of humans. *Gastroenterology*, **86**, 892–6

60. Sundler, F., Alumets, J., Hakanson, R., Ingemansson, S., Fahrenkrug, J. and Schaffalitzky de Muckadell, O. (1979). VIP innervation of the gallbladder. *Gastroenterology*, **72**, 1375–7

61. Alumets, J., Schaffalitzky de Muckedell, O., Fahrenkrug. J., Sundler, F., Hakanson, R. and Uddman, R. (1979). A rich VIP nerve supply in characteristic of sphincters. *Nature (London)*, **280**, 155–6

62. Fujita, T. and Kobayashi, S. (1979). Proposal of a neurosecretory system in the pancreas. An electron microscope study in the dog. *Arch. Histol. Jpn.*, **42**, 277–95

8

Microanatomy of the liver: physiopathological, clinical, and surgical aspects

L. J. A. DIDIO, E. GAUDIO and S. CORRER

The liver joins the pancreas in its classification as an amphicrine* organ, a structure functioning simultaneously as an exocrine and an endocrine gland. The angioarchitecture of the liver, including both vessels and biliary ducts parenchymal distributions, provides the morphological background for understanding hepatic physiopathology. The liver receives: (1) a relatively large volume of blood from **visceral** organs, such as those of the digestive system (oesophagus, stomach, intestines and pancreas) and the spleen, and (2) a small volume of blood from **parietal** organs, such as adjacent or neighbouring perihepatic structures. More blood arrives at the liver by means of the portal vein and its branches (representing vasa publica) than by means of the hepatic artery and its branches (representing vasa privata). The venous blood, rich in nutritional substances absorbed at the level of the digestive system, and the arterial blood, needed to supply the liver, circulate and are scrutinized in the hepatic parenchyma which is drained by the hepatic veins (right, intermediate and left) and by the caudate lobe (segment) veins. The liver is, then, the repository of a dense vascular network situated between digestive organs and spleen on the one hand and the heart and the general circulation on the other.

The hepatic vascular network is mainly capillary and more venous than arterial; it corresponds to an area of venous capillarization, that is, the interposition of capillaries between two sets of venules, one at each extremity (portal circulation), similar to that found in the hypophyseal area. Such a capillary network between venules provides the background for characteristic hepatic physiopathological events. As the branches of the portal vein and hepatic artery run together and are joined by biliary ducts, they form triads (tetrads if one adds lymph vessels, and pentads if one also adds nerves), the vessels and ducts of which come from or lead toward the porta hepatis (Figure 1), respectively. The triads are located at each angle of the polygonal (e.g. pentagonal or hexagonal) lobules, whereas the central venule is situated, as the name indicates, in the centre of each lobule. The biliary ducts convey the bile or exocrine secretion

and excretory substances away from the liver and toward the hepatic hilum; on the other hand, the central venules are the rootlets of the central veins and drain the blood in an opposite direction, toward the sulcus venae cavae. The confluence of these veins ultimately forms the hepatic and caudate lobe (segment) veins that drain the blood into the inferior vena cava, just inferior to the level of the right atrium of the heart.

Considering that 'at any moment form is the plastic image of function or dysfunction,' the above simplified morphological background is a clue to the most important roles played by the liver, which are as follows:

(1) Metabolism of nutrients, except lipids (these are components of the chyle, conveyed directly to the lymphatic ducts).

(2) Detoxification of poisonous substances absorbed with nutrients.

(3) Action on venous blood from the spleen, pancreas, gall bladder and abdominal wall.

(4) Secretion of bile to participate in intestinal, mainly duodenal, digestion.

(5) Excretion of degraded substances, as products of detoxification, by means of the bile, and further expulsion by the intestines.

(6) Synthesis of blood plasma proteins.

(7) Storage of carbohydrates as glycogen.

(8) Release of glucose and control of glycaemia.

The parenchyma of the liver (Figure 2a) is the cellular substance of the gland, as distinguished from the connective tissue, blood and lymph vessels, and nerves. It consists of hepatocytes, that is, etymologically, liver cells, which are epithelial cells having a polyhedral shape defined by six or more sides. Such cells have a diameter of approximately 20–25 μm and, since each of these cells is capable of performing all the functions carried out by the organ as a whole, each may be considered a miniature liver (see Chapters 1 and 9).

Under light microscopy, the hepatocyte resembles an ordinary cell, containing a centrally placed nucleus, having a diameter of about 8–9 μm and possessing 1–4 strongly basophilic nucleoli (Figure 2b).

* amphicrine, from the Greek, *amphi* = both; and *krinein* = to separate, secrete.

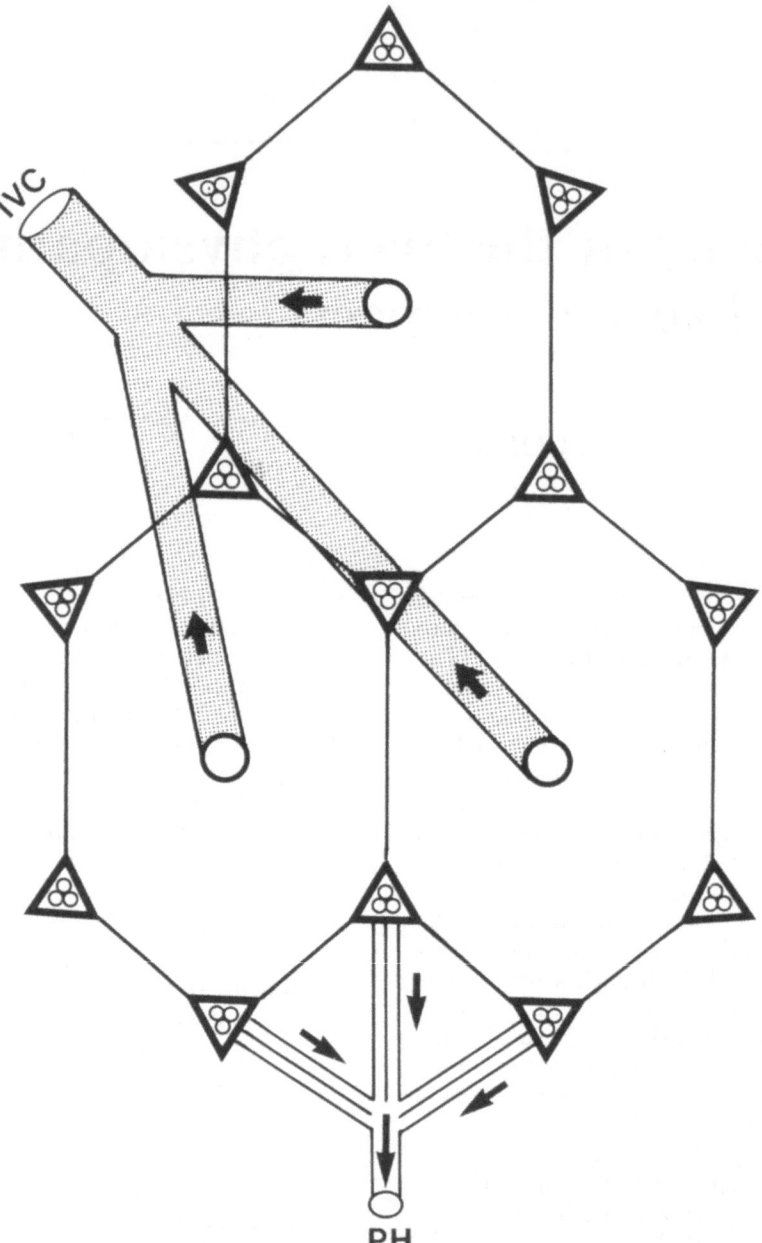

Figure 1 Diagram of the hepaton (microscopic liver lobule) from the anatomicosurgical standpoint. The figure illustrates 3 hepatons, each represented by a hexagonal liver lobule, the angles of which are occupied by triads (triangles containing 3 small circles). The large circle within each hepaton indicates the central venule, the confluence of which leads ultimately (arrows) to the inferior vena cava (IVC). The components of the triads run together, the vessels (branches of the portal vein and of the hepatic artery) toward the parenchyma and biliary ducts lead to the hilum or porta hepatis, from which they can be traced

The fetal or neonatal hepatocyte is diploid, while that of the adult is tetraploid[1].

The nucleus is voluminous, with scarce clusters of heterochromatin, mostly about the periphery, and abundant euchromatin dispersed within the karyoplasm. The size of the nucleus increases with age, probably due to increased DNA ploidy and content.

During the ageing process, in fact, there is probably an increase in nuclear endomitoses. For this reason, the liver contains more DNA than other tissues, due to the presence of numerous tetraploid nuclei, which contain double the amount of DNA contained in diploid nuclei. Up until six years of age, the liver contains only diploid nuclei, which, as already mentioned, decrease with age. The

quantity of DNA present in a tissue is useful as a reference substance, being indicative of the chemical composition of such a tissue.

In the liver, in fact, profound dietary alterations, such as fasting and protein deficiency, or pathological conditions, like fatty degeneration, while significantly modifying other parameters, do not significantly alter the quantity of DNA. Adult hepatocytes (which number about 10^8/g) do not normally proliferate; they remain quiescent during the G_0 phase of the cell cycle. Only about one in 2000 is able to enter the S-phase (semi-conservative DNA replication), while one in 20 000 is found in phase M (chromosome segregation). Among the factors that stimulate hepatocyte proliferation, are insulin, glucagon and EGF (Epidermal Growth Factor). The latter is produced in the duodenum by Brunner's glands and by the submandibular glands. Such factors, in appropriate contribution, act synergistically to allow commencement of DNA synthesis in hepatocytes; this takes place about 16 h after such stimulation. These proliferative effects can take place, however, only in environmental conditions of nutritional excess; that is, only in the presence of high levels of aminoacids and other nutritional factors. On the other hand, it should not be overlooked that unbalanced cellular proliferation can lead to carcinogenic phenomena, with loss of control over proliferation and over the steady state.

The abundant cytoplasm is characterized, under light microscopy, by the presence of numerous granules (Figure 2c) composed of organelles having a distinct structure and immersed deep within a cytoplasmic medium rich in water (85%) and proteins, and, in other regions, in glycogen or lipids.

The appearance of the cytoplasm varies according to the amount of water and fat contained therein.

When these glycogen-rich cells are treated with the most common stains, i.e. haematoxylin and eosin, the cytoplasm appears pale but has a dense distinct border. The quality of the glycogen present within the cells varies according to their functional state.

Moreover, the cells' glycogen content has also been shown to vary, increasing during the day[2,3]. The numerous intracytoplasmic granules observed by light microscopy are actually composed (see Chapter 1) of organelles including smooth and rough endoplasmic reticulum; ribosomes, either gathered into rosettes or dispersed in single units, the Golgi apparatus, lysosomes, and aggregates of peroxisomes and mitochondria interspersed among the RER and pigment granules. The latter may be divided into exogenous and endogenous pigments.

The most important exogenous pigment is carotene, which is dissolved within the lipid fraction and gives the liver its characteristic colour. The endogenous pigments include: the lipofuscins, produced by the oxidation and polymerization of unsaturated fatty acids which accumulate in avitaminosis E and in hypometabolic conditions (ageing, chronic malnutrition, debilitating diseases); the haemofuscins, which are probably of a lipofuscin-like nature; haemosiderin, which is demonstrable by common methods when present in quantities greater than 0.1% (viral hepatitis, haemochromatosis, cirrhosis, nutritional deficiency, transfusions).

Histochemical studies[4] involving hepatocytes have demonstrated the activity of numerous enzymes, such as alkaline phosphatase, 5'-nucleotidase acidase, acid phosphatase, pseudocholinesterase, β-glucuronidase, leucine aminopeptidase, γ-glutamyltranspeptidase, etc.

The most recent immunohistochemical techniques have demonstrated hepatocyte immunoreactivity for cytokeratin A, which seems to form the only type of intermediate filament present. Furthermore, with regard to microfilaments[5-8], either actin (F and G) or myosin are present, especially in those cytoplasmic regions immediately below the cell membrane, particularly towards the biliary pole. Further, recently it has been possible, through employment of immunological techniques adapted to light microscopy, to localize fibronectin within the cytoplasm of hepatocytes. The presence of collagen

types I and IV within hepatocytes has not been clearly proven[9]. Even hepatocytes having a high water content appear pale, but these have an indistinct border.

During fixation and preparation for light microscopy, the fat droplets present in the cytoplasm dissolve, leaving in their place some well-delineated vacuoles. In normal cells, these vacuoles have a diameter measuring less than 4 μm and are usually found near the free margin of the hepatocyte. The increase in the amount of fat present within the cells is dependent upon an equilibrium between the quantity of fat transported to the liver from the intestine and the degree of fat catabolism within the liver. The fat droplets become larger, and the entire cytoplasm is eventually occupied by droplets of various sizes[3].

In steatosis, only a single large fat droplet forms, displacing the nucleus towards the periphery of the cell. In more serious cases, droplets from adjacent cells apparently unite to form cysts.

The nucleoproteins present within the hepatocyte cytoplasm, which stain blue with haematoxylin, diminish under conditions of fasting or cell damage.

The cells near the centrolobular vein contain abundant lipofuscin granules; this pigment is found in progressively smaller amounts as one moves farther away from the vein.

Furthermore, especially during cholestasis, granules of bilirubin are present in the central region. Most of the haemosiderin is present within hepatocytes situated around the branches of the portal vein. The hepatocytes are arranged in interconnected laminae.

These plates radiate from central venules, the smallest rootlets of the hepatic veins and caudate lobe (segment) veins. On each side of the laminae, the blood flows in parallel canals, named hepatic sinusoids, which have intercommunications through holes or fenestrations.

With respect to normal capillaries, sinusoids are characterized by the following features: (1) tortuosity (sinuosity); (2) a large luminal diameter; (3) discontinuity of their wall (fenestrations); and (4) absence or wide discontinuity of the supporting basal membrane.

Besides the presence in the sinusoids of classic endothelial cells, which are flattened and have a chromophilic nucleus which protrudes into the lumen[10], two other types of cell must be taken into consideration: the Kupffer cells and the Ito cells (Figure 3a). (See Chapters 2 and 3.) The Kupffer cells, first described by von Kupffer[11] in livers impregnated with gold chloride, show a pronounced phagocytic activity in relation to substances injected into the circulation, and may be seen either within the sinusoidal lumen, overlapping the endothelium, or even between endothelial cells. Kuppfer cells contain an irregular or oval nucleus and possess more or less abundant cytoplasm, depending upon the functional activational state, which is rich in organelles and/or phagosomes of various forms and dimensions. In fact, these cells have both amoeboid and phagocytic activities[12] and currently are considered as part of the monocyte–macrophage system. They are especially numerous in the periportal zone where they carry out intense migratory activity.

The Ito cells[13], which we now relate to the 'Sternzellen' originally described by von Kupffer, in 1876[14], in the extrasinusoidal space, are characteristically gathered in the subendothelial region. They have a generally triangular shape and are provided with characteristic intra-

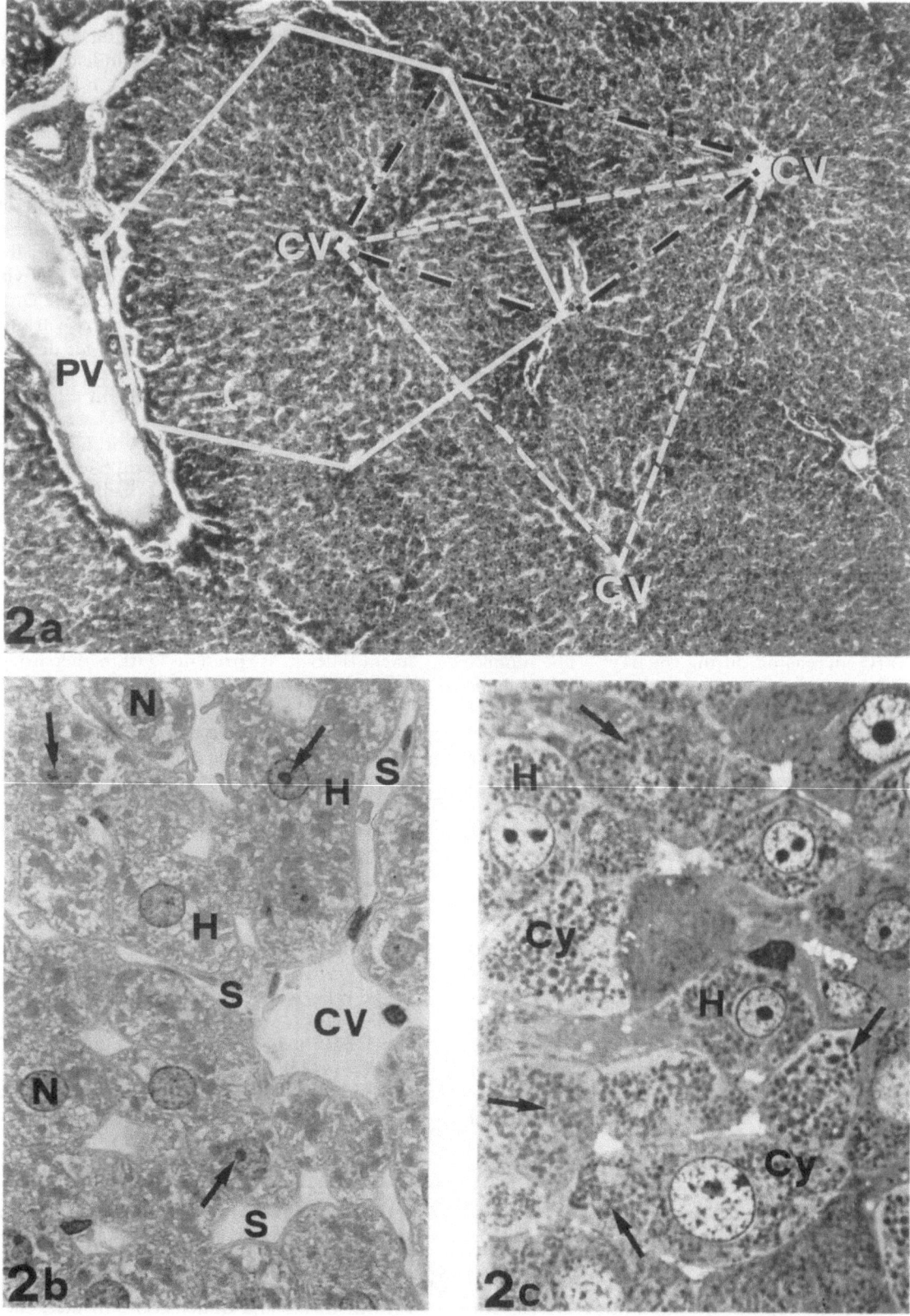

Figure 2   (a) Photomicrograph of human liver illustrating different concepts of liver units. _ Traditional hepatic lobule; _._. Hepatic acinus according to Rappaport; _ _ _ _ Portal lobule; CV = Central vein; PV = Portal vein. (Azan – Mallory; × 70)

(b) Photomicrograph of rat liver, showing the confluence of numerous sinusoids (S) with the central vein (CV). H = Hepatocytes; N = Nucleus; → = Nucleolus. (Eosin and Methylene blue; × 630)

(c) Photomicrograph of rat liver, showing hepatocytes (H) at the periphery of a traditional lobule with abundant cytoplasm (Cy) characterized by the presence of numerous granules (→). (Methylene blue; × 1000)

cytoplasmic lipid accumulations, which have earned them the name 'fat-storing cells'. These were formerly called pericytes, are of mesenchymal origin, and, in physiological conditions, they are capable of vitamin A accumulation[15]. (See Chapter 3.)

Recent studies have demonstrated that they are regularly disposed at intervals of 30–35 μm throughout the lobule, approximately 60 per 1000 hepatocytes, and that they surround, by means of their cytoplasmic processes, the entire sinusoidal structure.

In addition, even in physiological conditions, they are often seen associated with collagen fibres. Immunohistochemical studies have shown strong staining of such cells due to the presence of collagen types III and IV, and, to a lesser degree, of type I collagen and fibronectin[9]. They contribute, then, in normal conditions, to the formation of the delicate reticular and argyrophilic network supporting the hepatocyte plates and sinusoids (Figures 3b and c) while, in pathological conditions, they are capable of explicating remarkable fibrillogenic activity similar to that of fibroblasts.

Recently, a fourth type of sinusoid-associated cell has been described in the rat as well as in the human liver, whose nature and function is now related to natural killer cells, the so-called 'pit cells' situated in the sinusoidal spaces, with short stocky cytoplasmic prolongations and small dense granules dispersed in the cytoplasm[16].

The stroma of the liver comprises a connective tissue capsule (of Glisson) made up of collagen fibres and fibroblasts covered with a membrane of mesothelial cells. In addition, the stroma includes the capsular extensions from the hilum to the parenchyma.

Each liver lobule (or small lobe) in man is not separated from its neighbours by connective tissues partitions, making the parenchyma appear **continuous**. Each microscopic lobule (Figures 2a and 4) has a central venule (vein) and is surrounded at a distance by portal canals, areas, tracks, triads (tetrads or pentads). A portal triad belongs to more than one liver lobule, actually to three or more. When portal areas are not present, imaginary lines can be drawn to limit a typical liver lobule.

A portal lobule can be compared to a unit of an endocrine gland, which is, however, separated by septa from neighbouring units. The secretion of each unit is drained into a duct which joins others to form larger and larger ducts. The portal lobule, instead of surrounding the central venule, is the portion circumjacent to the portal triad, which contains the bile duct, where the external secretion and excretion are conveyed. Whereas the hepatic lobule is, at least, an imaginary polygonal (pentagonal or hexagonal) area, the portal lobule is triangular (Figures 2a and 4). The angles of the hepatic lobules contain the triads, while those of the portal lobules contain the central venules. If one considers portal lobules as the units of liver architecture, the central venules should be renamed 'angular' venules and the portal areas should be designated 'central' areas or 'portal centres'.

Since the portal lobule is not the minimum amount of parenchyma able to function as the entire liver, the concept of hepatic acinus was proposed by Rappaport *et al.*[17].

Hepatic acini are rhomboid or diamond-shaped areas, the extremities of which are determined by the central venules of two adjacent hepatic lobules (Figures 2a and 4). This rhomboid is divided into two triangles (united by their bases) by branches of the portal venule and hepatic arteriole emanating from one or two portal triads. Rappaport *et al.*[17] considered the liver functional unit as the mass of parenchyma associated with the most distal branches of the portal vein and of the hepatic artery, as well as the first rootlets of the biliary ductules. These small branches originate from the venules and arterioles at intervals and are accompanied by the fine rootlets that join the bile ductule at the same level. The direction of these branches and rootlets is perpendicular to the axis of each component of the triad and to the central venule. The hepatic acinus, smaller than the liver lobule and the portal lobule, is composed of portions of two adjacent liver lobules. It is defined as the amount of parenchyma supplied by a terminal branch of the portal vein and by a terminal branch of the hepatic artery and drained by a rootlet of the biliary ductule.

The boundaries of the hepatic acinus extend peripherally to adjacent central venules and neighbouring acini, making the parenchyma continuous and thus allowing collateral supply and drainage where and when necessary (for example, after failure of one or more acinar unit of supply and drainage).

Each triangle of the rhomboid hepatic acinus is divided into three zones: Zone 1 has a base formed by the plane that contains the canals of the triad and has a truncated apex which corresponds to the base of Zone 2. This zone also has a truncated apex which corresponds to the base of Zone 3, which, in turn, has an apex represented by the central venule. According to the direction of the blood flow, in the portal branch and in the hepatic arterial branch, the cells of Zone 1 are supplied with most of the incoming oxygen and nutrients. These fresh supplies are reduced in Zone 2 and are further lessened in Zone 3.

The architecture of the liver was considered, until recently, as a solid or three-dimensional network of cords of trabeculae; that is, cylinders made up of two rows of cells[18].

In order to conform with the microscopic images of sections of hepatic parenchyma, at least three concepts of cord-like arrangements were accepted, all with reservations. Although denied by Hering (1866)[19], none of these concepts could explain all findings, particularly the liver cell continuum and net-like pattern of silver-impregnated bile ductules[18]. The study and reconstruction of numerous sections of hepatic tissue and the presentation of three-dimensional illustrations, showing a framework of broad sheets, led Elias[20,21] to name the liver system of interconnected walls muralium. Because the hepatic parenchyma is made up of cells, it was called muralium cellulosum, the walls (laminae hepatis) of which enclose interconnecting spaces (lacunae hepatis) forming a labyrinthus hepatis.

The following definitions are given by Elias and Sherrick[18] in order to properly interpret microscopic images of liver tissue sections:

(I) Muralium simplex is a tunnelled continuum constituted of one-cell-thick hepatic laminae (the plates are two cells thick up to about the fifth year of life),

(II) Hepatic lacunae are tunnels or spaces in the muralium that form the labyrinth,

(III) Hepatic sinusoids are capillaries that form a three-

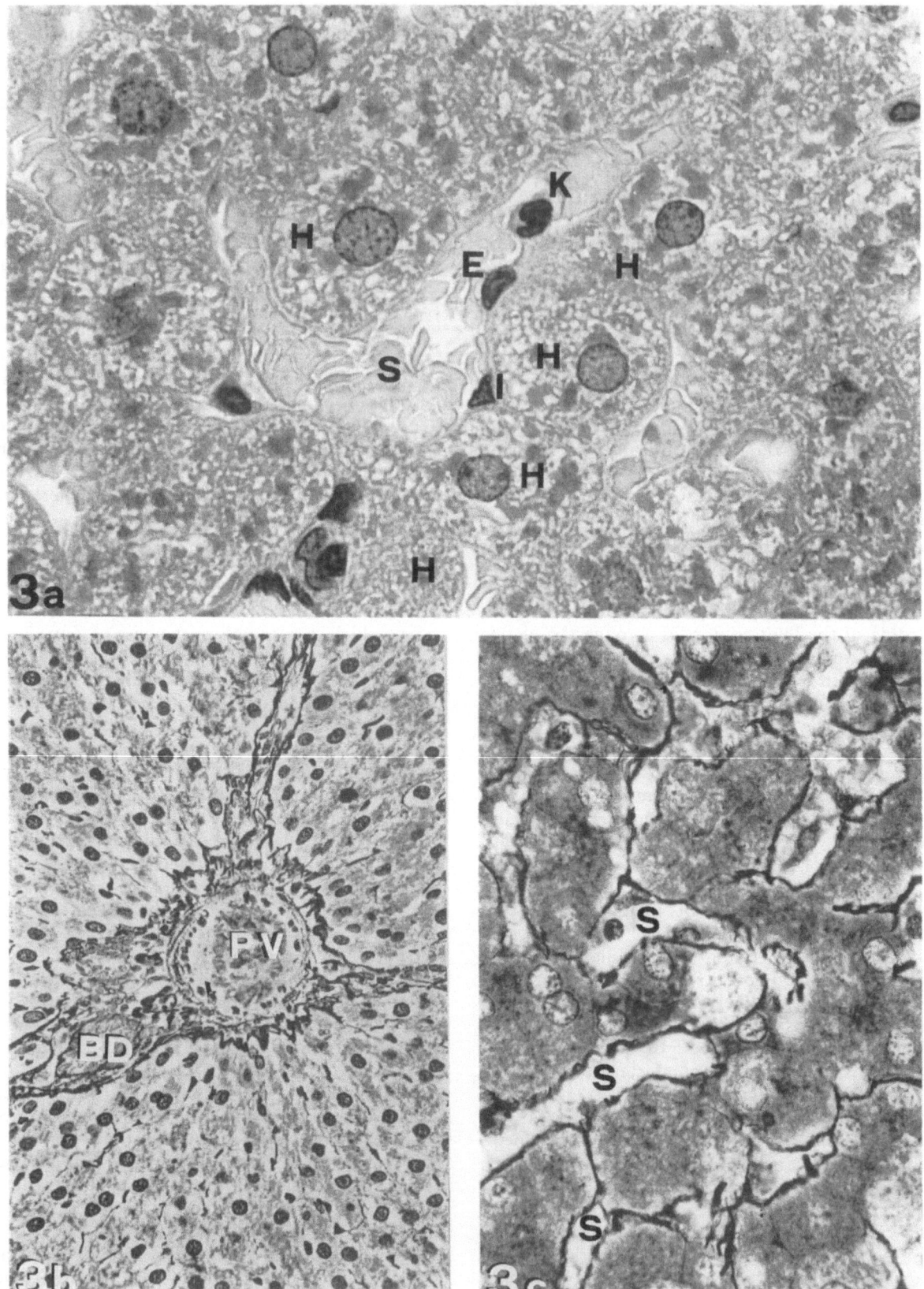

Figure 3 (a) Photomicrograph of rat liver illustrating plates of liver cells (H) and hepatic sinusoids (S). Endothelial cells (E), Kupffer cells (K) and Ito cells (I) are evident. (Haematoxylin and eosin; × 1260)

(b) Low power light microscopic appearance of hepatic reticular network in periportal zone. PV = Portal vein; BD = Bile duct. (Gomori staining; × 240)

(c) Photomicrograph of rat liver for demonstrating argyrophilic reticular network supporting the hepatocyte plates and sinusoids (S). (Pap's silver method; × 600)

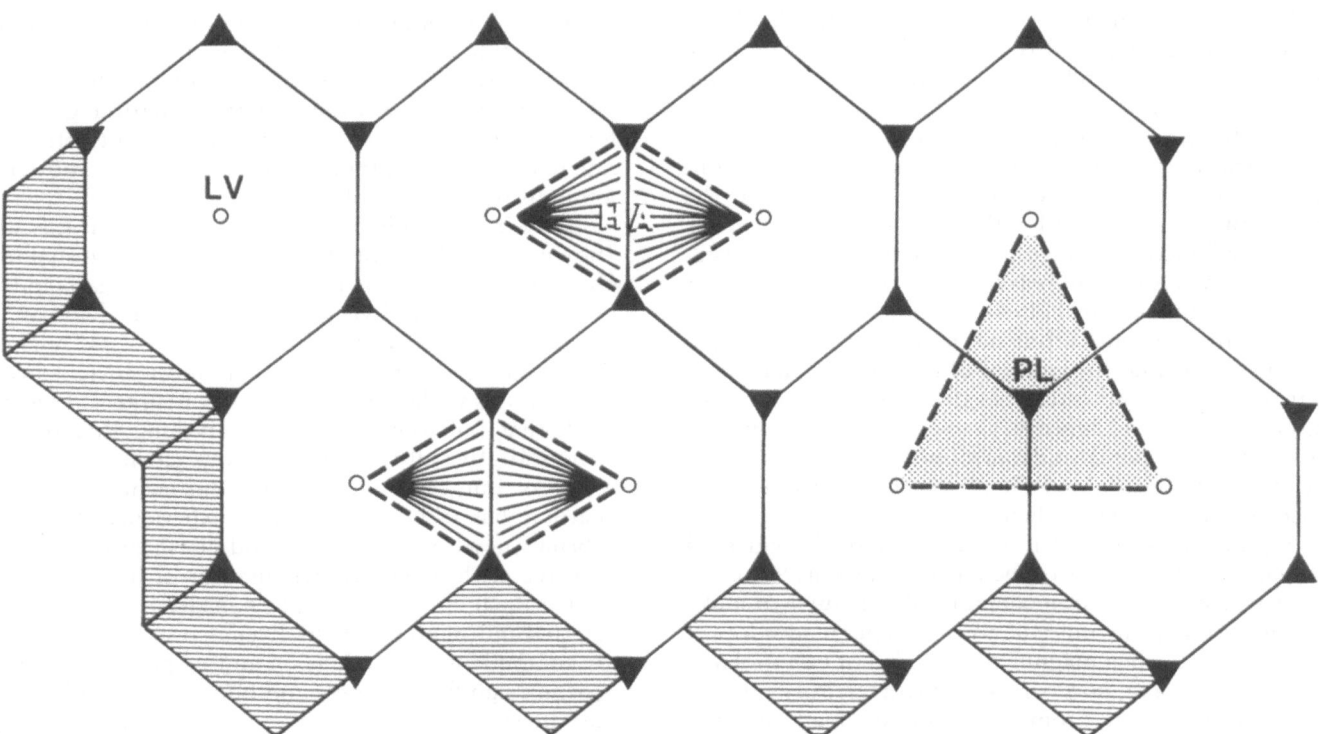

Figure 4 Diagram to illustrate different concepts of liver units. A microscopic liver lobule (LV), seen as a hexagonal unit, corresponds to the hepaton from the anatomicosurgical standpoint. The portal lobule (PL) is represented by the equilateral triangle (dotted), drawn between three central venules (circles) and containing, in its centre, a triad. Two hepatic acini (HA) are drawn as rhomboids or diamond-shaped areas between two central venules and two triads; the line linking the two triads divides each rhomboid into two triangles

dimensional network. Each sinusoid is suspended in a lacuna and the sinusoidal network is suspended in the lacunar labyrinth.

The authors emphasize that the lacuna is not a sinusoid, as the sinusoid occupies its central portion, and that the periphery of the lacuna has the perisinusoidal space (Disse's space), also called pericapillary space. The sinusoid is a capillary lined by littoral cells or Kupffer cells which act as endothelial cells and phagocytes.

They summarize their concept by stating that the lacuna is limited by hepatic cells and is divided, by flat littoral cells, into the sinusoid and the pericapillary space. In view of the recognition and descriptions of the classical lobule, portal lobule and liver acinus, Matsumoto *et al.*[22,23] studied the angioarchitecture and its relationship to the parenchymal structure of the normal human liver.

According to Greep and Weiss[24], 'The classical lobule, the portal lobule, and the acinus should not be considered as conflicting concepts of liver structure, but as complementary ones. Because of the complexity of the function of the liver, it is sometimes useful to think in terms of one and at other times in terms of another.' Matsumoto *et al.*[22] stated, then, that 'the concept of lobulation is an expression of what one means by basic organ structure' and, with this in mind, they studied the human liver by means of stereoscopic angiography and reconstruction from histological serial sections. They divided the portal tree into a conducting and a parenchymal portion, the first starting in the hilum, and the second being subdivided

into three steps: first, second (secondary or classical lobule), and third (having the septal branch).

The authors were led to expect from the typical lobular pattern, seen in histological sections, that the principal part of intralobular sinusoids arises from the marginal zone of the lobule and then converges toward the centrolobular area. They stated, however, that since the evidence of this expectation has been hitherto wanting, an attempt was made to clarify the three-dimensional angioarchitecture mediating the flow of blood from the parenchymal portal vein to the radial sinusoids. The marginal zone, according to the authors, demarcates the lobule and is divided into a septal and a portal zone. The septal branches (third-step branches) of the parenchymal portion supply and support the septal zone as a vascular skeleton. The portal zone is supplied by short venules given off by the portal tract or by each primary septal branch. 'The sinusoidal beds of the septal zone and those of the portal zone together constitute a synthetic functional unit: a high-potential pool from which portal blood pours uniformly into the radial sinusoids. This pool space appears as a sickle-shaped area on such sections as meet the parent portal tract transversely.' The authors called this area the sickle-zone and the most elementary cone shaped parenchymal unit the primary lobule, adding that six to eight primary lobules constitute a classical (secondary) lobule. Matsumoto *et al.*[22], after discussing the statement 'every organ has its characteristic structural unit,' indicated that metabolic phenomena, such as peripheral fatty change and glucose-6-phosphatase activity, do not conform with the acinus diagram, but, instead, with the sickle-zone pattern. They emphasize the determining role of the portal venous 'system' in forming the parenchymal angioarchitecture which characterizes the liver as a portal organ.

The different concepts and descriptions of the morphological and/or physiological units of the liver probably reflect anatomical variations depending upon the species of animal, or, within the same species, depending upon the functional stage at which they are observed. There is, then, sufficient reason for Elias' statement[25] that the liver lobule is an ephemeral expression of a field of pressure gradient. From the preceding discussion, it becomes clear that the concept of hepaton, analogous to that of nephron and osteon, as the minimum amount of parenchyma able to function as the entire liver is difficult to define. For practical and mnemonic purposes, however, it can be applied to an oversimplified classic 'liver lobule', since its morphology, when magnified, corresponds to the segmental arrangement of the organ, the background for partial hepatectomy or, better, for segmentectomy. In other words, the hepaton contains all structures to make it a morphological unit; it gives a general idea of its function, and, when magnified, extended or extrapolated to the entire organ, may correspond to a territory suitable for surgical removal. From the mnemonic standpoint, the hepaton (Figure 1) is the miniature of a liver anatomicosurgical segment[26], the components of the triads being traceable in the porta hepatis (pedicle) and the hepatic veins at their termination in the inferior vena cava.

The portal vein, the hepatic artery, the biliary duct, the lymphatic vessels and the nerves, together enter or exit from the liver through the hepatic hilum or porta hepatis, constituting the hepatic pedicle. The branches and rootlets of these vessels, ducts and nerves run jointly in the liver parenchyma, forming portobilioarterial pedicles for each homonymous anatomicosurgical segment. As already mentioned, at the microscopic level, these elements are seen in the triads, tetrads or pentads peripherally located in the angles of each hepaton.

The venous drainage of each hepaton is carried out by the central venule, far from the triads, an indication that the confluence of this venule with other central venules interdigitates with the portobilioarterial pedicles. The central venules ultimately lead to the hepatic veins and to the caudate lobe (segment) veins, tributaries of the inferior vena cava. There are, then, two sets of intertwined anatomicosurgical segments: portobilioarterial segments and hepatic venous (drainage) segments. Whereas the portobilioarterial segments possess pedicles that can be traced from the porta hepatis, the hepatic veins are found between these segments. The right, intermediate and left hepatic veins, as well as the caudate lobe (segment) veins, can be traced away from or toward the liver parenchyma from their termination in the inferior vena cava. The hepatic veins can also be traced in the liver parenchyma by making deepening incisions along the boundaries between adjacent portobilioarterial segments.

These intersegmental limits are identified, for example, during surgery, when one or more components of the portobilioarterial segmental pedicle or the entire segmental pedicle is, or are, temporarily or permanently ligated[26].

The old morphological division of the liver took into consideration landmarks on the hepatic surface provided by peritoneal relationships and grooves. The resulting lobes were named after their relative situation, geometric form or resemblance to a tail-like form: right, left, quadrate (anterior or quadrangularis), and caudate (posterior, minimus or exiguus) lobes.

In order to establish the transition between this well-known and still-helpful division, based on external morphological features for topographical purposes, and the modern segmental division of the liver, it seems appropriate to quote Leriche[27].

Anatomy 'is unquestionably the most ancient instrument of knowledge and is the base of surgery. One may think that [anatomy] did say everything that it could have said after all the time that was spent in dissecting cadavers. But, each time surgery approaches a new field, anatomy has to be reviewed and experience shows that it brings new, precise details and clarifications.' As has occurred with other parenchymatous or hollow viscera, such as the lungs, kidneys, spleen, heart and stomach, the external morphology of the liver is not a reliable guide for anatomicosurgical division and/or partial resection.

Many significant papers and books were published on the division of the liver[28–59]. These numerous contributions are an indication of the steady work on liver segmentation and its application to surgery for almost one century. In 1963, the successful performance of a liver transplantation[60,61] brought a new dimension to the study of applied anatomy of the liver and a promising development in hepatic surgery. In fact, it comprises the surgical removal of the normal liver from an individual (donor) and that of the pathological liver from a patient (recipient) as well as the implantation of the former to replace the latter. In other words, normal hepatic anatomy has to be known, not only because it is the pattern with which pathological anatomy has to be compared, but because it is itself subject to a surgical procedure that amounts to mere dissection. Finally, at least for the time being, liver transplantation may disregard the multiple concepts of the hepatic unit.

As happened to the nomenclature of the segments of the lung and of the kidney, several sets of terms, based on different criteria and the incidence of variations according to the populations examined, are available for the division of the liver. Most of the differences in terminology occurred because the segments were studied and designated in the isolated liver, in situ, in the anatomical position for description, or in other positions, considering the middle plane of the organ (gallbladder–inferior vena cava) or the sagittal plane of the human body as the major reference[26].

A comprehensive analysis of these proposed terminologies led us to consider Couinaud's[40] nomenclature and numbering of the sectors and segments of the liver, as the most acceptable. In fact, one of our colleagues[53,54] confirmed Couinaud's data in 52 specimens and we[62] were able to duplicate his findings in eight additional corrosion casts (Figure 3). Variations did occur in our cases, when compared with Couinaud's standard pattern (statistically the most frequent), but they were more in size than in location or number, thus confirming the validity of his description and terminology.

The nomenclature of liver segments proposed by Couinaud[40] and adopted here with minor modifications and a few additions, is based upon the embryogenesis, morphology, comparative anatomy of the organ and its components, variations, anomalies and surgical considerations.

Using an enlarged diagram of the classic lobule of the liver as the mnemonic figure to describe the division of the viscus, one is led to another two intertwined segments: a portobilioarterial and a hepatic (drainage) venous segment, the former corresponding to the triads and the latter to the central venule; similar to an open umbrella (according to the concept one wishes to adopt, the handle represents the portal or the central venule). Considering that the portal branch is the main essential component of the triad (or pentad), and considering that the portal vein is the leading directing element, being accompanied by the other elements (except the central venules and larger venous drainage vessels) Couinaud[40] named 'portal' the corresponding segments which we called portobilioarterial segments (disregarding lymphatic and neural components which join the elements of the pedicles). The hepatic venous segmentation corresponds to the areas of the liver drained by the hepatic veins, coming from the confluence of the central venules and veins, the position of which is more constant than that of the portal segments[40].

The portal (portobilioarterial) segmentation can be presented by following the hilar division of the portal vein (joined by the other components of the pedicle of the liver) into a right and left branch, resulting in a division of the organ into two hemilivers. The implantation (or peritoneal reflection) of the falciform ligament on the diaphragmatic surface of the liver is located to the left of the median (in the isolated organ), main, central, or principal fissural plane. This fissure is a constant one and corresponds to the plane that passes through (a) the centre of the cystic fossa (dividing the gallbladder into right and left halves) and (b) the left contour of the inferior vena cava, at the caval entrance site of the left hepatic vein[45]. In Couinaud's[40] words, 'the liver opens as a book and an excellent view of the superior aspect of the hilar plaque ... ' is obtained by making an incision along the principal fissural plane in the diaphragmatic surface. On the visceral surface of the liver, this plane corresponds to the middle of the gallbladder fossa, sections of the middle of the hilum, and reaches the left contour of the interior vena cava.

The right and left branches of the portal vein, accompanied by the other structures of the liver pedicle, supply the right and left hemiliver, respectively. Each hemiliver has, then, a pedicle of its own.

The right branch of the portal vein divides into two narrower branches, one for each of the following sectors: a right medial sector, juxtaposed and on the right side of the principal fissural plane, and a right lateral sector. The right lateral sector is separated from the medial sector by the right paramedian (paraprincipal, paracentral) fissural plane, which runs from a point located between the median fissural plane and the right hepatic 'angle' (one-third of the distance from the angle) and the termination of the right hepatic vein.

The left branch of the portal vein splits into two narrower branches at the left extremity of the hilum or porta hepatis, one for each of the following sectors: left lateral sector (posterior half of the left lobe) and left paramedian (paracentral) sector. These sectors are separated by the left paramedian (paracentral) fissural plane, which cuts the left lobe of the liver almost transversely. This plane describes a curve, having the concavity toward the left and posteriorly; the curve possesses a transverse anterior portion and a sagittal posterior portion. The extremities of this curve are as follows: the anterior corresponds to a point in the inferior margin of the liver, midway between the incisura of the round ligament and the left hepatic 'angle'; the posterior extremity corresponds to a point just left of the entrance of the left hepatic vein in the inferior vena cava.

The caudate lobe and the infrajacent hepatic parenchyma correspond to the dorsal sector, situated posteriorly to the trunk of the portal vein, from which it receives caudate lobe (sector, segment) branches.

There are, then, 5 sectors (Figure 5):

(a) The dorsal, posterior, belonging to both hemilivers;
(b) The two paramedian (right and left); and
(c) The two lateral (right and left).

The dorsal and the left lateral are unisegmental and the others are bisegmental.

Similar to the manner of indicating pulmonary segments, it is convenient to add numbering to the nomenclature of portal and hepatic venous (drainage) segments with Roman and Arabic numbers, respectively, considering the viscus within the body in the standard anatomical position for description. The numbering and nomenclature are valid whether the organ is isolated or not, regardless of the prone or supine position of the body, and obviously in any position required for clinical, radiological and surgical purposes.

The sectors comprise 8 segments (Figure 6), which are numbered clockwise with Roman numbers when the diaphragmatic aspect of the liver is observed from an anterosuperior view. They are named after taking into account that the organ is divided into two by a median plane, as follows:

(I) dorsal

(VIII) right posterior medial	
(VII) right posterior lateral	(II) left lateral
(VI) right anterior lateral	(III) left anterior
(V) right anterior medial	(IV) left medial

The (I) dorsal segment (lobe, sector) is visible only on the visceral aspect of the liver and the (VIII) right posterior medial segment is visible only on the diaphragmatic aspect (Figure 6).

Each pedicle is named after the sector or the segment to which it belongs.

The hepatic venous segmentation is so called because it comprises the veins that result from the confluence and affluence of central venules and veins to drain the blood from the liver in to the inferior vena cava. It could be named venous drainage segmentation of the liver.

There are 4 segments of hepatic venous drainage (territories drained by corresponding veins), numbered clockwise with Arabic numbers (Figure 7) when looking at the diaphragmatic aspect from an anterosuperior view, as follows:

(1) dorsal

(4) right   (2) left

(3) intermediate

The numbering of both the hepatic venous segments and portal segments (Figure 8) is anticlockwise when the liver is reflected upward to show the visceral aspect of the organ.

(1) The dorsal hepatic venous (caudate lobe, sector) segment is drained by caudate segment veins directly into the inferior vena cava. It is separated by the dorsal fissural plane from the remaining parenchyma of the right and left hemilivers.

(2) The left hepatic venous segment (left lobe) is drained by the left hepatic vein. This segment is separated from the intermediate one (3) by the left (hepatic venous) fissural plane and comprises portal segments II and III (sometimes part of IV). The left hepatic vein does not always follow the fissural plane.

(3) The intermediate hepatic venous segment is limited on each side by the left and right (hepatic venous) fissural planes and is located between homonymous segments. It is drained by the intermediate hepatic vein, the two roots of which join each other in the median fissural plane. This vein drains most of the portal segments IV, V and VIII.

(4) The right hepatic venous segment corresponds to the right one-third portion of the liver and is drained by the right hepatic vein, the roots of which have a confluence in the right paramedian fissural plane. This vein drains portal segments V, VI, VII and VIII.

On each aspect of the liver, the comparison between the hepatic venous segments and the portobilioarterial segments is the following:

A. Visceral aspect
Dorsal hepatic venous segment (1) = portal dorsal segment I; that is, dorsal sector (caudate lobe). It is seen only in this aspect of the liver.
Left hepatic venous segment (2) = portal segments II and III; that is, left lateral and left anterior segments, respectively.
Intermediate hepatic venous segment (3) = part of the left medial sector (portal segment IV) and of the right medial sector (portal segment V).
Right hepatic venous segment (4) = right lateral sector (portal segments VI and VII; that is, right anterior lateral and right posterior lateral) and part of the right medial sector (part of segment V or right anterior medial segment).

B. Diaphragmatic aspect
Dorsal hepatic venous segment (1) does not appear in this aspect of the liver.
Left hepatic venous segment (2) = left lateral sector (portal segment II or left lateral segment) and part of the left medial sector (portal segment III or left anterior segment).
Intermediate hepatic venous segment (3) = same as the visceral aspect.
Right hepatic venous segment (4) = portion of the right medial sector (lateral portions of portal segments V and

VIII, that is, right anterior medial and right posterior medial segments, respectively) and the right lateral sector (portal segments VI and VII, that is, right anterior lateral and right posterior lateral segments, respectively).

The correlation between the morphological lobes and he anatomicosurgical (portal and hepatic venous) segments of the liver shows the following:

A. With portal segmentation
Left lobe = left lateral sector plus a portion of the left medial sector.
Left lobe = portal segment II (left lateral segment) plus portal segment III (left anterior segment).
Right lobe = right hemiliver plus a portion of the left medial sector (except quadrate lobe).
Right lobe = portal segments IV (part), V, VI, VII, VIII; that is, left medial (except quadrate lobe), right anterior medial, right anterior lateral, right posterior lateral, and medial, respectively.
Caudate lobe = 'dorsal' sector, dorsal segment I and 1 (portal and hepatic venous).
Quadrate lobe = portion of the left medial sector or portion of the left medial segment (IV) seen from the visceral aspect of the liver.

B. With hepatic venous segments
Caudate lobe = dorsal segment 1.
Left lobe = segment 2.
Right lobe = most of segment 3 and segment 4.
Quadrate lobe = less than half of segment 3.

The correlation between the fissural planes of the portal and hepatic venous segmentations in the diaphragmatic aspect shows the following:

(A) The dorsal fissural plane is the same in both segmentations, separating segment I or 1 from the remaining liver parenchyma.

(B) The left hepatic fissural plane coincides posteriorly with the left paramedian fissural plane[40,52]; it separates segment II and the posterior portion of segment IV. Anteriorly, it coincides with the left anterior sagittal intersegmental fissural plane (between segments III and IV).

(C) The right hepatic fissural plane is found between the right paramedian and the median fissural plane.

In the visceral aspect, the correlation is as follows:

(A) The left hepatic fissural plane corresponds to the anterior and posterior left sagittal intersegmental fissural planes and to the left longitudinal sulcus (between segments II and III on one side and IV on the other).

(B) The right hepatic fissural plane is found between the right paramedian and the median fissural plane.

APPLIED ANATOMY

The segmentation of the liver is important especially for the performance of partial hepatectomy, as segmentectomy involves the surgical removal of one or more damaged, injured or diseased areas of the organ, and preserves those which are performing their functions well. Isolated cases of hepatic resection have been recorded

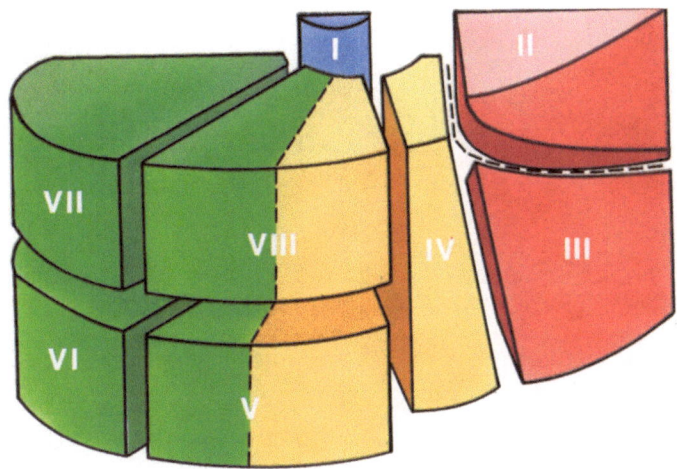

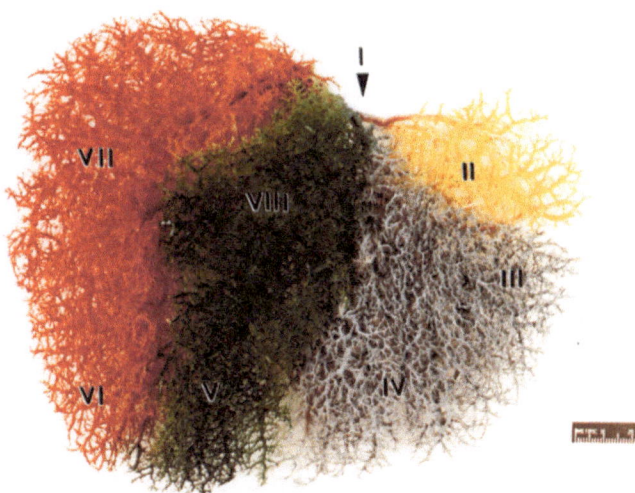

Figure 5 Diagram to illustrate the **sectors** and **segments** of the liver and the fissural planes. The 5 sectors are the dorsal (I), the left lateral (II), the left paramedian (III+IV), the right paramedian (V+VIII) and the right lateral (VI+VII). The **portal** or **portobilioarterial segments** are numbered I to VIII and named: dorsal (I), left lateral (II), left anterior (III), left medial (IV), right anterior medial (V), right anterior lateral (VI), right posterior lateral (VII) and right posterior medial (VIII). The **hepatic venous (drainage) segments** are: 1 or dorsal (blue, I), 2 or left (pink, II+III), 3 or intermediate (yellow, IV + parts of V and VIII) and 4 or right (green, VI+VII + parts of V and VIII)

Figure 6 Corrosion cast of **4 portal sectors** and 7 **portal segments** from a human liver injected with coloured vinyl acetate, seen from the diaphragmatic aspect of the organ. Dorsal sector (segment I) corresponds to the caudate lobe and is not seen (arrow indicates its posterior location). The left lateral sector is unisegmental (II, yellow), the left paramedian is bisegmental (III+IV, grey), the right paramedian is bisegmental (V+VIII, green) and the right lateral is bisegmental (VI+VII, red)

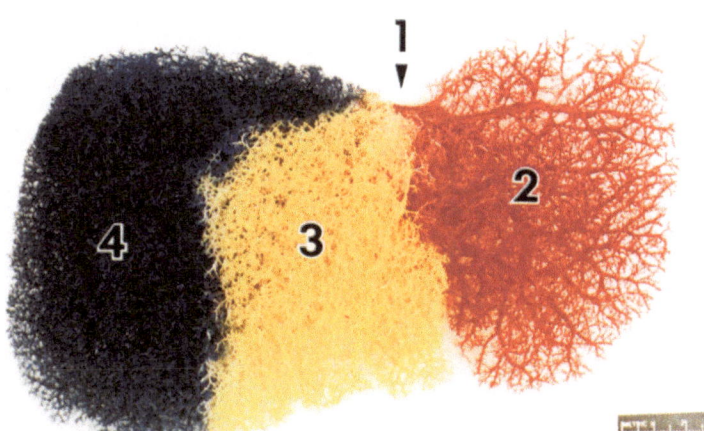

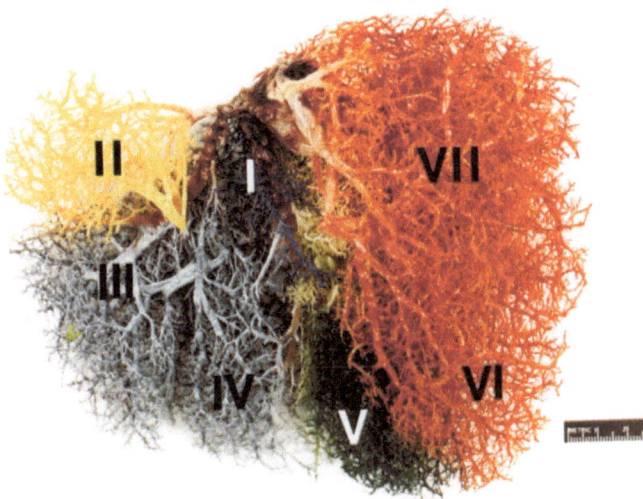

Figure 7 Corrosion case of 3 **hepatic venous (drainage) segments** from a human liver after retrograde injection with coloured vinyl acetate through the inferior vena cava, hepatic and caudate veins. The dorsal hepatic venous segment (1) is not seen (arrow indicates its posterior location as it corresponds to the caudate lobe). The left hepatic venous segment (2) appears red, the intermediate (3) appears yellow, and the right (4) appears blue. Diaphragmatic aspect of the liver

Figure 8 Corrosion cast of the 5 **portal sectors** and 7 **portal segments,** seen from the visceral aspect of the human liver (as in Figure 6). All 5 portal sectors are seen except portal segment VIII (right posterior medial) which cannot be observed from this aspect of the viscus. Because the view is from the visceral aspect of the liver, the numbering is anticlockwise

since 1716[63] but the successful removal of the right hemi-liver and a portion of the left hemiliver (segment IV or left medial segment), performed by Lortat-Jacob et al.[3,5], established the procedure as a viable surgical technique. In fact, up to 80% of liver parenchyma can be resected with little alteration in hepatic function[64].

Localized pathological lesions may be eliminated by segmentectomy, thus preserving the healthy remaining hepatic parenchyma. The conservative or limited resection is obviously preferable to more extensive mutilating surgery, since it restricts ablation to the segment or territory containing the lesion, maximally respecting the integrity of the organ's structure and function. Subsegmental hepatectomy is indicated for biopsy and in cases of cysts or benign tumours[63].

Identification of liver sectors and segments, as well as their pedicles, led to the standardization of surgical procedures for the performance of typical or 'réglées' segmentectomies[36]. Following the ligation of a segmental pedicle, haemostasis is produced. In one case of malignant cholangioma, Alves[48] had to keep ligated, for as long as 9 min, the pedicles of segments II and III (left lateral and left anterior, respectively) before successfully performing the segmentectomies. The ligation of each segmental pedicle is followed by the incision of the liver parenchyma along the corresponding fissural planes, indicated by discoloration caused by the ischaemia resulting from the obliteration of the vascular pedicular components. The hepatic vein(s) or tributaries that drain the segment(s) are ligated and the denuded surface is covered with peritoneum, for example, with the falciform ligament[63].

Partial hepatectomy, sectoriectomy or segmentectomy may follow portal or hepatic venous (drainage) segmentation, the vascular ligation always preceding parenchymal resection[40,65].

Based upon portal segmentation, the following surgical interventions can be performed: right or left hemihepatectomy, sectoriectomy (right lateral or medial, left medial, lateral, and dorsal), segmentectomy (one or more of the portal segments, except V, VII and VIII), extended hemihepatectomy or sectoriectomy, and associated segmentectomy.

Based upon hepatic venous (drainage) segmentation, simple or multiple segmentectomies can be performed. Among the simple segmentectomies, the following can be mentioned: ablation of segment 1, associate segmentectomy (II and III or 'left lobectomy') or ablation of segment 2, resection of segment 3 (intermediate), or of segment 4 (right hepatic venous segment). Multiple segmentectomies correspond to those in which more than one segment is resected.

As usual, several cases of lobar variations have been found to correspond to portal or hepatic venous segments that became separated also on the surface, thus isolating an independent area that has its own pedicle and is more easily removed surgically.

Laparoscopy or peritoneoscopy is used to study a structure endoscopically by means of an optical device introduced in the abdomen through an orifice made in the abdominal wall. This technique gives access to several organs[66], such as the round and falciform ligaments, liver, gallbladder, and other viscera, and provides the possibility of performing hepatic biopsy. Although it yields valuable information, the technique is not completely accident free; therefore, it requires extreme caution.

Angiography is frequently utilized to explore the vascular architecture of the liver because of the alterations resulting from almost all hepatopathies[67]. In addition to the diagnostic value, hepatic angiography can be applied for therapeutic purposes.

Biopsy of the liver can be percutaneously (IX right intercostal space) performed by needle puncture and suction of a fragment of the viscus or during laparoscopy or laparotomy. Liver biopsy allows diagnosis, monitoring and evaluation of hepatopathies, based upon alterations in the hepatic structure. According to Gayotto's[68] study, hepatocytes represent 80% of the volume of the liver, the remaining 20% comprising other cells, vessels and ducts. Pathologists consider the different concepts of a liver structural unit for their interpretation of the different hepatic diseases: acute hepatitis, chronic hepatitis and types of cirrhosis, cholestasis, hepatopathies (caused by alcohol, drug addiction, iatrogenic or therapeutic means), tumours and systemic diseases.

The first orthotopic hepatic graft in man was performed in 1963 by Starzl[69,71], and, in the subsequent 20 years, 540 livers were transplanted[71]. Immunosuppressive and technical advances made liver transplantation a feasible surgical therapy for patients afflicted by chronic, irreversible and progressive liver disease[71].

Liver transplantation has several limitations, among them, the absence of disease in other organs. For example, extrahepatic metastases from liver cancer or hepatic location of metastases from a malignancy elsewhere would preclude the adoption of radical surgical therapy. A viable donor is, for example, a young individual in the terminal stage of a non-malignant disease, who has suffered irreversible encephalic injury and whose circulation may be temporarily maintained by artificial means. Once this step is successfully reached, a series of tests will determine compatibility. Administration of drugs which decrease ischaemia by stabilizing plasmalemmas and avoiding disruption of lysosomal envelopes, cooling and perfusion of the liver are recommended. The dissection of the pedicle of the liver, for the surgical removal of the viscus, has been described as dissection of the 'portal triad'. Such an expression should be avoided for description of the major macroscopic components, both vascular and ductal (disregarding neural and lymphatic ones), and should be reserved only for the structure seen at microscopic level.

After the proper selection of recipients, the donor operation is performed, then the recipient surgical intervention, and the follow-up[60]. Liver transplant may be performed in children born with intrahepatic biliary atresia and patients presenting primary hepatic or unresectable malignancies, and serious cirrhosis[71,72]. The liver from the donor is isolated while maintaining the circulation by massaging the heart of the cadaver, is perfused, and is placed in a hyperbaric chamber. The liver is transplanted in the same site as the organ to be replaced (orthotopic, homotopic) or elsewhere (heterotopic), in addition to the recipient's pathological liver (which may be removed sooner or later).

In closing, it seems appropriate to quote Dr W. R. Waddell's statement, included in the foreword he wrote for Starzl and Putnam's books[73] on the subject: 'In clear relief against the background of clinical experience is shown the confluence of modern biology and medicine ranging from old and new anatomy to genetics, immunology, pharmacology, chemistry, microbiology, and more. As such, we have an outstanding example of what surgery is about and where it is going ... The consequence of the early failures was to stimulate the re-examination of the apparent problems in more detail and to evolve solutions. The course has been back and forth from the clinic to the laboratory with complete dissolution of the artificial barrier between "basic" and "clinical" sciences.'

References

1. Ranek, L., Keiding, N. and Jensen, S. T. (1975). A morphometric study of normal human liver cell nuclei. *Acta Pathol. Microbiol. Scand., Sect. A* 88, 467–476
2. Babcock, M. B. and Cardell, R. R. (1974). Hepatic glycogen patterns in fasted and fed rats. *Am. J. Anat.,* 140, 229–236
3. Schaffner, F. and Popper, N. (1986). In Berk, W. S. (ed.) *Bockus Gastroenterology*, 4th Edn., Vol. VI, pp. 2625–2658. (Philadelphia: W. B. Saunders Co.)
4. Oda, M. and Phillips, M. J. (1975). Electron microscopic chemical characterization of bile canaliculi and bile ducts in vitro. *Virchows Arch. (Cell. Pathol.),* 18, 109–118
5. Denk, H. and Franke, W. W. (1982). Cytoskeletal filaments. In Arias, L. M., Popper, H., Schachter, D. and Shafritz, D. A. (eds.) *The Liver: Biology and Pathobiology*, pp. 55–71. (New York: Raven Press)
6. French, S. W. and Davies, P. L. (1975). Ultrastructural localization of actin like filaments in rat hepatocytes. *Gastroenterology,* 68, 765–174
7. Fiskum, G., Craig, S. W., Decker, G. L. and Lehninger, A. L. (1980). The cytoskeleton of digitonin-treated rat hepatocytes. *Proc. Natl. Acad. Sci. USA,* 77, 3430–3434
8. Phillips, M. J., Oda, M., Mak, E., Fisher, M. M. and Jeejeebhoy, K. N. (1975). Microfilament dysfunction as a possible cause of intrahepatic cholestasis. *Gastroenterology,* 69, 48–58
9. Clement, B., Emonard, H., Rissel, M., Druguet, M., Grimaud, J. A., Herbage, D., Bourel, M. and Guillouz, A. (1984). Cellular origin of collagen and fibronectin in the liver. *Cell. Mol. Biol.,* 30(5); 489–496
10. Wisse, E. and Knook, D. L. (1982). Investigation of sinusoidal cells: a new approach to the study of liver function. *Prog. Liver Res.,* 6, 153–159
11. von Kupffer, C. (1899). Uber die sogenannten Sternzellen der Saugthierleber. *Arch. Mikr. Anat.,* 54, 254–262
12. Howard, J. G. (1970). The origin and immunological significance of Kupffer cells. In van Furth, R. (ed.) *Mononuclear Phagocytes*, pp. 178–199. (Oxford: Blackwell Scientific Publications)
13. Ito, T. and Shibasaki, S. (1968). Electron microscopic study on the hepatic sinusoidal wall and the fat-storing cells in the normal human liver. *Arch. Histol. Jpn.,* 29, 137–147
14. von Kupffer, C. (1876). Uber, Sternzellen der leber. *Arch. Mikr. Anat.,* 12, 353–368
15. Wake, K. (1980). Perisinusoidal stellate cells (fat storing cells, interstitial cells, lipocytes), their related structure in and around the liver sinusoids, and vitamin A storing cells in extrahepatic organs. *Int. Rev. Cytol.,* 66, 303–312
16. Kaneda, K., Dan, C. and Wake, K. (1983). Pit cells as natural killer cells. *Biomed. Res.,* 4, 567–576
17. Rappaport, A. M., Borowy, A. J., Lougheed, W. M. and

18. Lolto, W. N. (1954). Subdivision of hexagonal liver lobules into a structural and functional unit; role in hepatic physiology and pathology. *Anat. Rec.,* 119, 11–34
19. Elias, H. and Sherrick, J. C. (1969). *Morphology of the Liver*. (New York: Academic Press)
20. Hering, E. (1866). Über den Bau der Wirbeltierleber. *Sitzber. Akad. Wiss. Wien, Math. -Naturw. Kl.,* 54, 496–515
21. Elias, H. (1949). A re-examination of the structure of the mammalian liver. I. Parenchymal structure. *Am. J. Anat.,* 84, 311–334
22. Elias, H. (1949). A re-examination of the structure of the mammalian liver. II. The hepatic lobule and its relation to the vascular and biliary system. *Am. J. Anat.,* 85, 379–456
23. Matsumoto, T., Komori, R., Magara, T., Ui, T., Kawakami, M., Tokuda, T., Takasaki, S., Hayashi, H., Jo, K., Hano, H., Fujino, H., and Tanaka, H. (1979). Study on the normal structure of the human liver, with special reference to its angioarchitecture. *Jikeikai Med. J.,* 26, 1–40
24. Matsumoto, T. and Kawakami, M. (1982). The unit-concept of hepatic parenchyma. A re-examination based on angioarchitectural studies. *Acta Pathol. Jpn.,* 32 (suppl. 2), 285–314
25. Greep, R. O. and Weiss, L. (1977). *Histology*, 4th Edn. (New York: McGraw-Hill Book Co.)
26. Elias, H. (1955). Liver morphology. *Biol. Rev. Cambridge Philos. Soc.,* 30, 263–310
27. Motta, P. M. and DiDio, L. J. A. (1982). *Basic and Clinical Hepatology*. (The Hague: M. Nijhoff Publs.)
28. Leriche, R. (1951). *Philosophie de la Chirurgie*. (Paris: Flammarion)
29. Rex, H. (1888). Beiträge zur Morphologie der Saugerleber. *Morphol. Jahrb. Anat. Entwicklungsgesch.,* 14, 517–616
30. Hoche, M. L. (1925). Sur l'existence de territoires distincts dans le domaine de la veine porte Hépatique. *C. R. Soc. Biol.,* 92, 717–718
31. Hjortsjö, C. H. (1948). Die Anatomie der intrahepatischen Gallengänge beim Menschen; mittels Röntgen -und Injektionstechnik studiert nebst Beiträgen zur Kenntnis der inneren Lebertropographie. *Lunds Univ. Arsskr. Avd.,* 2, 44, 1–112
32. Hjortsjö, C. H. (1951). The topography of the intrahepatic duct systems. *Acta Anat.,* 11, 599–615
33. Hjortsjö, C. H. (1956). The intrahepatic ramification of the portal vein. *Lunds Univ. Arsskr. Avd.,* 2, 52, 1–30
34. Hjortsjö, C. H. (1957). *Leverns Segmentering*. (Uppsala: Lunds Universitet)
35. Elias, H. (1954). Segments of the liver. *Surgery,* 36, 950–952
36. Lortat-Jacob, T. C., Robert, H. G. and Henry, C. (1952). Un cas d'hépatectomie droite réglée. *Mém. Acad. Chir.,* 78, 244–250
37. Patel, J. and Couinaud, C. (1952). Les bases anatomiques des hépatectomies réglées. In *Proceedings of the 16th International Congress of Surgeons*, Copenhagen, pp. 1–18. (Bruxelles: Impr. Méd. Sc.)
38. Healey, J. E. and Schroy, P. C. (1953). Anatomy of the biliary ducts within the human liver. *Am. Med. Assoc. Arch. Surg.,* 66, 599–616
39. Healey, J. E., Schroy, P. C. and Sorensen, R. J. (1953). The intrahepatic distribution of the hepatic artery in man. *J. Int. Coll. Surg.,* 20, 133–148
40. Couinaud, C. (1954). Lobes et segments hépatiques. *Presse Méd.,* 62, 709–712

40. Couinaud, C. (1957). *Le Foie: Études Anatomiques et Chirurgicales*. (Paris: Masson et Cie.)

41. Elias, H. (1964). Zur chirurgischen Anatomie der Leber. *Verh. Anat. Ges., 59*. Vers. München (1963); *Ergeb. Anat. Anz., 113*, 235–252

42. Elias, H. (1970). Surgical anatomy of the liver. *Recent Results Cancer Res., 26*, 116–136

43. Healey, J. E. (1954). Clinical anatomic aspects of radical hepatic surgery. *J. Int. Coll. Surg., 22*, 542–549

44. Healey, J. E. (1970). Vascular anatomy of the liver. *Ann. NY Acad. Sci., 170*, 8–17

45. Gans, H. (1955). *Introduction to Hepatic Surgery*. (Amsterdam: Elsevier)

46. Gans, H. (1955). The intrahepatic anatomy and its repercussion on surgery. *Arch. Chir. Neerl., 7*, 131–146

47. Gans, H. and Bax, H. R. (1955). Partial resection of the liver in early carcinoma of the gall-bladder. In *Proceedings Congrés International de Chirurgie*, pp. 1–13. (Copenhagen)

48. Alves, J. R. (1957). Das Hepatectomias. *Rev. Bras. Cir., 34*, 23–31

49. Mancuso, M., Natalini, E. and Del Grande, G. (1955). Contributo alla conoscenza della struttura segmentaria del fegato in rapporto al problema della resezione epatica. *Policlinico Sez. Chir., 62*, apud Couinaud

50. Pinheiro, L. C. S. F. (1955). *Das Hepatectomias Regradas*, pp. 171. (Rio de Janeiro: Editora Gráfica Seleçóes Brasileiras)

51. Goldsmith, N. A. and Woodburne, R. T. (1957). The surgical anatomy pertaining to liver resection. *Surg. Gynecol. Obstet., 105*, 310–318

52. Couinaud, C. and Nogueira, C. E. D. (1958). The suprahepatic veins in man. *Acta Anat., 34*, 84–110

53. Nogueira, C. E. D. (1958). Pesquisas sôbre as *Venae Hepaticae* em relação aos planos divisores dos territórios anatomocirúrgicos no Homem. *Ph.D. dissertation, Surgery*, Fac. Med. Univ. Minas Gerais, pp. 95

54. Nogueira, C. E. D. (1958). Bases anatômicas das hepatectomias regradas. *Rev. Assoc. Med. Minas Gerais, 9*, 191–193

55. Michailov, S. S., Kagan, J. J. and Archipowa, S. E. (1966). Anatomische Untersuchungen über den Segmentaufbau der menschlichen Leber. *Anat. Anz., 119*, 317–336

56. Platzer, W. and Maurer, H. (1966). Zur Segmenteinteilung der Leber. *Acta Anat., 63*, 8–31

57. Mikhailov, G. A. (1970). Individual variations in hepatic lobes, segments, and vessels. In *Proceedings of the 9th International Congress of Anatomy*, Leningrad, pp. 1–5

58. Gupta, S. C., Gupta, C. D. and Gupta, S. B. (1981). Hepatovenous segments in the human liver. *J. Anat., 1*, 1–6

59. Nakamura, S. and Tsuzuki, T. (1981). Surgical anatomy of the hepatic veins and the inferior vena cava. *Surg. Gynecol. Obstet., 152*(1), 43–50

60. Starzl, T. E. (1964). Hepatic transplantation. In Schwartz, S. I. (ed.) *Surgical Diseases of the Liver*, Chap. 12. (New York: McGraw-Hill Book Co.)

61. Smith, B. (1969). Segmental liver transplantation from a living donor. *J. Pediatr. Surg., 4*, 126–132

62. DiDio, L. J. A. (1978). The anatomical background for partial hepatectomy. In *Proceedings of the 5th Pan American Congress of Anatomy*, São Paulo, Brazil, pp. 198–204

63. Schwartz, S. I. (1964). *Surgical Diseases of the Liver*. (New York: McGraw-Hill Book Co.)

64. Schwartz, S. I. (1979). *Principles of Surgery*. (New York: McGraw-Hill Book Co.)

65. Calne, R. Y. and Della Rovere, G. Q. (1982). *Liver Surgery*. (Padua: Piccin Medical Books)

66. Silva, A. O. and Cunha, A. C. F. (1980). Laparoscopia. Experiência em 230 casos. In Mello, J. B., Moraes, J. N., Nahas, P., Arruda, R. and Abrão, N. (eds.) *Capítulos de Cirurgia*, Chap. 13 (São Paulo: Abbott Labs.)

67. Mies, S. (1980). Valor diagnóstico da angiografia nas doenças do fígado. In Mello, J. B., Moraes, J. N., Nahas, P., Arruda, R. and Abrão, N. (eds.) *Capítulos de Cirurgia*, Chap. 14 (São Paulo: Abbott Labs.)

68. Gayotto, L. C. (1980). Importância da anatomia patológica na avaliação das doenças hepáticas. In Mello, J. B., Moraes, J. N., Nahas, P., Arruda, R. and Abrão, N. (eds.). *Capítulos de Cirurgia*, Chap. 12 (São Paulo: Abbott Labs.)

69. Starzl, T. E. (1981). The succession from kidney to liver transplantation. *Transplant. Proc., 13*, (1, suppl. 1), 50–54

70. Calne, R. Y. (1983). *Liver Transplantation*. (New York: Grune and Stratton)

71. Sherlock, S. (1983). Hepatic transplantation: The state of play. *Lancet, 1*, 778–779

72. Tolosa, E. M. C., Behmer, O. A. and Fujimura, I. (1978). Transplante de Orgãos. In Goffi, F. S. (ed.) *Técnica Cirúrgica*, Chap. 11. (Rio de Janeiro: Livraria Atheneu)

73. Starzl, T. E. and Putnam, C. W. (1969). *Experience in Hepatic Transplantation*. (Philadelphia: W. B. Saunders Co.)

9

Morphology of isolated and cultured hepatocytes from normal liver and in hepatocarcinogenesis

D. BERNAERT, R. MOSSELMANS, L. DE RIDDER and P. GALAND

This paper is dedicated to the memory of Professor P. Drochmans and Professor J.-C. Wanson.

INTRODUCTION

In a wide variety of experimental hepatocarcinogenic models, the administration of chemical carcinogens induces the same sequence of morphological and functional alterations preceding tumour development (see review in reference 1).

For example in the Scherer and Emmelot model used in our laboratory, one observes, following diethylnitrosamine (DENA) administration, the sequential formation of foci of altered hepatocytes after a few weeks, neoplastic nodules predominating after about 9 months, and of hepatocellular carcinomas after 12–15 months, yet with persisting foci and nodules (nomenclature is included in reference 2).

A lineage relationship between these lesions is suggested from their constant sequential appearance before that of tumours, and from the similarities in their morphological and metabolic alterations (reviewed in references 3–5).

The demonstration of the induction of foci and microcarcinomas within pre-existing foci following administration of a second carcinogen to DENA-treated rats reinforces this hypothesis[6].

Further support for this suggestion was given by the demonstration that hepatocytes from isolated neoplastic nodules had the ability to invade embryonic tissue in vitro[7], a widely accepted malignant characteristic[8].

However, a direct lineage between the lesions was never demonstrated and alternative origins for the ultimate hepatocarcinomas might be considered[9,10].

Oval cells have been proposed as precursors of the hepatocarcinomas that develop in response to various carcinogens[9,11]. However, proliferation of oval cells is not observed with DENA treatment (reference 12 and our own observations).

Abbreviations used: DENA = diethylnitrosamine; GGT = γ-glutamyltranspeptidase; G6Pase = glucose-6-phosphatase; AFP = α-fetoprotein; ATPase = adenosine triphosphatase; NNM = N-nitrosomorpholine.

Our approach for elucidating the lineage relationships between early focal lesions, neoplastic nodules and tumours, consists of comparing their morphofunctional properties with those of the hepatocarcinomas and of looking for the possible gradual appearance of characteristics of malignancy in the stepwise lesions. This involves the isolation of purified hepatocytic populations from foci, nodules and tumours, the comparison of their properties under primary culture conditions, and their response to in vitro testing of their potential expression of biological traits of malignancy.

NORMAL HEPATOCYTES IN CULTURE

Isolation of adult rat liver parenchymal cells can be achieved with a high yield by the enzymatic perfusion technique previously described[13-15].

Ultrastructural analysis shows that well-preserved monodispersed adult hepatocytes in culture are able to re-form anastomosing cell trabeculae (hepatic laminae), comparable to those seen in the intact liver parenchyma. After 24 h of contact, they reconstitute sinusoidal and interhepatocytic faces, attached by specific desmosomes and tight junctions enclosing reconstituted bile canaliculi. The hepatocytes have reorganized their intracellular biliary polarity of Golgi complexes close to the bile channel[16-18]. The functional character of the latter is indicated by the fact that galactosyl–bovine serum albumin, labelled with gold particles and added to the culture medium, appears in the bile canaliculi after 12 h incubation[19], confirming previous observations of transcellular fluorescein transport in hepatocyte monolayers[20].

Primary cultures of adult rat hepatocytes have been proven very useful for the investigation of specific parenchymal metabolic functions, such as albumin[21] or transferrin[22] synthesis and their regulation. This experimental model also proved appropriate for analysing endocytosis[19,23] and recycling of specific membrane receptors[24,25].

Addition of hormones to the culture medium enhances survival of the cells and induces specific differentiated functions. Insulin, for example, stimulates glycogenesis[26] and, like tri-iodothyronine, stimulates the phosphorylation of chromosomal non-histone proteins[27]. Glucocorticoids improve both survival and maintenance of polygonal shape of cultured hepatocytes[28]. These hormones or their analogues also modulate a series of hepatocytic activities[29,30]. A combination of several hormones is required for retention or induction of some specific enzymes, such as glucokinase, glycogen synthetase[31] and glucose-6-phosphatase (G6Pase)[32].

However, the purity of the experimental system is a major problem. Cultures of differentiated cells have a limited survival, lose their differentiated functions, and may progressively express various activities which are characteristic of the fetal period, e.g. γ-glutamyltranspeptidase (GGT) activity and production of α-fetoprotein (AFP)[33], or fetal-type isozymic forms[34]. The presence of a collagenous matrix and hormonally defined media appear to be essential for improving cell culture survival and prolonged retention of their differentiated state as expressed, for example, by specific mRNA translation[35-37].

The essential role of the biomatrix in cultures appears to be the preservation of the three-dimensional shape of the cells, sustained by an adequate cytoskeleton[38-40], which, through the so-called 'skeletal framework', might also play a role in the regulation of translation and transcription[39,41].

Adult hepatocytes in serum-free medium synthesize multiple collagen types[42] and fibronectin[43].

In regenerating liver and in pathological conditions, although not in normal liver, the hepatocytes play an important role in the production of extracellular components and even of a basement membrane[42,44]. Changes in the distribution of biomatrix components, such as a loss of fibronectin (observed in DENA-induced neoplastic nodules[45]) or a defect in collagen accumulation (seen in hepatocarcinoma cell culture[46]), seem to take place.

If cell purity is not an absolute requirement, the use of elaborated matrices can be valuably replaced by cocultures[18,36,47].

A major result that emerged from coculture models is that the loss of differentiated hepatocytic functions is a reversible phenomenon[36].

Proliferative activity of normal hepatocytes in cultures

Whereas prolonged survival of functional hepatocytes from normal adult animals has been obtained in several laboratories, cultures of such 'adult' hepatocytes that would exhibit proliferative activity and eventually become established seem more difficult to produce[35]. On conceptual grounds, one might, in fact, question attempts to obtain hepatocyte cell lines which could be propagated while still retaining normal traits. We do consider that, under normal conditions, hepatocytes do not proliferate in situ, except during post-traumatic liver regeneration. Central to this issue is the demonstration that the liver cells with which we begin are actually mature hepatocytes, and that the cells in culture express more than a few 'hepatocyte-like' functions. The autoradiographic labelling index (LI), after [³H]thymidine incorporation, is not a bona fide criterion for true proliferative activity, as illustrated by reports showing hepatocyte cultures with high frequencies of S-phase cells (i.e. high LI), without any change in cell numbers or detectable mitoses.

With these considerations in mind, we can compare them with reports in the literature that claim to have obtained proliferation of 'adult' hepatocytes in vitro, using various (and sometimes contradictory) hormonal climates and serum conditions. However, only two seem to fulfil the above requirements, indicating that, before ceasing to grow, the cultures had undergone 2–3 doublings[48,49]. In one work, mitoses (some of which were labelled by [³H]thymidine) were seen[50]. On the other hand, it has repeatedly been shown that, provided they were isolated at a time that corresponds to a high-frequency of S-phase cells, hepatocytes from regenerating adult liver do enter into S-phase in vitro, and incorporate [³H]thymidine[51].

However, whereas we could confirm these observations, we did not detect any evidence of subsequent division of the cells thus labelled (Galand and Bernaert, unpublished).

In summary, although it seems that hepatocytes from normal adult animals can undergo partial or a limited number of cell cycles under appropriate conditions in vitro, thus possibly fulfilling some operational purposes, obtaining truly normal propagative lines of such cells remains an unachieved (and perhaps utopian) goal.

Possible applications offered by cultured hepatocytes

Endowed with numerous pathways for procarcinogen metabolism, cultured hepatocytes seem to represent a useful tool for screening drugs for their potential carcinogenic properties. This is, however, limited to short-term cultures, since several drug-metabolizing properties of liver cells drastically decrease within 24 h in primary cultures[52]. On the other hand, established lines of liver epithelial cells are not fully representative of mature hepatocytes since they do not possess the same level of microsomal metabolizing functions[53]. Moreover they often undergo spontaneous transformation after a series of subcultures[54].

Cultures of parenchymal cells on floating collagen retained their drug-metabolizing enzymes and the inducibility of different types of cytochromes and mono-oxygenase activities for more than 10 days[53]. Therefore, these cultures are suitable for investigating the enzymatic activation of procarcinogens and the repair of the resulting structural alteration of DNA[54].

Hepatocyte cultures are also successfully used to assess their metabolic effects on new anticancer drugs[55]. In the same way, the transforming ability of viral or cellular DNA can be studied by transfection in that system[56].

Isolated hepatocytes may also be useful for hybridome production, as shown by experiments in which hybrids of isolated normal rat hepatocytes and AFP-producing mouse hepatoma cells were used to investigate gene regulation mechanisms and rat gene mapping[57].

HEPATOCYTES FROM PRENEOPLASTIC AND NEOPLASTIC LIVER

The rats are treated according to the Scherer–Emmelot model[58]. This consists of administering DENA intragastrically to young adult female Sprague–Dawley rats, up to a final dose of 70 mg kg⁻¹ body weight, given in 10 daily doses, starting 24 h after partial hepatectomy.

Liver parenchymal cells are isolated afterwards by collagenase perfusion, as described above[14].

During a period of about 8 months after carcinogenic treatment, all parenchymal cells dissociate under these conditions. By contrast, neoplastic nodules are not readily dissociated by the enzymatic perfusion, so that entire nodules, 1.5–5 mm in diameter, separated from the surrounding cell suspension, can be collected by filtration on Perlon with 200 μm pore size.

Isolation of hepatocytes from liver with foci

Whole parenchymal population

Foci in situ are composed of hepatocytes with an increased cytoplasmic volume, containing tremendous amounts of glycogen, lipid vacuoles or/and proliferated smooth endoplasmic reticulum (SER). Less frequently, stacks of scattered rough endoplasmic reticulum (RER) are observed. Mitoses are seen. The cells show enlarged nuclei with a hypertrophied nucleolus[1,5,59]. The nucleus sometimes has an indented shape (Figure 2b); this becomes more frequent in later stages of carcinogenesis.

In early foci, in this model, all hepatocytes appear to be positive for GGT activity. Most of them have deficient bile canalicular ATPase and G6Pase activities, contrasting with the homogeneous activity of the surrounding normal parenchyma[60].

At the early stages (1–6 months), glycogen is retained in the lesions after fasting of the animal, revealing a dysfunction in glycogen phosphorylase[1] and also reflecting the observed deficiency in G6Pase.

The frequency and degree of some phenotypic alterations increase, while others decrease with the growth of the foci and in neoplastic nodules.

At later stages of hepatocarcinogenesis, the glycogen level in the lesions is significantly reduced. A gradual recovery in G6Pase activity is then observed[1,10].

Neoplastic nodules and hepatocarcinomas often display GGT-positive cells distributed at their periphery, whereas the majority of other altered hepatocytes do not show any GGT activity.

During the nodular stage of the carcinogenic process, an increasing number of phenotypically altered hepatocytes show a positive reaction for G6Pase. This is observed in persistent foci and, to various degrees, in the neoplastic nodules, which display significant heterogeneity in the levels of this enzyme (Figure 5a).

The glycogen-rich foci, deficient in G6Pase and glycogen phosphorylase activity, also exhibit a progressive increase in G6P-dehydrogenase activity, suggesting a predominance of the pentose–phosphate pathway[5]. In neoplastic nodules, hepatocytes maintain high levels of G6P dehydrogenase and also show increased activity of the glycolytic enzyme, glyceraldehyde-3-phosphate dehydrogenase, indicating that transformed cells may develop alternative pathways of carbohydrate metabolism[5].

A broad alteration in membrane component(s), involved in enzyme insertion could be the origin of the various altered phenotypes associated with membrane-bound enzymes, as suggested by Glueckson-Waelsch and Cori[61] to explain the pleiotropic effects of radiation-induced lethal mutations in mice; G6Pase, for example, is indeed highly labile in the free state[62].

On the other hand, the importance of membrane fluidity in the regulation of cellular functions, including several membrane-integrated enzymes and receptors[63], is well documented. A decrease in membrane fluidity after liver injury[64] and an increase in microsomal membrane fluidity at birth have been reported[65]. The latter was suggested as partially responsible for the changes in enzymatic activities observed during the perinatal period[65]. UDP-glucuronyltransferase and G6Pase activities, both of which play a role in these changes, were shown to be influenced by such alterations in membrane properties[66]. Similar mechanisms might be involved in the G6Pase deficiencies seen in altered hepatocytes.

However, defective transcriptional activity of the encoding gene in carcinogen-treated altered hepatocytes might also be the cause of the enzyme deficiency observed in carcinogenesis.

Among the isolated hepatocytes from DENA-treated liver, G6Pase-deficient cells, having a large average size, can be recognized (Figure 2a) and probably correspond to the altered cells from foci. Their activity contrasts markedly with that of isolated normal cells (Figure 1a).

When placed in culture, parenchymal cells isolated 10 months after DENA treatment, representing a mixture of normal and altered hepatocytes deriving from persistent foci, reform trabeculae, integrating hepatocytes with altered ultrastructural phenotypes and deficient in G6Pase, as well as ultrastructurally and cytochemically normal parenchymal cells (Figure 3a). The altered phenotypes, as seen in the cultured cells, include the proliferation of the SER (a frequent and persistent phenotype during hepatocarcinogenesis) and disorganized RER with either unfolded areas or whorled structures (Figure 3b).

Enrichment in hepatocytes from DENA-induced foci

Centrifugal elutriation, performed as previously reported, to fractionate normal adult hepatocytes[67], was applied to isolated hepatocytes from DENA-treated livers 2 or 6 months after carcinogen treatment.

The population of hepatocytes obtained after enzymatic perfusion in these two instances exhibited much heterogeneity in size compared with hepatocytes from normal livers (Figures 1b and 2c).

From this starting material, five distinct subpopulations were separated by counterflow centrifugation. These were subjected to morphometric measurements using a Coulter Channelyzer and a Zeiss TGZ3 particle size analyzer.

Large hepatocytes concentrated in the elutriated fractions IV and V, in proportions that varied with the time since application of the carcinogenic treatment. This included a significant shift towards lower size classes, with a doubling in the relative proportion of cells in fraction I, 6 months after DENA treatment (Table 1).

Cytophotometric quantitation of DNA content was performed in the total populations from normal liver and from DENA-treated parenchymal cells, 2, 6 or 15 months after treatment (Table 2).

Ploidy distribution examined in each elutriated fraction showed that the diploid cells were concentrated in fraction I, while the majority of octoploid and polyploid cells are found in fractions IV and V.

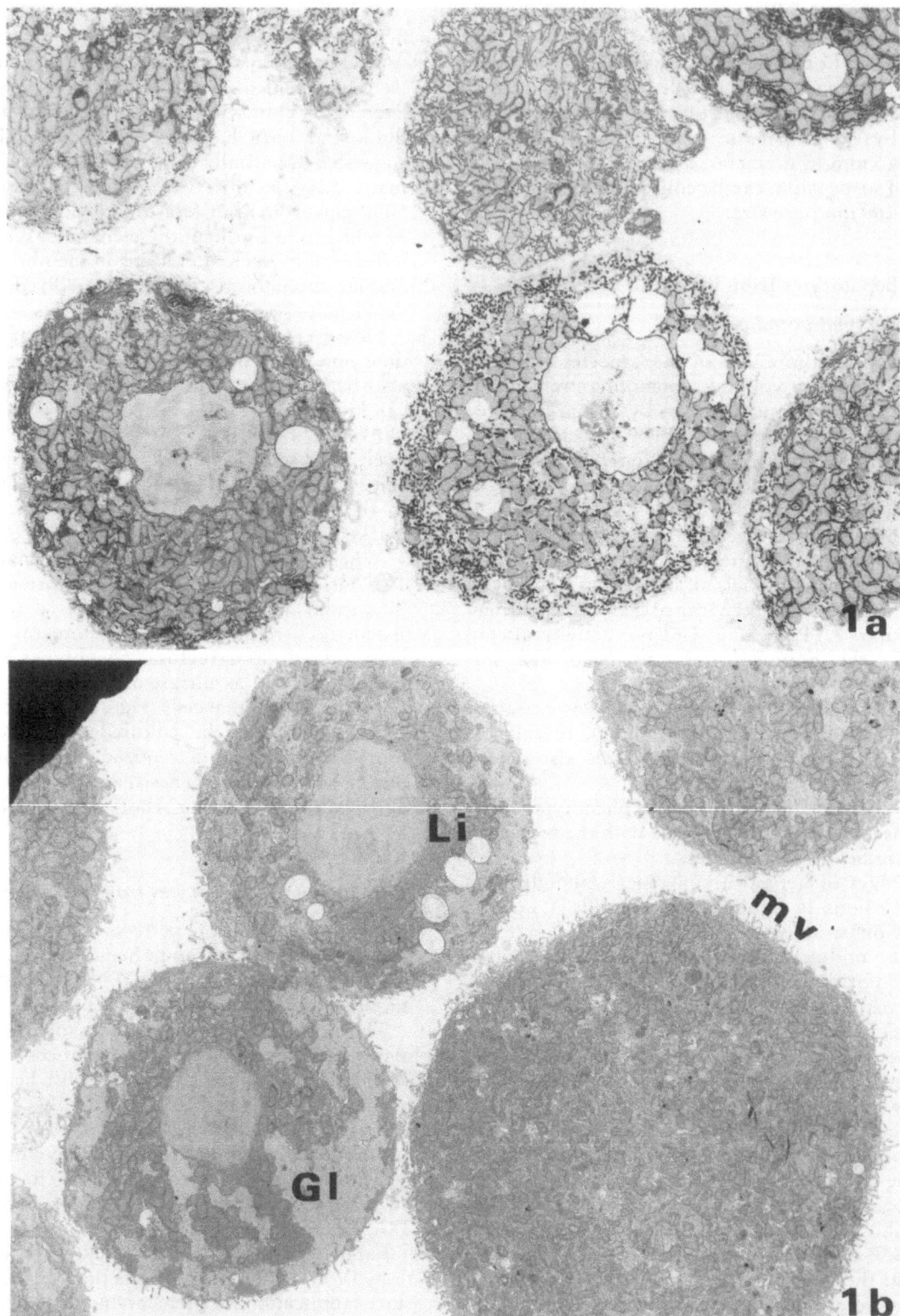

Figure 1a   Electron micrograph of isolated normal adult rat hepatocytes. Frozen sections of sedimented cells, entrapped in fibrin, were treated for cytochemical demonstration of G6Pase activity. Note, in all the cells, homogeneous lead phosphate deposits on smooth and rough ER and in the nuclear envelope. × 3100

Figure 1b   Isolated hepatocytes from a DENA-treated rat (2 months post-induction) illustrating heterogeneity in cell size and other phenotypes, such as abnormally high storage of glycogen (Gl). Numerous microvilli (mv) cover the entire cell surface Li: lipid droplets. × 2900

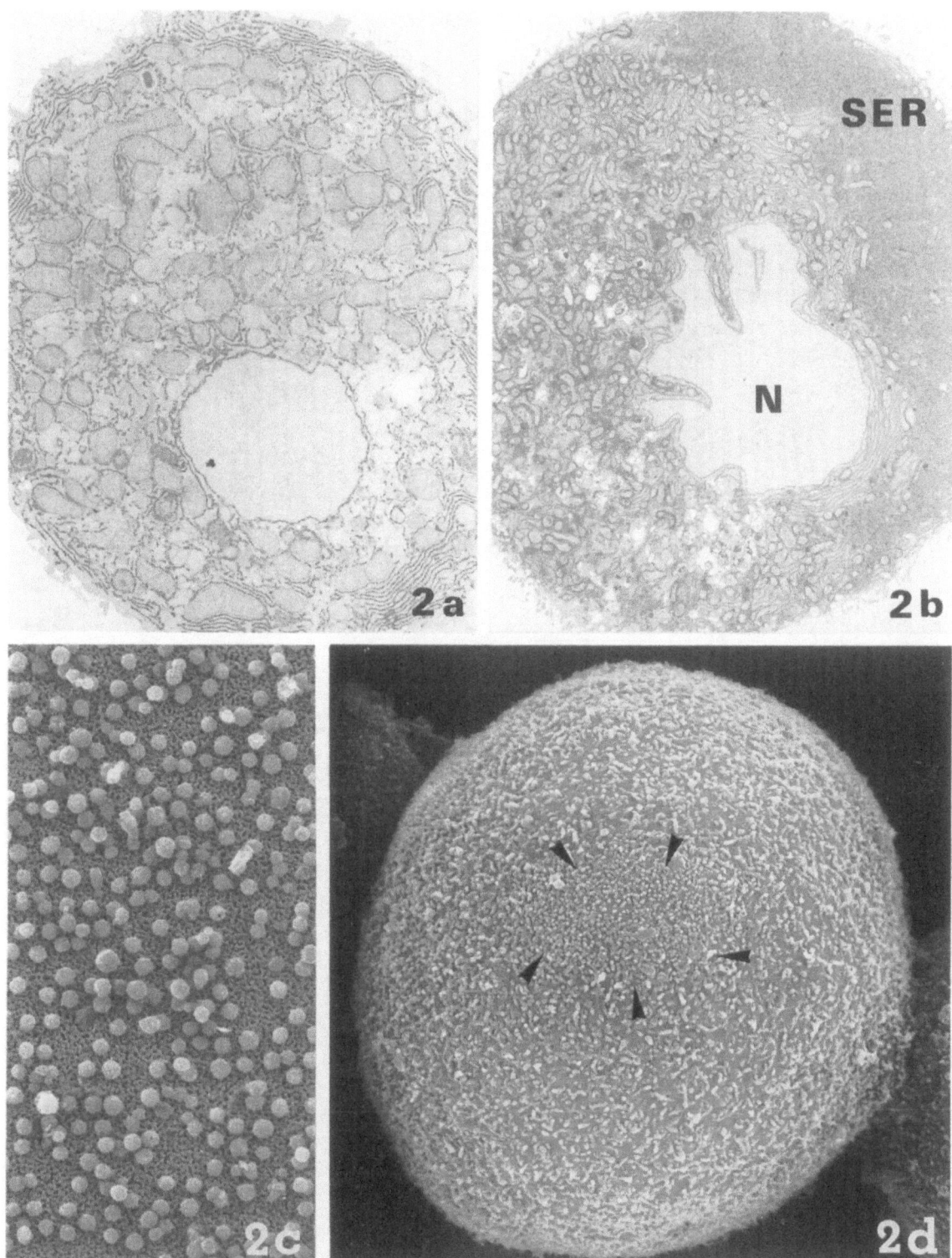

Figure 2a Isolated hepatocyte from a DENA-treated rat (6 months after treatment) exhibiting weak and heterogeneous G6Pase reaction in the cisternae of the reticulum and in the nuclear membrane. This corresponds to the G6Pase deficiency found in situ in the DENA-induced foci of altered phenotypes. × 6500

Figure 2b Isolated liver cell from a DENA-treated rat (2 months after treatment). This hepatocyte is from an elutriated fraction of cells enriched with large cells exhibiting typical phenotypic alterations encountered in the foci in situ; note the markedly hypertrophied SER and the indented nucleus (N). × 5000

Figure 2c Scanning electron micrograph showing heterogeneity in cell size of isolated hepatocytes from a 6 months DENA-treated rat. × 200

Figure 2d Enlarged cell from the same population as in Figure 2c showing an area of densely packed short microvilli (arrowheads). Such an altered pattern was never observed in normal liver cells. × 3800

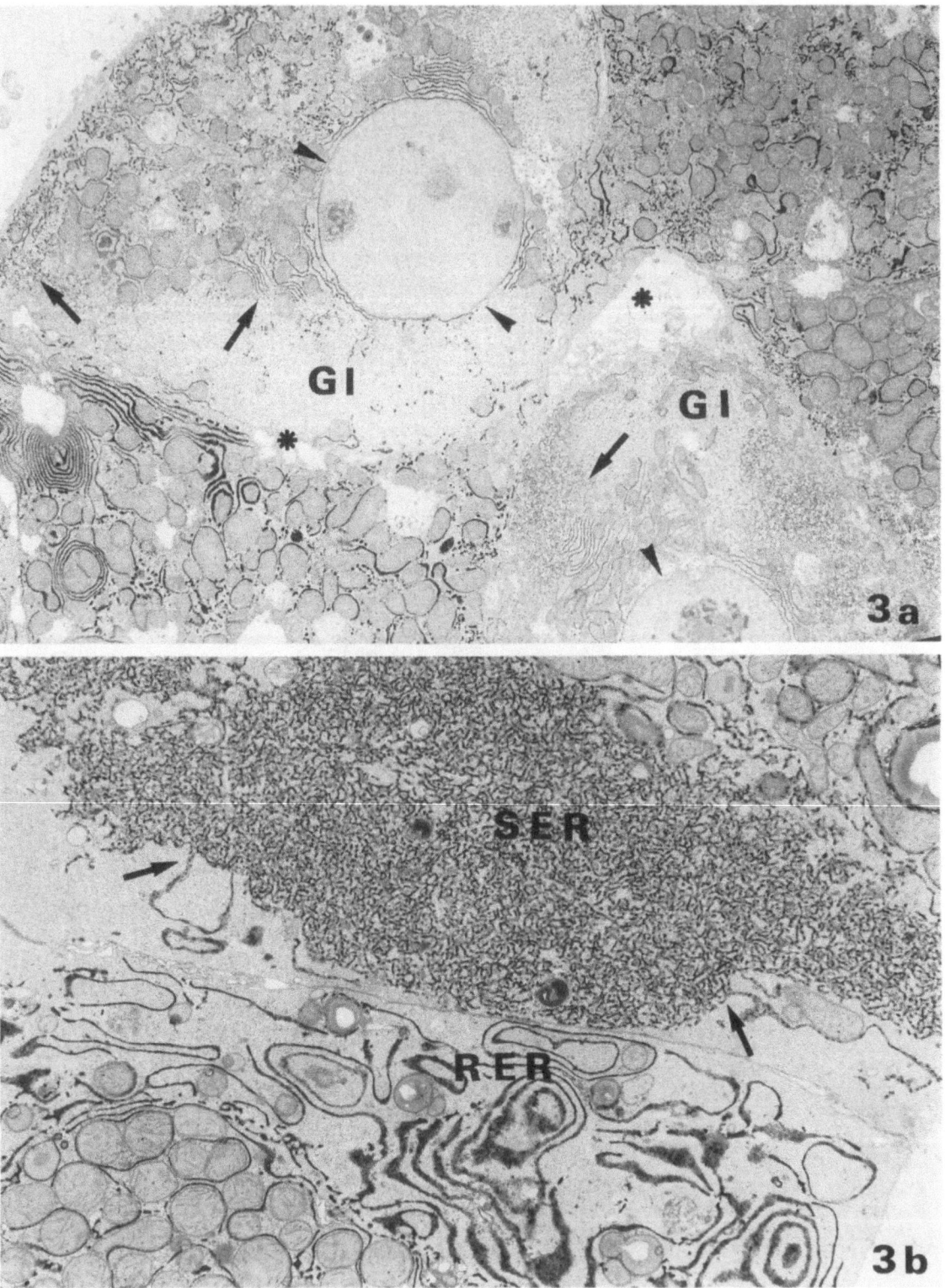

Figure 3a Newly reformed laminae in a 24 h culture of hepatocytes from a 10 months DENA-treated rat, staining for G6Pase activity. Note loose cell contacts (asterisks) between reassociated normal and altered cells. Two hepatocytes with a high glycogen content (GI) display weak and heterogeneous G6Pase activity (as in Figure 2a) while the neighbouring cells are homogeneously stained (arrows: ER with a dotted pattern; arrow-heads: discontinuous lead phosphate deposits in nuclear envelope). × 3600

Figure 3b Typically altered hepatocytes from late stages of DENA treatment (10 months). One cell exhibits a proliferated SER, with a highly positive G6Pase reaction. Rough endoplasmic cisternae show local contacts with the SER tubules (arrows). The adjacent cell displays a disorganized RER with unfolded or concentrically arranged cisternae. × 8600

Table 1 Cell size of hepatocytic elutriated fractions

Cell subfraction	Control		DENA 2 months		DENA 6 months	
	$\bar{D}(\mu m)$	%IC	$\bar{D}(\mu m)$	%IC	$\bar{D}(\mu m)$	%IC
OP	20.9 ± 0.2		22.1 ± 0.1		21.0 ± 0.1	
I	17.5 ± 0.3	11.6	17.5 ± 0.2	7.2	18.2 ± 0.2	16.9
II	19.9 ± 0·2	35.6	19.3 ± 0.1	18.7	19.1 ± 0.2	24.3
III	20.8 ± 0·2	48.6	20.6 ± 0.1	41.7	20.7 ± 0.2	33.7
IV	23.1 ± 0·3 (24.6)	4.2	23.2 ± 0.2 (24.2)	22.4	23.0 ± 0.3	18.1
V	—	—	24.8 ± 0.1 (27.6)	10.0	25.1 ± 0.1	7.0

OP: original population of hepatocytes; IC: isolated cells; $\bar{D}$: mean diameter
The percentage of hepatocytes recovered in each fraction only represents the isolated cells, contaminating doublets deduced. Values in parentheses correspond to the corrected ones obtained with the Zeiss analyser TGZ3, the Coulter counter being unable to discriminate between large isolated cells and doublets of small cells. Values are means ± SE of 8 experiments for control, 6 experiments for DENA 2 months and 4 experiments for DENA 6 months

Table 2 Histophotometric determinations of DNA content in isolated cells (IC) or nuclei (IN) from whole liver or from nodules

Fractions		2N	4N	6N	8N	>8N
Control IC		32	62	2	4	—
DENA-treated						
Treatment duration (months)						
2	IC	18.2	53.0	7·6	16.7	4.5
6	IC	37.9	44.8	—	13.8	3.4
15 Nodules	IN	44.0	45.0	—	3.0	—
15 Adjacent parenchyma	IC	16.0	71.0	—	13.0	—
	IN	13.0	77.0	—	10.0	—

Values, expressed in % of ploidy classes are means of 8 control experiments, 6 experiments for DENA 2 months, 4 experiments for DENA 6 months and 3 experiments for DENA 15 months

There was a marked increase in octoploid cells, from 4% in control to 16.7% after 2 months of treatment; this was maintained at 6 months, but the liver, in this case, also showed a higher proportion of diploid cells.

Similar observations were previously reported in the case of N-nitrosomorpholine (NNM)-treated hepatocytes[68].

At a later stage in hepatocarcinogenesis (15 months), isolated cells from liver parenchyma adjacent to nodules showed proportions of diploid and octoploid cells similar to those found 2 months after DENA treatment. In the nodule, a higher proportion of diploid nuclei and a very low level of octoploid nuclei were found, very similar to the situation seen in controls. This is in accordance with in situ observations by Emmelot and Scherer, who described large nuclei in hepatocytes of early foci and a progressive reduction in the nuclear size towards a diploid-type diameter with the growth of the foci in the neoplastic nodules and in the hepatocarcinomas[1].

In the starting population of isolated hepatocytes, the large cells exhibit the same altered ultrastructural phenotypes seen in the focal areas in situ (Figures 1b and 2a). Elutriation fractions IV and V contained a high proportion of cells with glycogen accumulation, not seen in similar fractions from normal livers. Some cells in these fractions showed a pronounced proliferation of SER, associated or not with other altered phenotypes, such as an indented nucleus (Figure 2b), not infrequently

encountered in early foci but never observed in normal parenchymal cells. This suggests that we have indeed obtained fractions enriched with cells from the DENA-induced foci.

Under the scanning electron microscope (SEM), all isolated cells from normal liver display homogeneously distributed microvilli covering the entire cell surface. By contrast, hypertrophied hepatocytes isolated from DENA-treated rats exhibit a heterogeneous pattern of microvilli, with areas of the cell surface showing short closely packed microvilli (Figure 2d). The same disturbed arrangement of cell surface microvilli was observed on large hepatocytes induced after either DENA or NNM treatment[68-70].

Using the Solt–Farber model of hepatocarcinogenesis, Evarts et al.[71] showed that early lesions were deficient in asialoglycoprotein (AGP) receptors and G6Pase activity, which only partially coincided with the GGT-positive areas. Centrifugal elutriation allowed them to separate the parenchymal cells into a small- and a large-cell fraction. The latter contained a majority of AGP-receptor-deficient cells, GGT positive or GGT negative, which did not attach to asialofetuin.

Several techniques for fractionating liver cell suspensions into metabolically distinct classes of hepatocytes are now available[72] (review in reference 73).

A three-step procedure was proposed consisting of anterograde or retrograde enzymatic perfusion of the

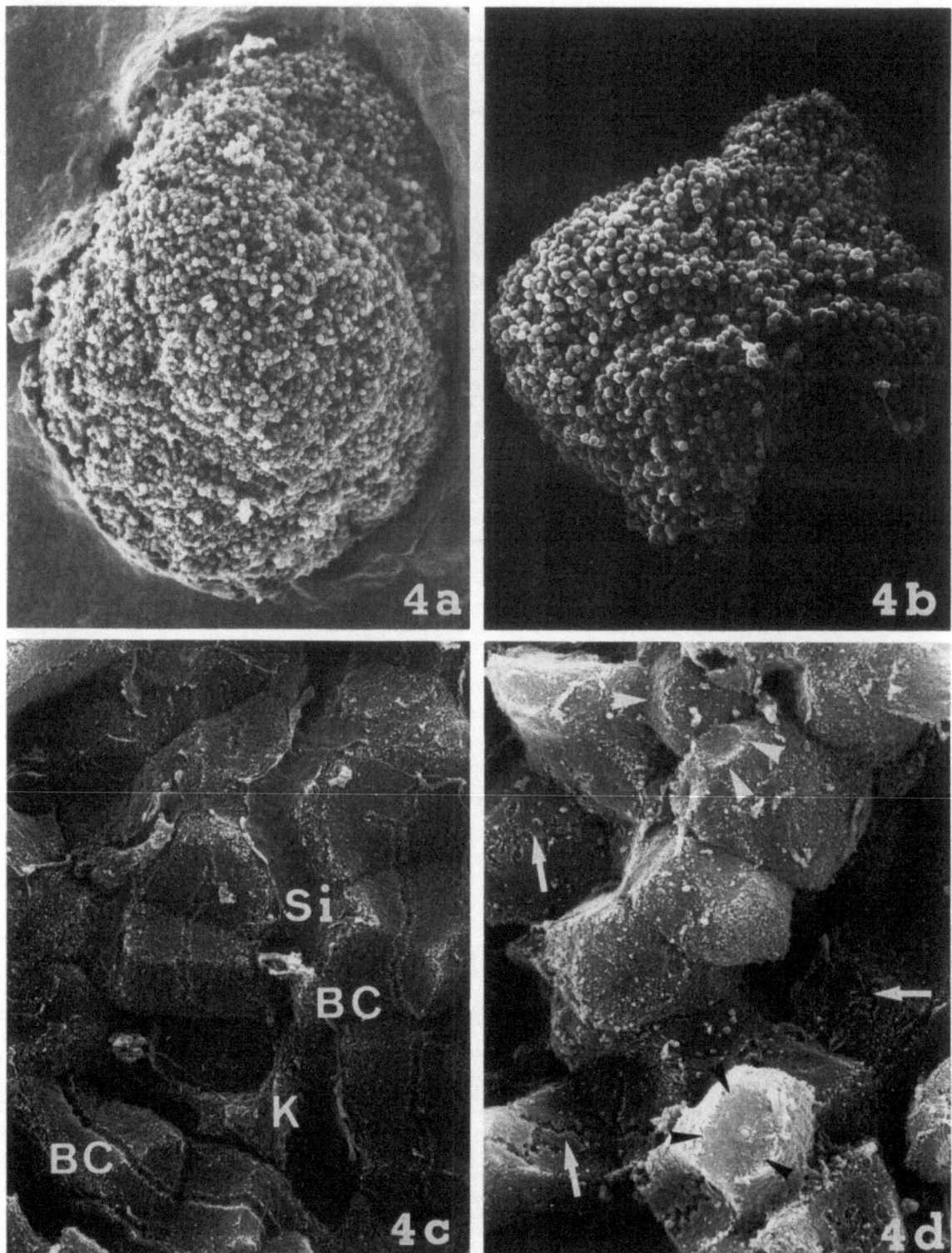

Figure 4   Scanning electron micrographs from normal liver and from DENA-treated liver at the stage of neoplastic nodules.
Figure 4a   Cryofracture of a nodule in situ (DENA treatment: 11 months) emerging from the surrounding parenchyma. × 80
Figure 4b   One of the neoplastic nodules, isolated after collagenase dissociation of the liver parenchyma. × 120
Figure 4c   Cryofracture from a control liver, showing regular polyhedral hepatocytes limited by sinusoids (Si). The bile canaliculi (BC) run linearly and are uniformly bordered by microvilli. K: Kupffer cell. × 1600
Figure 4d   Cryofracture inside an isolated neoplastic nodule revealing irregularly shaped hepatocytes with reduced smooth inter-hepatocytic faces (arrowheads). Bile canaliculi are distorted and are bordered by scarce and short microvilli (arrows). × 1600

liver, centrifugation in Percoll density gradients and finally centrifugal elutriation of the resulting hepatocytes into five fractions[74]. Determination of cytochrome P-450 levels after phenobarbital induction (known to act predominantly on distal zone[75]) and selective prelabelling with acridine-orange were used as criteria for acinar origin of the fractions.

Oval cells have also been isolated from carcinogen-treated livers by elutriation[11,76].

Based on their biochemical properties, which are intermediate between those of biliary and parenchymal cells[11,76], and on their patterns of specific antigens[77], it was proposed that oval cells represent a stem cell population which can differentiate into transitional hepatic cells and further evolve into mature biliary or hepatocytic cells.

Neoplastic nodules

Isolation and culture

Neoplastic nodules constitute the predominant lesions in the liver at about 9 months after DENA treatment. These are large (1.5–5 mm in diameter), well-delineated but not encapsulated lesions, and they induce important distortions of the parenchyma, compressing the surrounding normal hepatic laminae[59]. Within the nodule, thickened trabeculae formed by joint cell laminae, exhibit a disorganized pattern and are separated by dilated sinusoids. Several nodules are protruding at the surface of the liver. This is illustrated in Figure 4a, showing, under SEM, a cryofracture of a peripheral nodule surrounded by the smooth capsule of Glisson. As for the nodules in situ, cryofractures performed through an isolated nodule reveal cell trabeculae, lined by endothelial cells and consisting of hepatocytes more rounded in shape than in the normal counterparts; this corresponds to decreased cell contacts (Figure 4d). Reduced interhepatocytic faces and branched sinuous bile canaliculi, bordered by few and short microvilli[70], contrast with the situation in normal liver (Figure 4c). Bile canaliculi, some of which are distended, frequently exhibit very weak ATPase activity. The sinusoidal endothelia within the neoplastic nodules in this experimental system, appear fenestrated and devoid of an underlying basement membrane. Kupffer cells can be detected in the lumen of the sinusoids (Figure 5a).

Nodule hepatocytes display most of the ultrastructural phenotypes characterizing the foci, as well as additional alterations. They are heterogeneous in size and in the relative proportions of their different phenotypes. The smallest cells in these lesions are basophilic. Most of the larger cells are characterized by extensive development of the SER; they often present an unfolded RER and accumulated lipid droplets; a few of these cells retain a large amount of glycogen. One or more hypertrophied nucleoli are frequently observed. Most of the nodular hepatocytes are deficient in bile canalicular ATPase, whereas G6Pase activity is partially normal (Figure 5a).

Small fragments of isolated nodules plated in collagen-coated Falcon dishes in Dulbecco's medium, supplemented with fetal bovine serum and insulin, attached to the bottom after a delay of 48 h. Cells then migrated out of the tissue pieces which, after 3 days, were surrounded by flattened cells. These may show undulating

membranes or, at the front of migration, develop elongated cytoplasmic extensions. A few hepatocytes lose all contact with the tissue fragment (Figure 6a).

With time, the area of flattened cells increases in size and the cells pile up in multiple layers. Labelling with [³H]thymidine and observation of mitotic cells among peripheral hepatocytes indicate that this is not caused just by migration and spreading of the cells.

Under the same conditions, normal liver fragments never show any signs of proliferative activity. Fibroblasts and endothelial cells can be recognized in the nodular culture, perhaps explaining the prolonged (up to 30 days) survival of what is better considered a co-culture.

Throughout their survival, the cultured nodular hepatocytes reveal ultrastructural phenotypes similar to those observed in situ. The nuclei show great heterogeneity in size and often present prominent nucleoli. Indented nuclei are encountered. Some hepatocytes are multinucleated. The RER which presents unfolded cisternae and sometimes whorl-like structures (Figure 6c), lies closely connected to the SER, as in normal cells. The SER in many cells occupies an increased proportion of the cytoplasm; it is associated with glycogen particles and, more frequently, with lipid droplets (Figure 6d). Differentiated junctions, such as tight junctions or desmosomes are preserved, as are bile canaliculi not possessing microvilli. Cells at the periphery of the outgrowth exhibit large undulating membranes underlined by a cytoskeletal structure of microfilamentous bundles and generally poor in cell organelles, except for endocytic vesicles. Peripheral hepatocytes also develop many folds in the region of the undulating membrane. Parallel-oriented microfilaments, with small organelles lined-up between them, run within the folds (Figure 6b).

Nodule hepatocytes in culture present a particular phenotype: they often send long and narrow cytoplasmic extensions into areas of loose cell contacts. These extensions insert between the adjacent cells (Figure 5b) in a manner similar to that observed in the invasive process (see below).

Cultures of hepatocarcinoma fragments seem to display phenotypic stability and survival for about 1 month, and a behaviour comparable to that of samples from neoplastic nodules.

In vitro *invasion test*

The possibility of isolating and culturing fragments from DENA-induced nodules and tumours allowed us to test whether hepatocytes from these neoplastic lesions had acquired the ability to invade a host tissue. Therefore, we used the experimental model elaborated by Mareel et al.[8].

Fragments of isolated nodules or hepatocarcinoma and associated precultured embryonic chick heart tissue attach to each other within 2–4 h of contact in a semisolid medium. The confronting tissues are then further incubated in Dulbecco's medium which has been supplemented with 5% fetal calf serum and insulin (2 mU/ml) in a gyratory shaker and are examined daily up to 15 days as described[7].

The hepatocytes attach like a cap at one pole of the cardiac tissue (Figure 7a) and completely surround it within 24 h. Then, from day 4 of incubation on, increasing

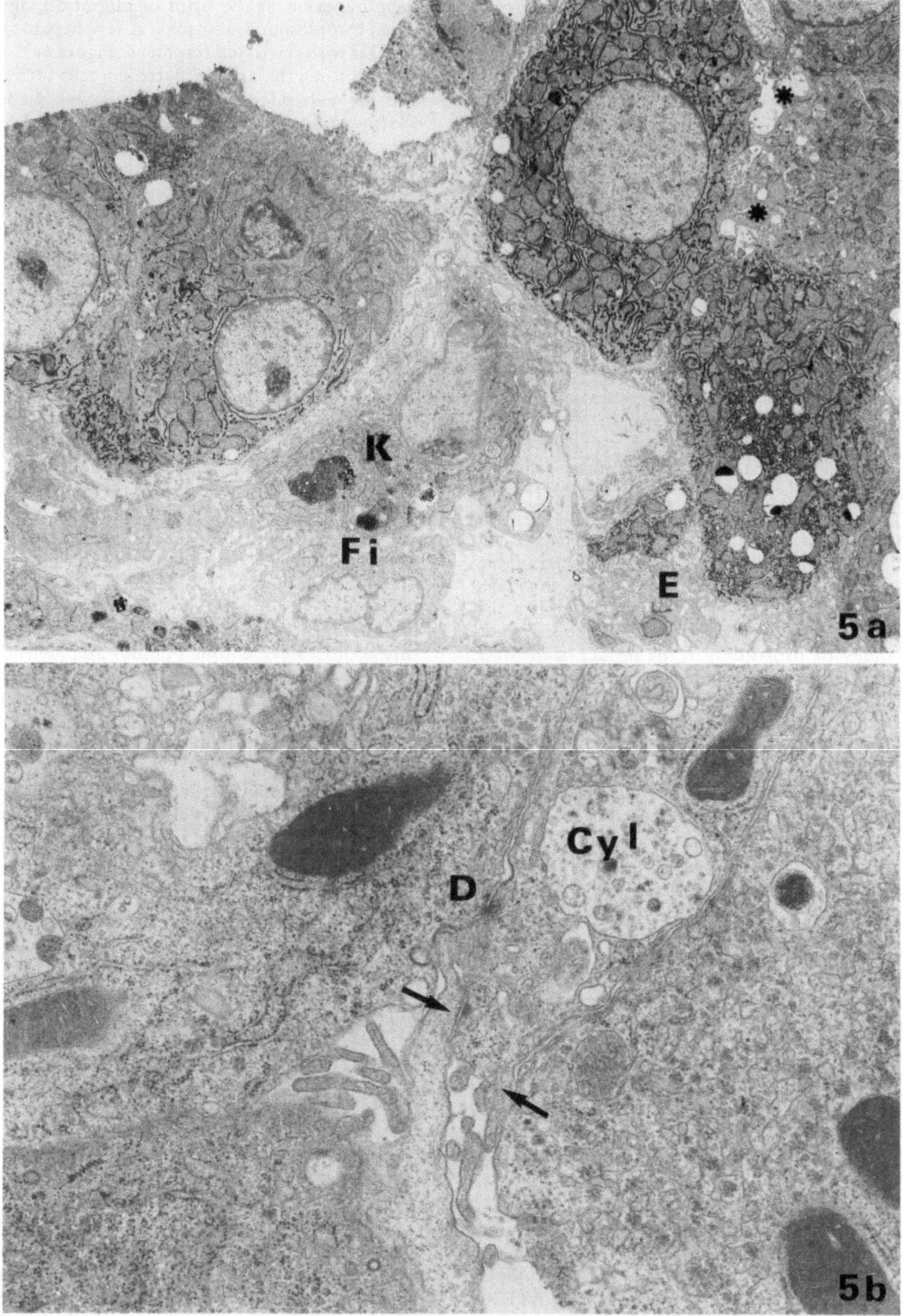

Figure 5a   G6Pase reaction in an isolated nodule showing, as in situ, high inter- and intracellular heterogeneity of enzymatic activity; poorly reactive hepatocytes may present regions of loose cell contacts with the neighbouring parenchymal cells (asterisks). Kupffer cells (K), endothelial cells (E) and fibroblasts (Fi) are also present. × 3800

Figure 5b   Fragment of a neoplastic nodule at 6 days of culture. Some hepatocytes in areas of loose cell contacts present long and narrow cytoplasmic extensions which insinuate between the adjacent cells (arrows). D: desmosome; Cyl: cytolysome. × 25 500

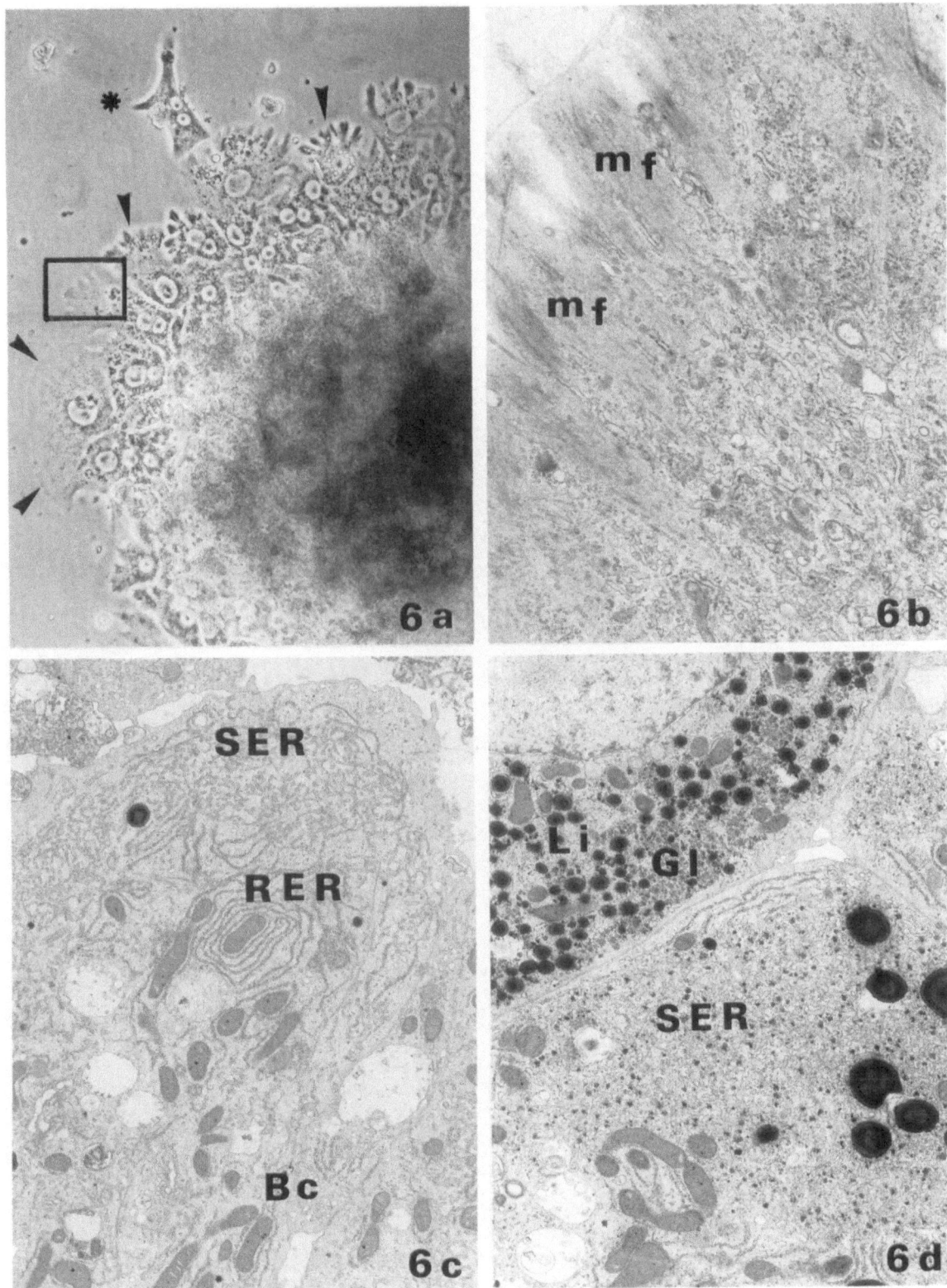

Figure 6   Cultured fragments from neoplastic nodules.
Figure 6a   3 day culture: the peripheral cells of the outgrowth exhibit undulating membranes (arrowheads), suggesting a migratory process; one cell is detached from the tissue fragment (asterisk). × 320
Figure 6b   Enlargement at EM level of an area similar to the rectangle in Figure 6a: the undulating membrane of a flattened hepatocyte forms folds with parallel-oriented microfilaments (mf) and small organelles lined up between them. × 10 800
Figures 6c and d   Ultrastructural phenotypes of nodular hepatocytes established in culture for at least 8 days: a proliferated SER, unfolded or whorled RER, and, in some cases, numerous lipid droplets (Li). Gl: α-glycogen rosettes; Bc: dilated bile canaliculus. Figure 6c: × 8500. Figure 6d: × 8200

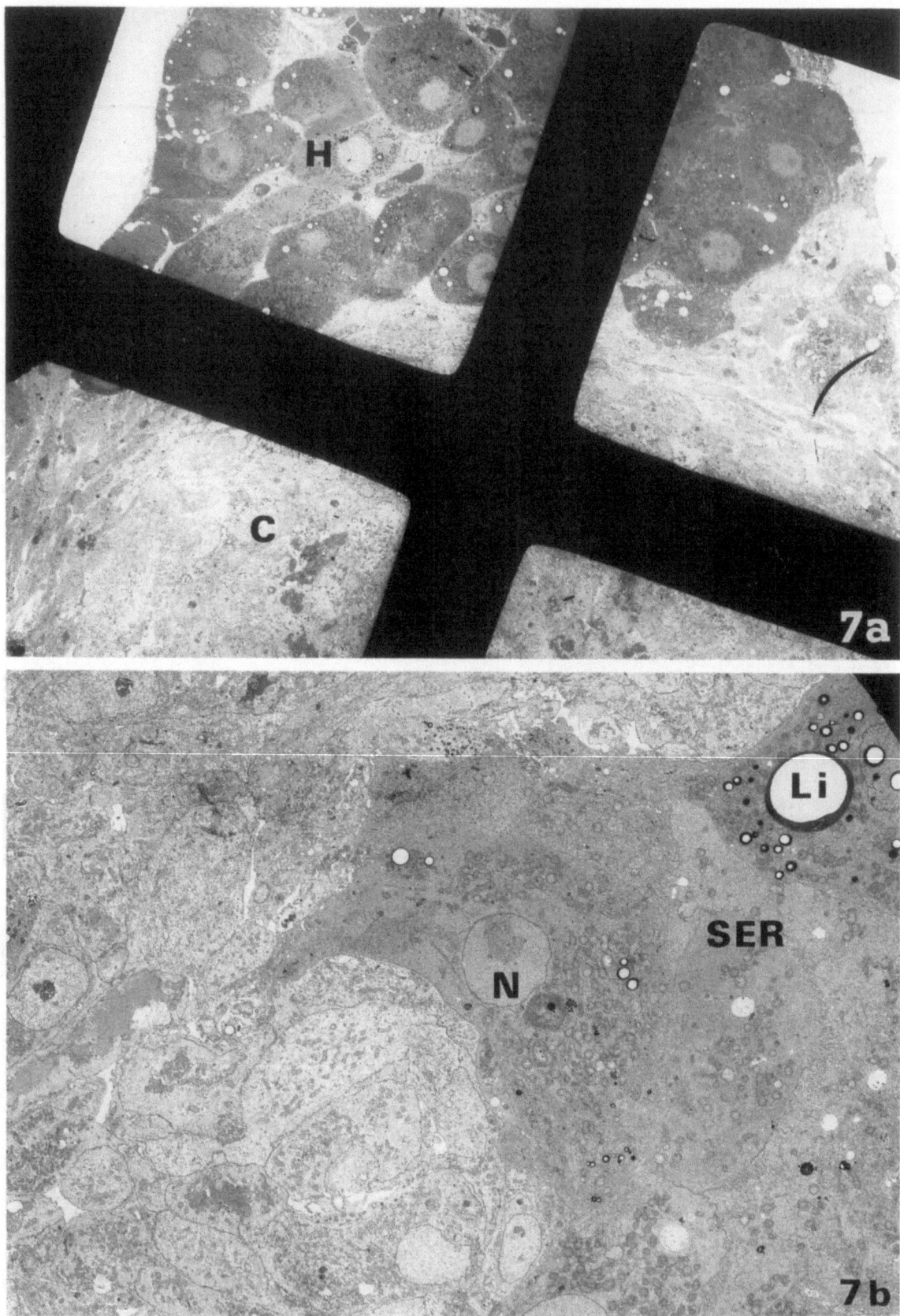

Figure 7a   First step of the *in vitro* invasion test: attachment between chick embryonic heart tissue (C) and the tested tissue sample (here a hepatocarcinoma fragment, H), after 2 h of confrontation. × 1100

Figure 7b   A 10-day coculture showing a group of hepatocarcinoma cells having invaded the cardiac tissue. The ultrastructural phenotypes are similar to those seen in nodule cells: large nuclei and nucleoli (N), development of SER and high content of lipid droplets (Li). × 2000

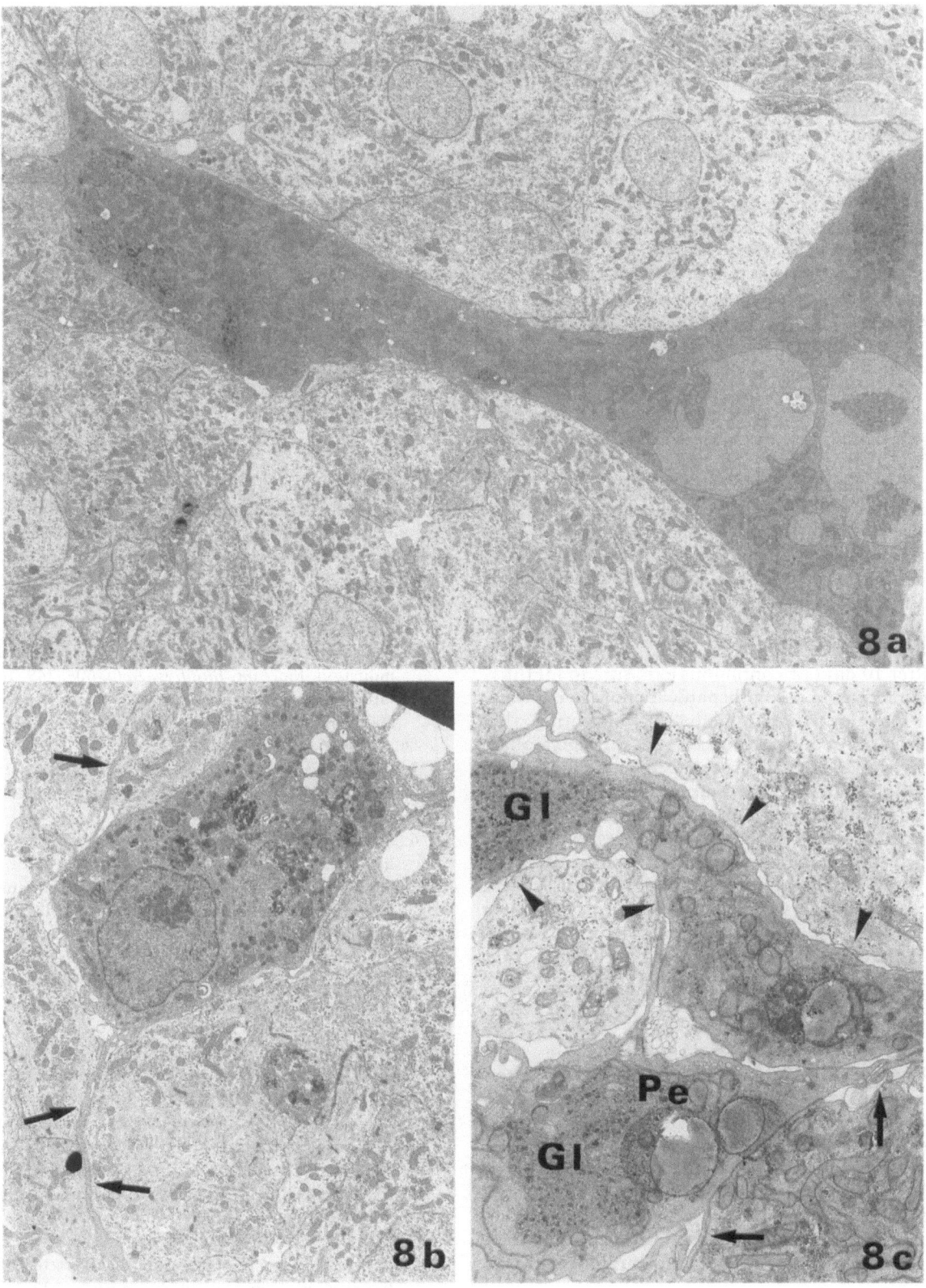

Figure 8a A 14-day confronting culture of a neoplastic nodule fragment; hepatocytes, like this one, present long cytoplasmic extensions and are found inside the chick heart tissue. × 2700

Figure 8b Same observation as in Figure 8a, but here in a hepatocarcinoma cell that has invaded the cardiac tissue and exhibits long cytoplasmic extensions (arrows) infiltrating between the myocytes which otherwise present firm contacts. × 3300

Figure 8c A 6-day coculture, illustrating the high deformability of invasive nodular hepatocytes. The figure also shows zones of small contacts between the two cellular types (arrowheads) and microvilli insinuating between folds of neighbouring cells (arrows). The well-preserved hepatocytes can be clearly recognized by their characteristic α-glycogen particles (GI) and peroxisomes (Pe). × 10 900

numbers of hepatocytes are found within the heart tissue sample. This is observed in 10 out of 12 samples from hepatocarcinoma (the 2 negative being necrotic at the start), and only in 13 of 36 fragments from neoplastic nodules. In positive samples from hepatocarcinoma and nodules, mitotic activity is detected in the hepatocyte populations, and ultrastructural observations reveal the presence among the cultured hepatocytes of a high degree of polymorphism. Some cells (Figure 8) are elongated and develop important cytoplasmic extensions that infiltrate between the myocytes (Figure 8b and c). All this is strongly suggestive of locomotive behaviour and active invasion, with the extensions detaching the myocytes from each other. During the invasion process, the neoplastic cells maintain well-differentiated hepatocytic structures, such as peroxisomes and α-glycogen particles (Figure 8c).

From day 10 of incubation, we observed a progressive replacement of the host tissue by hepatocarcinoma cells (Figure 7b). This was not observed with nodules. After 14 days of confrontation, the cytoplasm of the myocytes occasionally showed signs of lysis in regions of contact between the two cell types. Invading hepatocytes exhibited ultrastructural phenotypes corresponding with those found in situ or in culture: unfolded RER cisternae, accumulation of lipid droplets, hypertrophied nuclei, etc. No particular ultrastructural phenotype seems to be linked with invasiveness[78].

Even after 10 days of continuous exposure to [3H]thymidine, numerous invading hepatocarcinoma cells were found to have remained unlabelled, indicating that invasion does not require that a cell goes through S phase and cell division. This is in accordance with experiments demonstrating that, for MO4 mouse fibrosarcoma, cell invasion and proliferation can be dissociated[79].

The fact that some nodular hepatocytes express the same invasiveness shown by hepatocarcinoma cells in the in vitro assay lends support to the hypothesis that a lineage relationship between neoplastic nodules and liver tumours exists. This finding also indicates that cells in the nodules have taken at least one step in the multistage carcinogenic process.

CONCLUSION

The close analogies between the morphofunctional alterations and the stages observed in human liver carcinogenesis[5,80] and in experimental hepatocarcinogenic systems support the relevance of the latter as a model.

The demonstration that hepatocytes from neoplastic nodules express the malignant property of invasiveness warrants further investigation into the possible presence of other malignant properties, not only in those lesions, but also during earlier stages in the carcinogenic progression.

Cell isolation and elutriation seem to offer a way of obtaining tissue subpopulations enriched with cells originating from the foci of altered phenotypes, thus opening perspectives for such studies. These subpopulations might be transplanted into isogeneic rats in order to check for their possible evolution towards hepatocarcinoma, as has been done for cells of nodular origin[81,82].

As we have shown here, primary cultures of selected subpopulations constitute a useful system for parallel analyses of ultrastructural and biochemical alterations as well as malignant characteristics.

Such an integrative approach could be adapted to studies of other pathological situations, not only in experimental models, but also in clinical settings.

As shown here for hepatocarcinogenesis, ultrastructural investigations of isolated and purified populations of altered cells, combined with cytochemical and biochemical analyses, appear to be essential to the proper definition of the cell type involved, as well as for trying to find morphological correlates of the functional alterations thus observed.

Acknowledgements

We gratefully acknowledge the excellent technical assistance of J. Lemaire and J. Rummens and are indebted to Mrs Y. Bauwens for having typed this manuscript.

References

1. Emmelot, P. and Scherer, E. (1980). The first relevant cell stage in rat liver carcinogenesis. A quantitative approach. Biochim. Biophys. Acta, 605, 247–304
2. Squire, R. A. and Levitt, M. H. (1975). Report of a workshop on classification of specific hepatocellular lesions in rats. Cancer Res., 35, 3214–23
3. Farber, E. (1980). The sequential analysis of liver cancer induction. Biochim. Biophys. Acta, 605, 149–166
4. Pitot, H. C. and Sirica, A. E. (1980). The stages of initiation and promotion in hepatocarcinogenesis. Biochim. Biophys. Acta, 605, 191–215
5. Bannasch, P., Mayer, D. and Hacker, H. J. (1980). Hepatocellular glycogenosis and hepatocarcinogenesis. Biochim. Biophys. Acta, 605, 217–45
6. Scherer, E. (1984). Neoplastic progression in experimental hepatocarcinogenesis. Biochim. Biophys. Acta, 738, 219–36
7. Wanson, J.-C., de Ridder, L. and Mosselmans, R. (1981). Invasiveness of hyperplastic nodule cells from diethylnitrosamine-treated rat liver. Cancer Res., 41, 5162–75
8. Mareel, M., Kint, J. and Meyvisch, C. (1979). Methods of study of the invasion of malignant C3H-mouse fibroblasts into embryonic chick heart in vitro. Virchows Arch. (Cell Pathol.), 30, 95–111
9. Sell, S. and Leffert, H. L. (1982). An evaluation of cellular lineages in the pathogenesis of experimental hepatocellular carcinoma. Hepatology, 2, 77–86
10. Bannasch, P. (1976). Cytology and cytogenesis of neoplastic (hyperplastic) hepatic nodules. Cancer Res., 36, 2555–62
11. Yaswen, P., Hayner, N. T. and Fausto, N. (1984). Isolation of oval cells by centrifugal elutriation and comparison with other cell types purified from normal and preneoplastic livers. Cancer Res., 44, 324–31
12. Becker, F. F. and Sell, S. (1979). Differences in serum α-fetoprotein concentrations during the carcinogenic sequences resulting from exposure to diethylnitrosamine or acetylaminofluorene. Cancer Res., 39, 1437–42
13. Berry, M. N. and Friend, D. S. (1969). High-yield preparation of isolated rat liver parenchymal cells. J. Cell Biol., 43, 506–20
14. Drochmans, P., Wanson, J.-C. and Mosselmans, R. (1975). Isolation and subfractionation on Ficoll gradients of adult rat hepatocytes. Size, morphology and biochemical characteristics of cell fractions. J. Cell Biol., 66, 1–22

15. Seglen, P. O. (1976). Preparation of isolated rat liver cells. *Meth. Cell Biol.*, **13**, 29–83

16. Wanson, J. C., Drochmans, P., Mosselmans, R. and Ronveaux, M.-F. (1977). Adult rat hepatocytes in primary monolayer culture. Ultrastructural characteristics of intercellular contacts and cell membrane differentiations. *J. Cell Biol.*, **74**, 858–77

17. Wanson, J.-C., Bernaert, D. and May, C. (1979). Morphology and functional properties of isolated and cultured hepatocytes. In Popper, H. and Schaffner, F. (eds.) *Progress in Liver Diseases*, Vol. 6, pp. 1–22. (New York: Grune and Stratton, Inc.)

18. Wanson, J.-C., Bernaert, D., Mosselmans, R. and Penasse, W. (1982). Morphofunctional features of cultured liver cells. In Motta, P. M. and DiDio, L. J. A. (eds.) *Basic and Clinical Hepatology*, pp. 69–83. (The Hague/Boston/London: (Martinus Nijhoff Publishers)

19. Deschuyteneer, M., Prieels, J.-P. and Mosselmans, R. (1984). Galactose-specific adsorptive endocytosis: an ultrastructural qualitative and quantitative study in cultured rat hepatocytes. *Biol. Cell*, **50**, 17–30

20. Barth, C. A. and Schwarz, L. R. (1982). Transcellular transport of fluorescein in hepatocyte monolayers: evidence for functional polarity of cells in culture. *Proc. Natl. Acad. Sci. USA*, **79**, 4985–7

21. Guillouzo, A., Beaumont, C., Le Rumeur, E., Rissel, M., Latinier, M.-F., Guguen-Guillouzo, C. and Bourel, M. (1982). New findings on immunolocalization of albumin in rat hepatocytes. *Biol. Cell*, **43**, 163–72

22. Vassy, J., Rissel, M., Kraemer, M., Foucrier, J. and Guillouzo, A. (1984). Ultrastructural indirect immunolocalization of transferrin in cultured rat hepatocytes permeabilized with saponin. *J. Histochem. Cytochem.*, **32**, 538–40

23. Mosselmans, R., Deschuyteneer, M. and Wanson, J.-C. (1984). Membrane recycling after endocytosis of cationized ferritin in cultured rat hepatocytes. *J. Submicrosc. Cytol.*, **16**, 447–58

24. Deschuyteneer, M., Prieels, J.-P., May, C., Perraudin, J.-P. and Wanson, J.-C. (1982). Studies on the liver galactose and fucose recognition systems in cultured and isolated adult rat hepatocytes. *Biol. Cell*, **44**, 15–24

25. Zeitlin, P. L. and Hubbard, A. L. (1982). Cell surface distribution and intracellular fate of asialoglycoproteins: a morphological and biochemical study of isolated rat hepatocytes and monolayer cultures. *J. Cell Biol.*, **92**, 634–47

26. Bernaert, D., Wanson, J.-C., Drochmans, P. and Popowski, A. (1977). Effect of insulin on ultrastructure and glycogenesis in primary cultures of adult rat hepatocytes. *J. Cell Biol.*, **74**, 878–900

27. Guguen-Guillouzo, C., Tichonicky, L., Glaise, D. and Kruh, J. (1982). Insulin and triiodothyronine induce changes in chromatin phosphorylations characteristic of the cell differentiation state in fetal and adult rat hepatocytes. *Biol. Cell*, **44**, 101–10

28. Laishes, B. A. and Williams, G. M. (1976). Conditions affecting primary cell cultures of functional adult rat hepatocytes. II. Dexamethasone enhanced longevity and maintenance of morphology. *In Vitro*, **12**, 821–32

29. Redshaw, J. C. (1980). Adenylate cyclase and phosphodiesterase activities in rat hepatocytes cultured in the presence and absence of dexamethasone. *In Vitro*, **16**, 377–83

30. Yamada, S., Otto, P. S., Kennedy, D. L. and Whayne, T. F. Jr. (1980). The effects of dexamethasone on metabolic activity of hepatocytes in primary monolayer culture. *In Vitro*, **16**, 559–70

31. Schudt, C. (1980). Influence of insulin, glucocorticoids and glucose on glycogen synthetase activity in hepatocyte cultures. *Biochim. Biophys. Acta*, **629**, 499–509

32. Spagnoli, D., Dobrosielski-Vergona, K. and Widnell, C. C. (1983). Effects of hormones on the activity of glucose-6-phosphatase in primary cultures of rat hepatocytes. *Arch. Biochim. Biophys.*, **226**, 182–9

33. Sirica, A. E., Richards, W., Tsukada, Y., Sattler, C. A. and Pitot, H. C. (1979). Fetal phenotypic expression by adult rat hepatocytes on collagen gel/nylon meshes. *Proc. Natl. Acad. Sci. USA*, **76**, 283–7

34. Guguen-Guillouzo, C., Tichonicky, L., Szajnert, M.-F., Schapira, F. and Kruh, J. (1978). Changes of some chromatin and cytoplasmic enzymes in primary cultures of adult rat hepatocytes. *Biol. Cell*, **31**, 225–34

35. Reid, L. M. and Jefferson, D. M. (1984). Culturing hepatocytes and other differentiated cells. *Hepatology*, **4**, 548–59

36. Guguen-Guillouzo, C. and Guillouzo, A. (1983), Modulations of functional activities in cultured rat hepatocytes. *Mol. Cell. Biochem.*, **53/54**, 35–56

37. Jefferson, D. M., Clayton, D. F., Darnell, J. E. Jr. and Reid, L. M. (1984). Posttranscriptional modulation of gene expression in cultured rat hepatocytes. *Mol. Cell. Biol.*, **4**, 1929–34

38. Michalopoulos, G. and Pitot, H. C. (1975). Primary culture of parenchymal liver cells on collagen membranes. Morphological and biochemical observations. *Exp. Cell Res.*, **94**, 70–8

39. Ben-Zéev, A. (1986). The relationship between cytoplasmic organization, gene expression and morphogenesis. *TIBS*, **11**, 478–81

40. Gospodarowicz, D., Greenburg, G. and Birdwell, C. R. (1978). Determination of cellular shape by the extracellular matrix and its correlation with the control of cellular growth. *Cancer Res.*, **38**, 4155–71

41. Cervera, M., Dreyfuss, G. and Penman, S. (1981). Messenger RNA is translated when associated with the cytoskeletal framework in normal and VSV-infected HeLA cells. *Cell*, **23**, 113–20

42. Diegelmann, R. F., Guzelian, P. S., Gay, R. and Gay, S. (1983). Collagen formation by the hepatocyte in primary monolayer culture and in vivo. *Science*, **219**, 1343–5

43. Sudhakaran, P. R., Stamatoglou, S. C. and Hughes, R. C. (1986). Modulation of protein synthesis and secretion by substratum in primary cultures of rat hepatocytes. *Exp. Cell Res.*, **167**, 505–16

44. Clement, B., Grimaud, J. A., Campion, J.-P., Deugnier, Y. and Guillouzo, A. (1986). Cell types involved in collagen and fibronectin production in normal and fibrotic human liver. *Hepatology*, **6**, 225–34

45. Sell, S. and Ruoslahti, E. (1982). Expression of fibronectin and laminin in the rat liver after partial hepatectomy, during carcinogenesis, and in transplantable hepatocellular carcinomas. *J. Natl. Cancer Inst.*, **69**, 1105–14

46. Karasaki, S. and Raymond, J. (1981). Formation of intercellular collagen matrix by cultured liver epithelial cells and loss of its ability in hepatocarcinogenesis in vitro. *Differentiation*, **19**, 21–30

47. Wanson, J.-C., Mosselmans, R., Brouwer, A. and Knook, D. L. (1979). Interaction of adult rat hepatocytes and sinusoidal cells in coculture. *Biol. Cell*, **36**, 7–16

48. Leffert, H. L., Moran, T., Boorstein, R. and Koch, K. S. (1977). Procarcinogen activation and hormonal control of cell proliferation in differentiated primary adult rat liver cell cultures. *Nature (London)*, **267**, 58–61

49. Enat, R., Jefferson, D. M., Ruiz-Opazo, N., Gatmaitan, Z., Leinwand, L. A. and Reid, L. M. (1984). Hepatocyte proliferation in vitro: its dependence on the use of serum-free hormonally defined medium and substrate of extracellular matrix. *Proc. Natl. Acad. Sci. USA*, **81**, 1411–5

50. Parzefall, W., Galle, P. R. and Schulte-Hermann, R. (1985). Effect of calf and rat serum on the induction of DNA synthesis and mitosis in primary cultures of adult rat hepatocytes by cyproterone acetate and epidermal growth factor. *In Vitro Cell. Dev. Biol.*, **21**, 665–73

51. Richman, R. A., Claus, T. H., Pilkis, S. J. and Friedman, D. L. (1976). Hormonal stimulation of DNA synthesis in primary cultures of adult rat hepatocytes. *Proc. Natl. Acad. Sci. USA*, **73**, 389–93

52. San, R. H. C. and Williams, G. M. (1977). Rat hepatocyte primary cell culture-mediated mutagenesis of adult rat liver epithelial cells by procarcinogens. *Proc. Soc. Exp. Biol. Med.*, **156**, 534–8

53. Michalopoulos, G., Sattler, G., Sattler, C. and Pitot, H. C. (1976). Interaction of chemical carcinogens and drug-metabolizing enzymes in primary cultures of hepatic cells from the rat. *Am. J. Pathol.*, **85**, 755–71

54. Williams, G. M. (1976). The use of liver epithelial cultures for the study of chemical carcinogenesis. *Am. J. pathol.*, **85**, 739–54

55. Alley, M. C., Powis, G., Apple. P. L., Kooistra, K. L. and Lieber, M. M. (1984). Activation and inactivation of cancer chemotherapeutic agents by rat hepatocytes cocultured with human tumor cell lines. *Cancer Res.*, **44**, 549–56

56. Woodworth, C., Secott, T. and Isom, H. C. (1986). Transformation of rat hepatocytes by transfection with Simian virus 40 DNA to yield proliferating differentiated cells. *Cancer Res.*, **46**, 4018–26

57. Szpirer, J., Szpirer, C. and Wanson, J.-C. (1980). Control of serum protein production in hepatocyte hybridomas: immortalization and expression of normal hepatocyte genes. *Proc. Natl. Acad. Sci. USA*, **77**, 6616–20

58. Scherer, E. and Emmelot, P. (1975). Kinetics of induction and growth of precancerous liver-cell foci, and liver tumour formation by diethylnitrosamine in the rat. *Eur. J. Cancer*, **11**, 689–96

59. Wanson, J.-C., Bernaert, D., May, C., Deschuyteneer, M. and Prieels, J.-P. (1980). Isolation and culture of adult rat hepatocytes and preneoplastic nodules from diethyl-nitrosamine treated livers: Glucose-6-phosphatase distribution, albumin synthesis and hepatic binding protein activity. *Ann. NY Acad. Sci.*, **349**, 413–5

60. Wanson, J.-C., Penasse, W., Bernaert, D. and Popowski, A. (1981). Glucose-6-phosphatase distribution in isolated and cultured adult rat hepatocytes. *Eur. J. Cell Biol.*, **24**, 88–96

61. Glueckson-Waelsch, S. and Cori, C. F. (1970). Glucose-6-phosphatase deficiency: mechanisms of genetic control and biochemistry. *Biochem. Genet.*, **4**, 195–201

62. Burchell, A. and Burchell, B. (1980). Stabilization of partially-purified glucose-6-phosphatase by fluoride. Is enzyme inactivation caused by dephosphorylation? *FEBS Lett.*, **118**, 180–4

63. Sandermann, H. Jr. (1978). Regulation of membrane enzymes by lipids. *Biochim. Biophys. Acta*, **515**, 209–37

64. Schuller, A., Solis-Herruzo, J. A., Moscat, J., Fernandez-Checa, J. C. and Municio, A. M. (1986). The fluidity of liver plasma membranes from patients with different types of liver injury. *Hepatology*, **6**, 714–7

65. Kapitulnik, J., Tshershedsky, M. and Barenholz, Y. (1979). Fluidity of the rat liver microsomal membrane: increase at birth. *Science*, **206**, 843–4

66. Eletr, S., Zakim, D. and Vessey, D. D. (1973). A spin-label study of the role of phospholipids in the regulation of membrane-bound microsomal enzymes. *J. Mol. Biol.*, **78**, 351–62

67. Bernaert, D., Wanson, J. C., Mosselmans, R., De Paermentier, F. and Drochmans, P. (1979). Separation of adult rat hepatocytes into distinct subpopulations by centrifugal elutriation. Morphological, morphometrical and biochemical characterization of cell fractions. *Biol. Cell*, **34**, 159–74

68. Wanson, J.-C., Bernaert, D., Penasse, W., Mosselmans, R. and Bannasch, P. (1980). Separation in distinct subpopulations by elutriation of liver cells following exposure of rats to N-nitrosomorpholine. *Cancer Res.*, **40**, 459–71

69. Wanson, J.-C., Penasse, W., Bernaert, D. and Mosselmans, R. (1979). Cell surface properties of control and carcinogen-treated hepatocytes, isolated in subpopulations by elutriation. *SEM/1979/III*, SEM Inc., AMF O'Hare, Il 60666, USA, pp. 161–8

70. Wanson, J.-C., Penasse, W., Bernaert, D. and May, C. (1980). SEM study of adult rat hepatocytes from preneoplastic and hyperplastic foci induced in the liver by diethylnitrosamine. *SEM/1980/III*, SEM Inc., AMF O'Hare, Il 60666, USA, pp. 29–35

71. Evarts, R. P., Marsden, E., Hanna, P., Wirth, P. J. and Thorgeirsson, S. S. (1984). Isolation of preneoplastic rat liver cells by centrifugal elutriation and binding to asialofetuin. *Cancer Res.*, **44**, 5718–24

72. Sumner, I. G., Freedman, R. B. and Lodola, A. (1983). Characterization of hepatocytes subpopulations generated by centrifugal elutriation. *Eur. J. Biochem.*, **134**, 539–45

73. Jungermann, K. (1986). Functional heterogeneity of periportal and perivenous hepatocytes. *Enzyme*, **35**, 161–80

74. Gumucio, J. J., May, M., Dvorak, C., Chianale, J. and Massey, V. (1986). The isolation of functionally heterogeneous hepatocytes of the proximal and distal half of the liver acinus in the rat. *Hepatology*, **6**, 932–44

75. Baron, J., Redick, J. A. and Guengerich, F. P. (1981). An immunohistochemical study on the localizations and distributions of phenobarbital- and 3-methylcholanthrene-inductible cytochromes P-450 within the livers of untreated rats. *J. Biol. Chem.*, **256**, 5931–7

76. Hayner, N. T., Braun, L., Yaswen, P., Brooks, M. and Fausto, N. (1984). Isozyme profiles of oval cells, parenchymal cells and biliary cells isolated by centrifugal elutriation from normal and preneoplastic livers. *Cancer Res.*, **44**, 332–8

77. Hixson, D. C. and Allison, J. P. (1985). Monoclonal antibodies recognizing oval cells induced in the liver of rats by N-2-fluorenylacetamide or ethionine in a choline-deficient diet. *Cancer Res.*, **45**, 3750–60

78. de Ridder, L., Mosselmans, R., Bernaert, D. and Galand, P. (1987). Invasiveness, proliferative activity and ultrastructural phenotypes of hepatocytes from diethyl-nitrosamine-induced neoplastic nodules and hepatocarcinomas in vitro. *Int. J. Cancer*, **40**, 664–668

79. Mareel, M., Bruyneel, E., De Bruyne, G., Dragonetti, C.

and Van Cauwenberghe, R. (1982). Growth and invasion: separate activities of malignant MO4 cell populations in vitro. In Galeotti, T. *et al.* (eds.) *Membranes in Tumor Growth*, pp. 223–32. (New York: Elsevier Biomed. Press)

80. Fischer, G., Hartmann, H., Droese, M., Schauer, A. and Bock, K. W. (1986). Histochemical and immunohisto-chemical detection of putative preneoplastic liver foci in women after long-term use of oral contraceptives. *Virchows Arch. (Cell Pathol.)*, 50, 321–37

81. Laishes, B. A. and Rolfe, P. B. (1980). Quantitative assess-ment of liver colony formation and hepatocellular car-cinoma incidence in rats receiving intravenous injections of isogeneic liver cells isolated during hepatocarcinogenesis. *Cancer Res.*, 40, 4133–43

82. Bernaert, D., Mosselmans, R., Penasse, W., Reith, A., Laishes, B. A. and Wanson, J.-C. (1985). Ultrastructural and cytochemical study of the early stages of liver col-onization by transplanted neoplastic hepatocytes. *J. Natl. Cancer Inst.*, 75, 545–59

10

The pathology of the liver: an ultrastructural approach

K. TANIKAWA

INTRODUCTION

Ultrastructural studies have become extremely important in the field of pathology, especially in combination with histochemical or histoimmunological techniques. In addition to experimental studies on the liver, various human liver diseases have been investigated extensively at the ultrastructural level, thanks to the relatively easy technique of liver biopsy. In this chapter, the fine structural changes encountered in human liver pathology are described, with special reference to pathogenesis and clinical manifestations. Possible diagnostic applications are also discussed.

VIRAL HEPATITIS

Viral hepatitis is the most common and important hepatic disease throughout the world. Three different types of viral hepatitis have been recognized so far, namely, Types A, B, and non-A, non-B. At present, however, only the viral aetiological agents of Types A(HAV) and B(HBV) hepatitis have been found. In fact, hepatitis Types A and B are readily diagnosed clinically, while the diagnosis of non-A, non-B hepatitis is made only by exclusion of the other two types. Under the electron microscope, HAV has often been found in the lysosomes of hepatocytes and Kupffer cells of the periportal zone[1,2] (Figures 1a and 1b). Such lysosomes are found only in biopsy specimens taken within 10 days of onset of the disease[3] and appear as particles having a diameter of approximately 27 nm; the particles, some of which appear empty, form clusters. Though most enteroviruses appear to be crystalloid when examined ultrastructurally, HAV shows a particulate structure. It is currently unclear why HAV particles are detected mostly in lysosomes; it has been suggested that they undergo a process of elimination from the infected host cell.

In Type A hepatitis, relatively few lymphocytes are seen in close contact with hepatocytes, and, under the electron microscope, it seems that, unlike Type B hepatitis, lymphocyte-mediated hepatocellular necrosis is not evident. A characteristic change noted in hepatocytes in hepatitis A is the appearance in the cytoplasm of numerous myelin figures which resemble lysosomes and which often contain HAV particles.

The most characteristic alterations seen in early hepatitis A are related to the Kupffer cells, which appear remarkably enlarged and enclose numerous electron-dense lysosomes (Figure 2), some of which contain HAV particles; and to organelles, whose changes are probably indicative of dysfunction[3]. Type A hepatitis is characterized clinically by high fever at onset and the occasional occurrence of extrahepatic manifestations, such as renal failure and high serum IgM levels. In type A hepatitis, our studies established the frequent occurrence at onset of transient endotoxaemia, high levels of serum immune complexes and high titres of IgM antibodies against enteric bacteria. Since endotoxins, immune complexes and bacteria derived from the intestinal region are taken up mainly by the Kupffer cells, these findings, not unexpected in the light of fine structural study results, are ascribable to Kupffer cell dysfunction and could indeed explain the characteristic clinical manifestations seen in Type A hepatitis.

Studies employing monoclonal antibodies against various lymphocytes have shown that most of the lymphocytes infiltrating the liver tissue are Leu 2a-positive; however, a considerable number of Leu 7-positive cells are also found, as opposed to the situation encountered in hepatitis B. From such fine structural and immunohistological studies, it has been speculated that three different mechanisms of hepatocyte necrosis are operating in Type A hepatitis, i.e. one involving the cytotoxic T cell, one related to the natural killer cell, and, finally, a mechanism involving Kupffer cell-mediated processes[4] (Figure 3).

In Type A hepatitis, portal duct or ductular alterations are occasionally prominent; such is not the case in acute hepatitis B. The cholestatic subtype of Type A hepatitis could be partly due to these changes.

In acute Type B hepatitis, HBV-associated antigens are hardly ever observed by electron microscopy in human specimens. However, in specimens taken by liver biopsy from healthy HBV carriers or chronic Type B hepatitis patients, HBs, HBc and Dane particles are often detected in hepatocytes examined by electron microscopy (Figures 4, 5, 6 and 7).

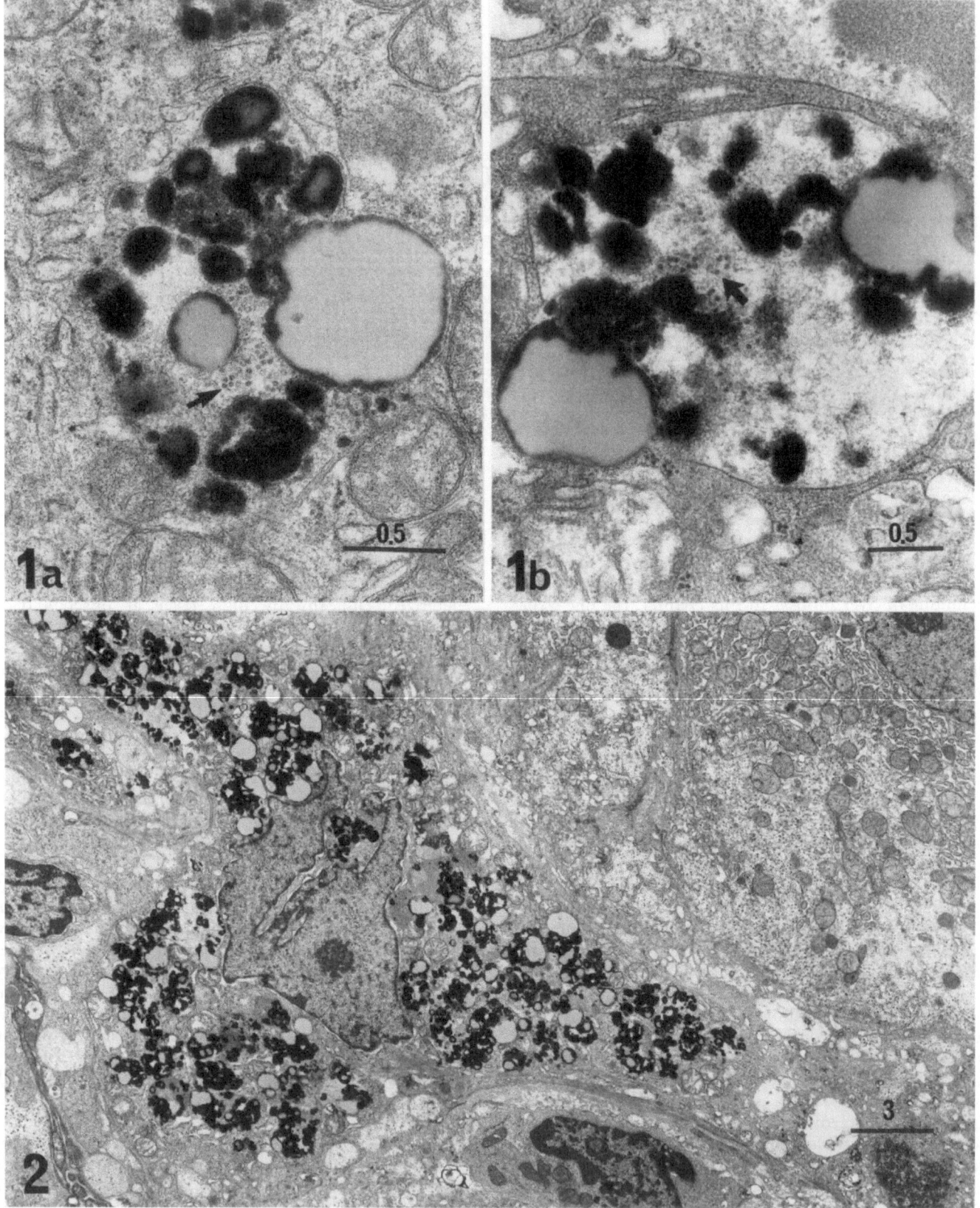

Figure 1   Hepatitis A virus in lysosomes of the hepatocyte (**1a**) and Kupffer cell (**1b**)

Figure 2   The Kupffer cell in Type A hepatitis appears to be markedly enlarged with numerous electron-dense granules and distorted organelles

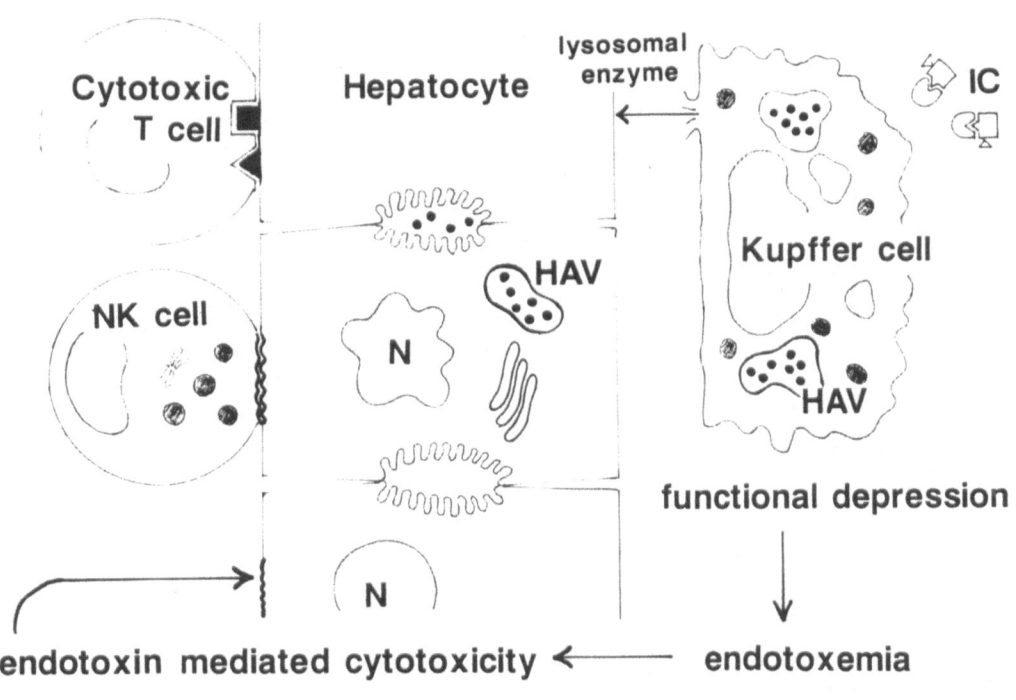

Figure 3 Possible mechanisms of hepatocyte damage in hepatitis Type A

Core antigens (HBc), which have a diameter of approximately 25 nm, are detected predominantly in the nucleus, although some may also be seen in the cytoplasm of the hepatocyte. Filamentous HBs antigens are seen in the dilated cisternae of the smooth endoplasmic reticulum (SER) (Figures 4a and 4b). Sometimes, such antigen-containing SER occupies most of the hepatocyte's cytoplasm. Dane particles (complete HBV) are rarely found in the cytoplasm. Morphologically speaking, the development of HBV particles seems to involve the envelopment of HBc antigens within the ER membrane, which is positive for HBs antigens[7] (Figure 5). A schematic representation of HBV-associated antigens in the hepatocyte may be seen in Figure 6.

In acute or chronic Type B hepatitis, degenerating or necrotic hepatocytes, having a shrunken electron-dense cytoplasm, often appear in close contact with lymphocytes (Figure 7a). Immunohistochemical studies using antibodies against various lymphocytes demonstrate that such lymphocytes usually prove Leu 2a-positive upon electron microscopic examination (Figure 7b); thus, a cytotoxic T cell-mediated mechanism seems to be important in hepatocellular necrosis. At present, it has not been elucidated which HBV-associated antigens represent targets for such lymphocytes; however, the HBc antigen associated with the hepatocyte's plasma membrane seems to be the most probable one[8]. A possible mechanism for hepatocellular necrosis is presented in Figure 8.

In non-A, non-B hepatitis, small fairly round particles, measuring about 20–27 nm in diameter, are often detected in the nucleus of the hepatocyte[9]. Although their significance remains unknown, they are probably non-specific. Chimpanzees, inoculated with sera of non-A, non-B hepatitis patients, show characteristic inclusions in the hepatocyte cytoplasm[10]; however, such inclusions have not been found in human cases.

Hepatic changes due to Epstein–Barr virus or cytomegalovirus infection are usually mild. In such cases of virus-induced hepatitis, the presence of numerous lymphocytes within the sinusoids may be noted, although it seems difficult to speculate from fine structural observations, through which mechanism hepatocellular damage occurs. Occasionally, virus-like particles, having a diameter of approximately 100 nm, are found in the cytoplasm of the hepatocyte, ductal cell or lymphocyte[11].

In general, fairly similar mechanisms of hepatic damage seem to be operant in the various forms of viral hepatitis. By electron microscopy, however, some differences among them are noted, and many problems in this field still remain unsolved. Electron microscopy, in its various forms, should be of considerable help in further studies on the pathogenesis of hepatitis.

ALCOHOLIC LIVER INJURIES

Both in alcoholics and alcoholic liver injuries, hepatocyte size is increased, with frequent occurrence of the so-called 'ballooning hepatocyte', which is probably due to an accumulation of export proteins and lipids, such as albumin, transferrin or VLDL. The accumulation of such proteins is most likely to be due to a reduction in the number of microtubules and Golgi complex-associated enzymes[12]. Mitochondrial size is also increased, accompanied by changes such as decreased matrix density and the appearance of large mitochondrial granules or distorted cristae. Giant mitochondria, similar in size to the nucleus, are also often seen. However, the cause of such large mitochondria is not clear; metabolic disorders,

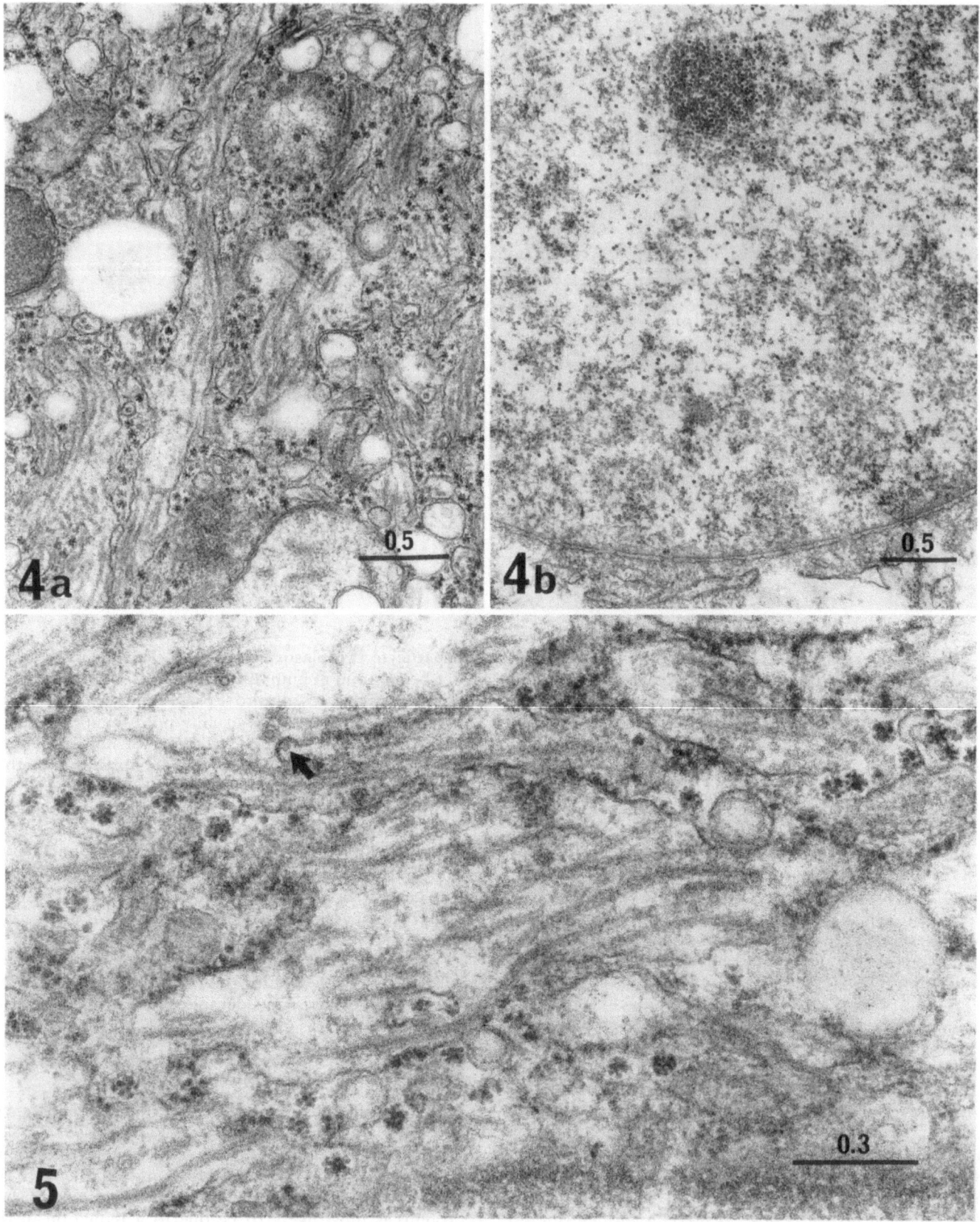

Figure 4   HBV-associated antigens in a hepatocyte of chronic Type B hepatitis. Filamentous HBs antigens (**4a**) appear to be abundant in the dilated cisternae of the ER, and numerous HBc antigen particles (**4b**) are scattered within the nucleus

Figure 5   A Dane particle appears to develop by HBc antigens being wrapped by ER membrane (arrow). Numerous Dane particles and filamentous HBs antigens are noted in the dilated ER cisternae

HBV in the hepatocyte

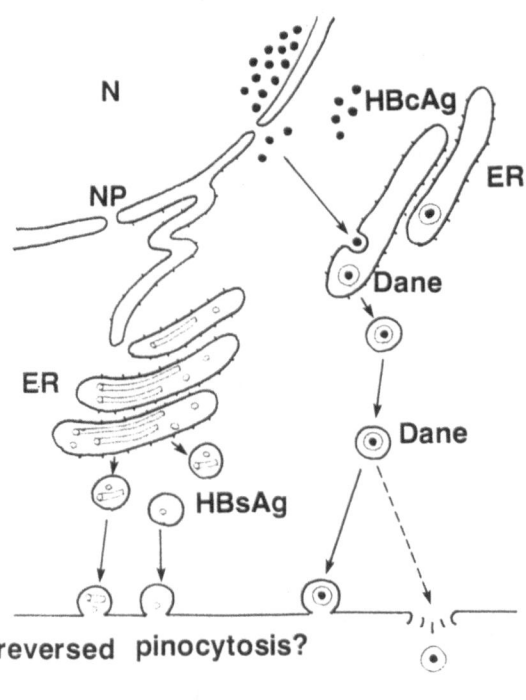

6

Figure 6 Schematic representation of HBV-associated antigen formation in the hepatocyte

such as riboflavin deficiency, might play a role since giant mitochondria frequently occur in riboflavin deficiency[13], a condition often encountered in alcoholism. The number of peroxisomes is also increased; this is probably an adaptive change induced by ethanol oxidation occurring in the hepatocyte. One of the more important changes seen in alcoholics is an increase in the amount of SER, a reflection of the activities of induced drug-metabolizing enzymes and the stimulation of the microsomal ethanol-oxidizing system.

As far as the aetiological factors of the alcoholic fatty liver are concerned, enhanced synthesis of triglyceride, decreased mitochondrial oxidation of fatty acids, increased fatty acid mobilization from the peripheral tissues to the hepatocyte and impaired secretion of lipoproteins have been documented. Electron microscopic examination of the alcoholic fatty liver shows numerous fat droplets of various sizes occupying most of the hepatocyte cytoplasm and deviation of the nucleus towards the periphery.

In the hepatocyte cytoplasm in such a fatty liver, amorphous materials, probably triglyceride in nature, accumulate within the dilated cisternae of the SER and in larger fat droplets. Membranous structures, some of which are continuous with the SER membrane, are occasionally seen at the periphery of the droplets; this suggests that ruptured SER membranes form larger fat droplets[14].

In alcoholic hepatitis, the histology of the liver is char-

acterized by the appearance of Mallory bodies in degenerating hepatocytes and by neutrophil infiltration. Mallory bodies, which appear under light microscopy as eosinophilic structures, are accumulations of fine fibrils measuring about 14–20 nm in diameter and lacking surrounding membranes. Immunological studies indicate that these fibrils originate from intermediate filaments. The fibrils appear to be slightly larger than the tonofilaments of normal hepatocytes and have a fuzzy, coat-like structure on the surface. Mallory bodies are ultrastructurally classified into three types. Type I has a structure consisting of parallel fibrils, 14.1 nm in diameter, occasionally having a lamellar arrangement. Type II, the most common one, has numerous fibrils, 15.2 nm in diameter, running irregularly. Type III is composed of granular or amorphous electron-dense materials, containing only scattered remains of fibrils. By electron microscopy, small accumulations of the above-mentioned fibrils are often noted in specimens in which Mallory bodies have not been observed previously under light microscopy. Thus, electron microscopy may be helpful diagnostically in differentiating viral hepatitis from alcoholic hepatitis.

Hepatocytes bearing Mallory bodies generally appear markedly altered, probably due to disruption of the order of the intermediate filaments, which are important components in the maintenance of cell shape. Such disruption results in ballooning of the hepatocyte and, ultimately, leads to cell necrosis.

Alcoholic liver injury is characterized by pericellular fibrosis and perivenular sclerosis. Pericellular fibrosis occurs mainly in the centrolobular area. From a morphological point of view, fat-storing cells and hepatocytes seem to participate in fibrogenesis. In the areas of perivenular sclerosis, myofibroblasts are increased in number and seem to be intimately associated with fibrogenesis in these regions.

The myofibroblast is spindle-shaped, has long bundles of microfilaments with dense areas along the plasma membrane, and is usually surrounded by connective tissue; this cell is also known as a 'contractile fibroblast'[16]. The myofibroblast possesses a well-developed RER, abundant free ribosomes and distinct Golgi complexes, along with numerous microtubules and pinocytotic vesicles. Nerve endings are also noted in close contact with the cell. These fine structural observations seem to indicate that this cell participates, not only in fibrogenesis in this area, but also in contraction of the central vein.

Although it has been accepted that Kupffer cell function is depressed in alcoholics and in alcohol-induced liver disease, no direct proof has so far been put forth. In cultured rat Kupffer cells incubated for one hour in a medium containing 50 mmol L^{-1} of ethanol or in cells taken from rats fed Lieber's liquid diet for a period of six weeks, marked inhibition of phagocytosis, together with swollen mitochondria and depletion of microtubules has been noted[18]. In addition, a decrease in the number of Fc receptors on the cell surface has been documented by electron microscopic methods[19] (Figures 9a–9d). Thus, a direct effect of ethanol on the phagocytic function of the Kupffer cell has now been well established; this may indeed explain the alcoholic's increased susceptibility to infections.

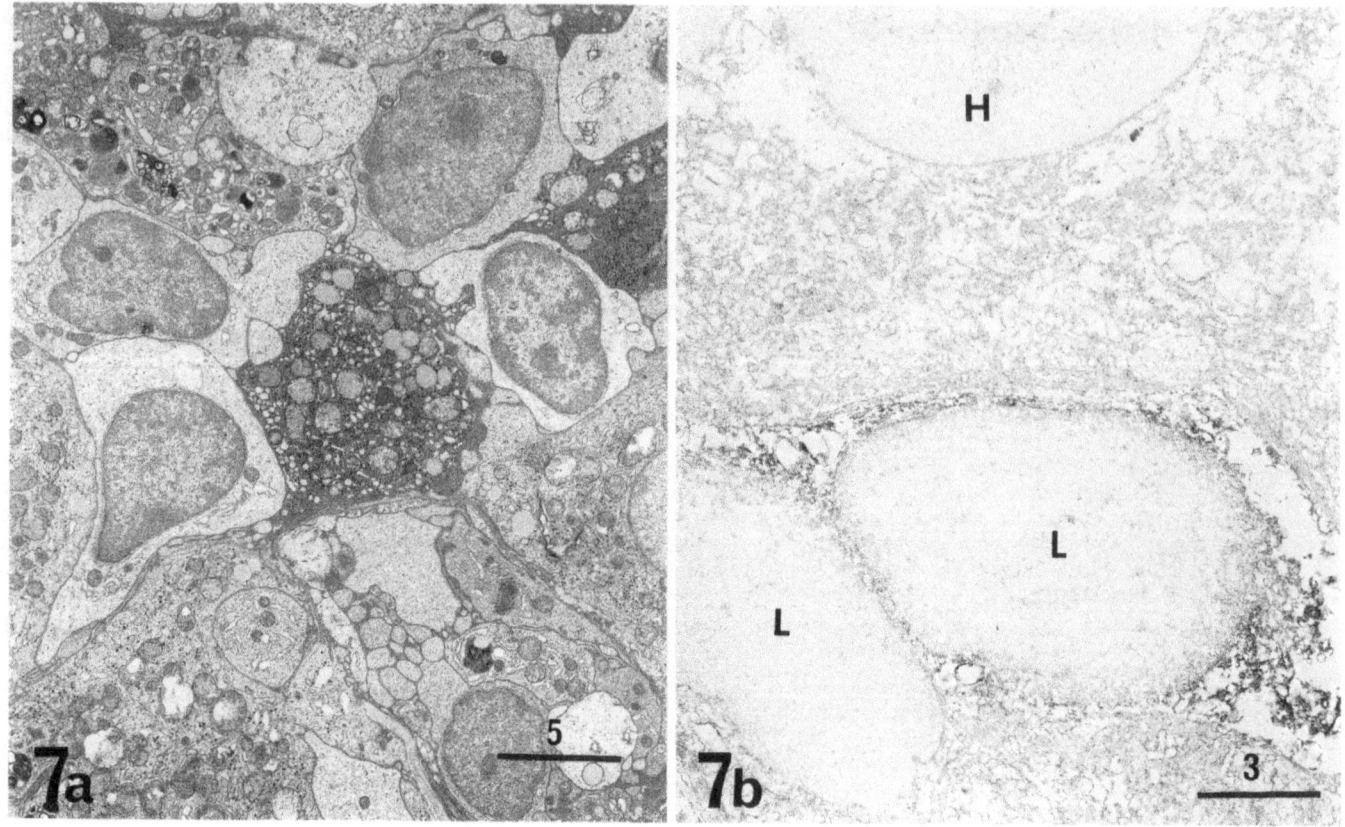

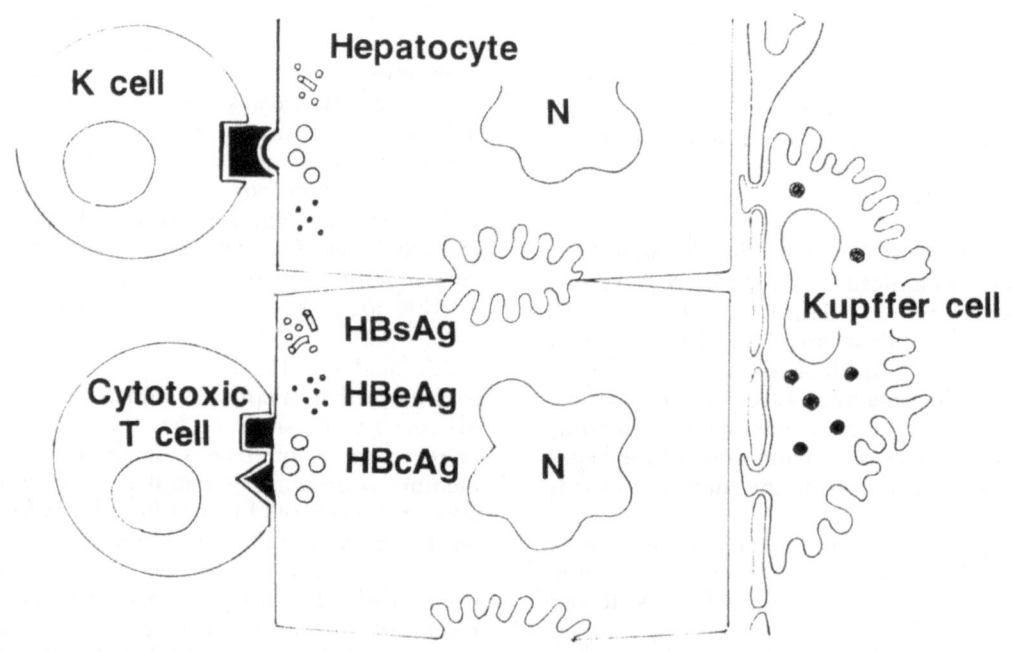

Figure 7   Lymphocyte-mediated hepatocyte damage in chronic Type B hepatitis.
Figure 7a: Lymphocytes (L) in close contact with an apparently degenerate hepatocyte.
Figure 7b: A Leu 2a-positive cell (L) is seen in close contact with the hepatocyte
Figure 8   Schematic representation of a possible mechanism of lymphocyte-mediated hepatocyte damage in Type B hepatitis

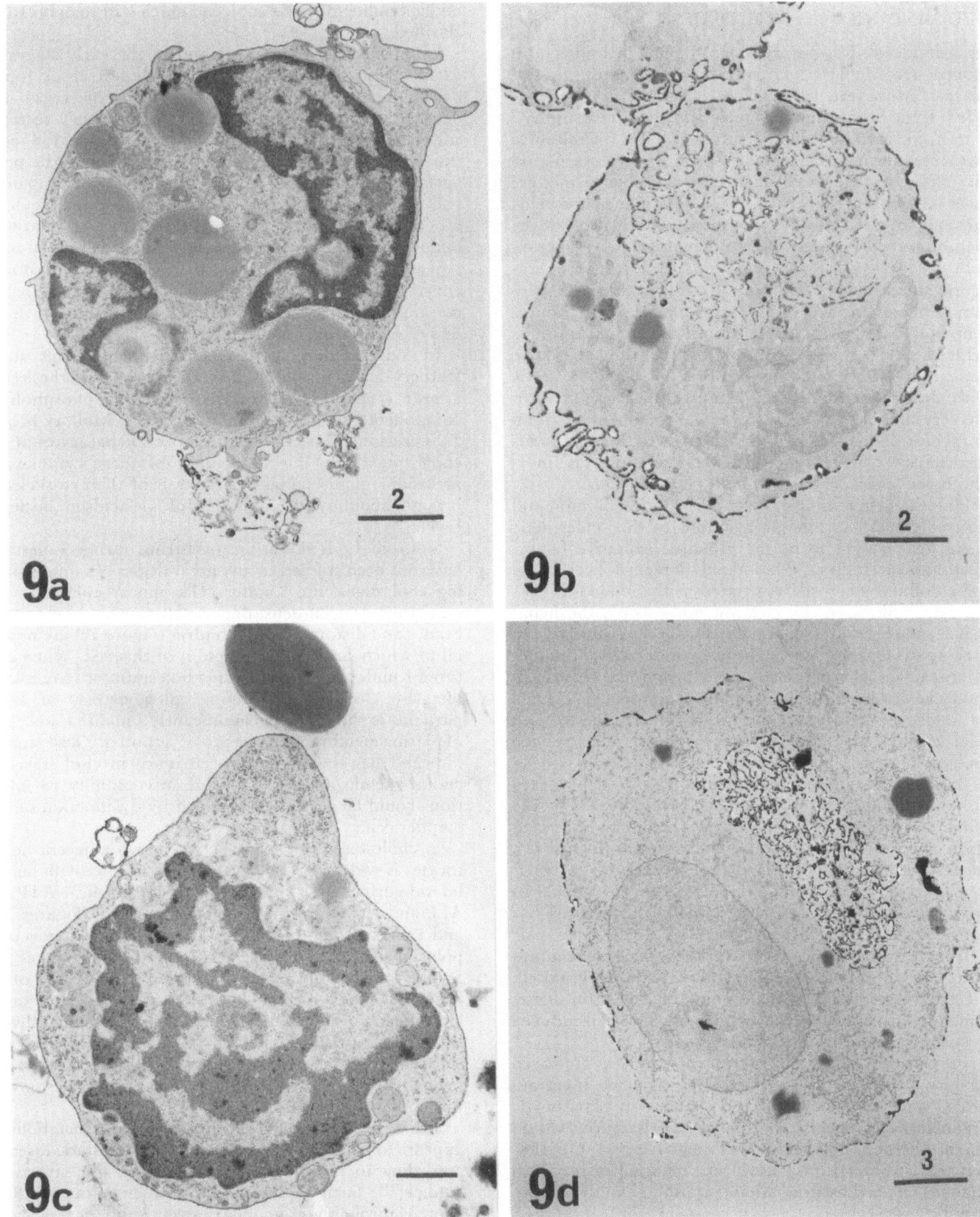

Figure 9 Phagocytotic study and Fc receptors in cultured rat Kupffer cells. Latex particles are well phagocytosed to the normal Kupffer cell (9a), which has abundant Fc receptors on the cell surface (9b). On the other hand, Kupffer cells taken from rats fed Lieber's diet for 6 weeks have a flattened cell surface and appear not to take up latex particles (9c). Fc receptors on the cell surface are decreased in number (9d)

DRUG-INDUCED LIVER INJURIES

Drug-induced liver injuries can be divided into two groups, according to their pathogenesis: hepatotoxic and allergic. Moreover, two clinical types have been recognized: toxic hepatocellular injury and cholestatic injury.

In toxic hepatocellular injury, reactive metabolites produced during drug metabolism in the hepatocyte are thought to be the most important aetiological factors: these metabolites react with macromolecular cell proteins through covalent binding, or induce peroxidation of the membrane lipids, resulting in hepatocyte dysfunction and, eventually, cell necrosis. One of the various therapeutic agents which induce such toxic injury is acetaminophen. In acetaminophen-induced liver injury, centrolobular necrosis without marked cell infiltration is evident. Under the electron microscope, the hepatocyte appears to be occupied by membranous clumps of SER with electron-dense deposits (Figure 10). These features are very similar to those observed in experimental carbon tetrachloride-induced liver injury; in fact, Trump and his associates[20-22] have described these features as morphological characteristics of lipid peroxidation.

Halothane liver injury is one of the most common and serious kinds, and allergic reactions to this anaesthetic agent are thought to be the principal causative factor. Histological studies of halothane-damaged liver show centrolobular necrosis associated with abundant lymphocyte infiltration. By electron microscopy, the hepatocyte's mitochondria characteristically show alterations, such as swelling and dense deposits or decreased number of cristae[23]; such alterations are similar to those seen in the Reye syndrome. The usually poor prognosis carried by halothane-induced liver injury might be due to such relatively selective changes in the mitochondria, which are crucial to cell integrity.

Another interesting fine structural feature encountered in halothane-induced liver damage is represented by the numerous infiltrating lymphocytes which may be seen in close contact with degenerating hepatocytes (Figure 11), suggesting a lymphocyte-mediated mechanism in hepatocellular necrosis. Though these lymphocytes appear to be of the cytotoxic T cell variety, their ultrastructure has not been studied extensively.

In some drug-induced liver injuries, marked accumulation of phospholipid within the hepatocyte is noted. Electron microscopy reveals numerous electron-dense, lamellar structures in the cytoplasm. Coralgil-induced liver injury is one such example[24,25].

In general, drug administration induces increased activity of hepatic drug-metabolizing enzymes. If certain drugs were to induce specific changes in hepatocytic organelles, such specific morphological alterations would be very helpful, both in clinical diagnosis and in pathogenetic considerations; however, most ultrastructural changes effected by drug administration seem to be nonspecific.

CHOLESTASIS

For years, mechanisms of jaundice and of intrahepatic cholestasis have been principal topics for clinicians and pathologists interested in liver diseases. Although electron microscopy has contributed greatly towards a better understanding of these subjects, much still remains to be clarified.

In intrahepatic cholestasis and in the early stages of extrahepatic obstructive jaundice, cholestasis is found predominantly in the centrolobular zone. This is probably due to the fact that bile acids are less actively secreted and sinusoidal oxygen tension is lower in the centrolobular zone, especially in comparison with the periportal region. Thus, micelle formation is easily impaired and susceptibility to monohydroxy bile acids, such as lithocholate, is rapidly increased even after relatively minor damage. In addition, hepatocytes in this zone possess abundant SER in which drug-metabolizing enzymes are found; consequently, these liver cells are continuously exposed to cytotoxic metabolites of drugs and of other foreign materials[26].

In long-standing cholestasis, the hepatocytes show feathery degeneration. By electron microscopy, these cells appear to be full of electron-dense bile-like phospholipid components, suggesting biliary necrosis. Mallory bodies are occasionally seen in the periportal hepatocytes of the cholestatic liver; the appearance of these cytoplasmic inclusions might signal dysfunction of the cytoskeleton brought about by accumulations of bile acids in the hepatocyte.

Sinusoidal cell alterations occurring during cholestasis have not been studied to any great degree. In long-standing cholestasis, the Kupffer cells appear enlarged, and numerous electron-dense deposits, flattened plasma membranes and distorted mitochondria (Figure 12) are noted, all of which suggests dysfunction of this cell. When cultured Kupffer cells taken from cholestatic rats are examined by electron microscopy, phagocytosis of latex particles is shown to be significantly impaired, and loss of plasma membrane Fc receptors[19] is noted. These studies indicate that the frequent occurrence in cholestasis of endotoxaemia and/or increased susceptibility to infections could be partially explained by dysfunction of the Kupffer cell.

In cholestasis, the space between two adjacent hepatocytes is widened. The development of microvilli on the lateral surface and increased activity of Mg^{2+} ATPase, ALP and γ-GTP on the basolateral surface (Figures 13a and 13b) is also noted. These findings indicate a reversed polarity of bile excretion in cholestatic hepatocytes[27,28]. Swollen mitochondria having curled cristae[29] are often observed in the cytoplasm of the hepatocyte in cholestasis, although their significance remains unknown. In Zellweger's disease, in which there is defective oxidation of the side chain of cholesterol, mitochondrial changes are prominent[30] and probably represent primary lesions of this cholestatic disease.

The SER, site of bile acid, lipid and drug metabolism, appears to be decreased in amount in cholestatic disease, according to morphometric analysis of fine structural studies[31,32]. Such a decrease in the hepatocyte's SER content, probably a secondary event, nonetheless accelerates the progression of cholestasis. The most prominent fine structural changes seen in the cholestatic liver are found at the level of the bile canaliculus, which appears dilated and possesses stunted microvilli (Figure 14a). Such dilatation of the canalicular lumen, especially in extrahepatic obstructive jaundice, is partly caused by increased intraluminal pressure. In intrahepatic chol-

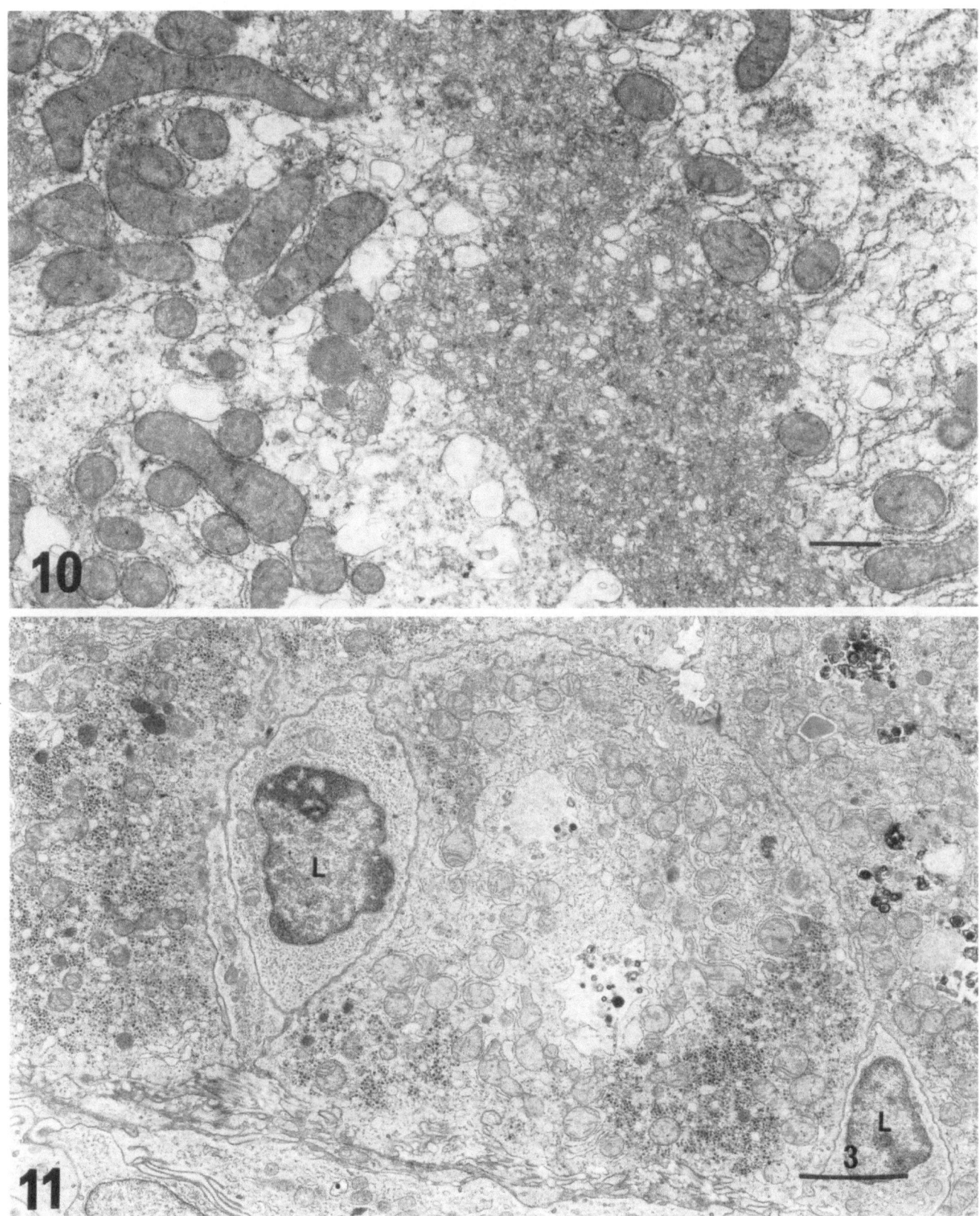

Figure 10 Acetaminophen-induced liver injury. The hepatocyte has clumps of membranous structures containing electron-dense deposits

Figure 11 Halothane-induced liver injury. Lymphocytes (L) are in close contact with the hepatocyte, which appears markedly altered with distorted mitochondria

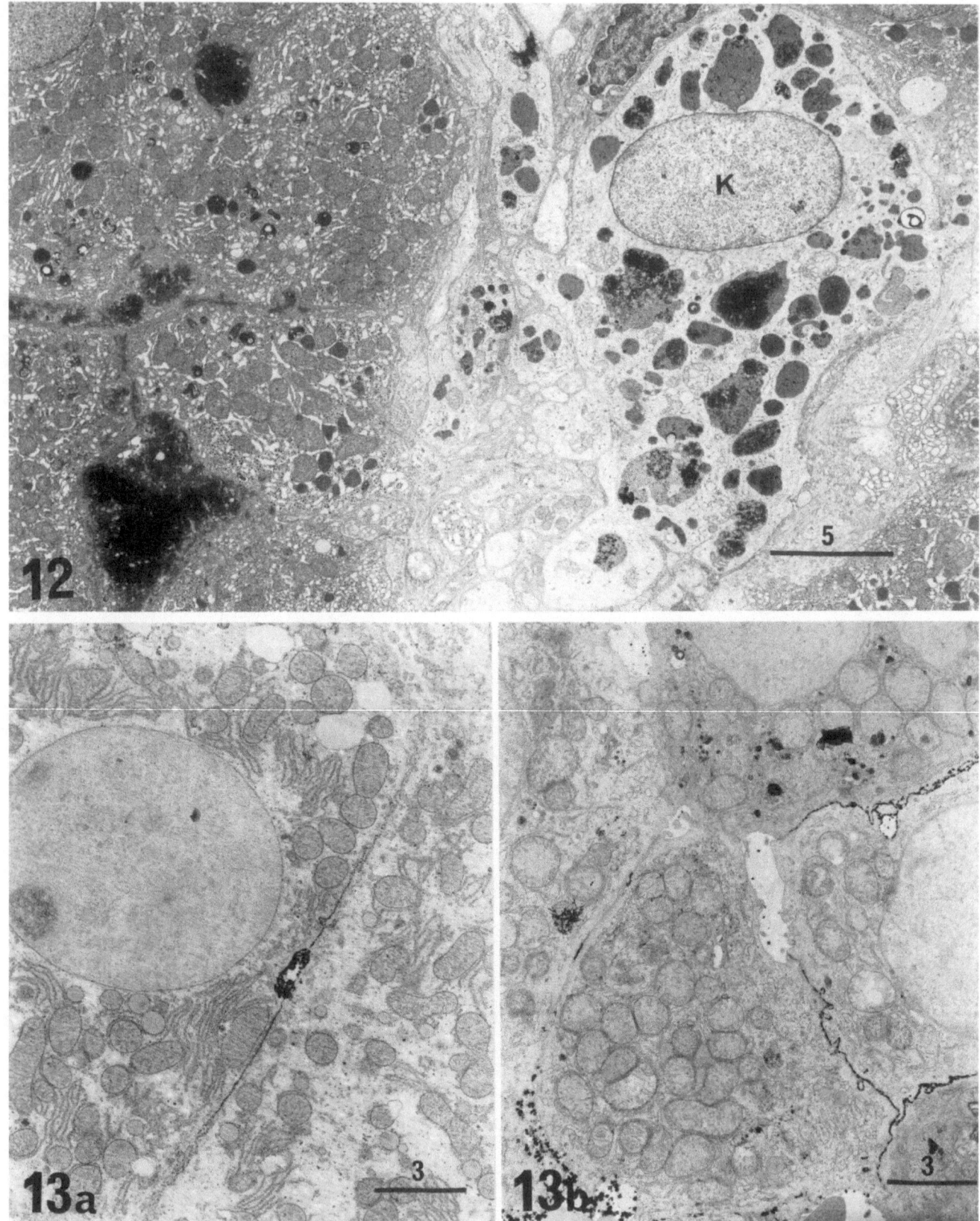

Figure 12   Kupffer cell in extrahepatic cholestasis. The Kupffer cell (K) appears to be enlarged and contains numerous electron-dense materials and flattened plasma membranes

Figure 13   Ultrastructural demonstration of alkaline phosphatase activity in experimental cholestasis in rats. In normal liver, alkaline phosphatase activity is observed on the canalicular membrane (**14a**). However, in extrahepatic obstruction, this enzyme's activity in the dilated canaliculus perishes and is shifted to the basolateral surface of the plasma membrane (**14b**)

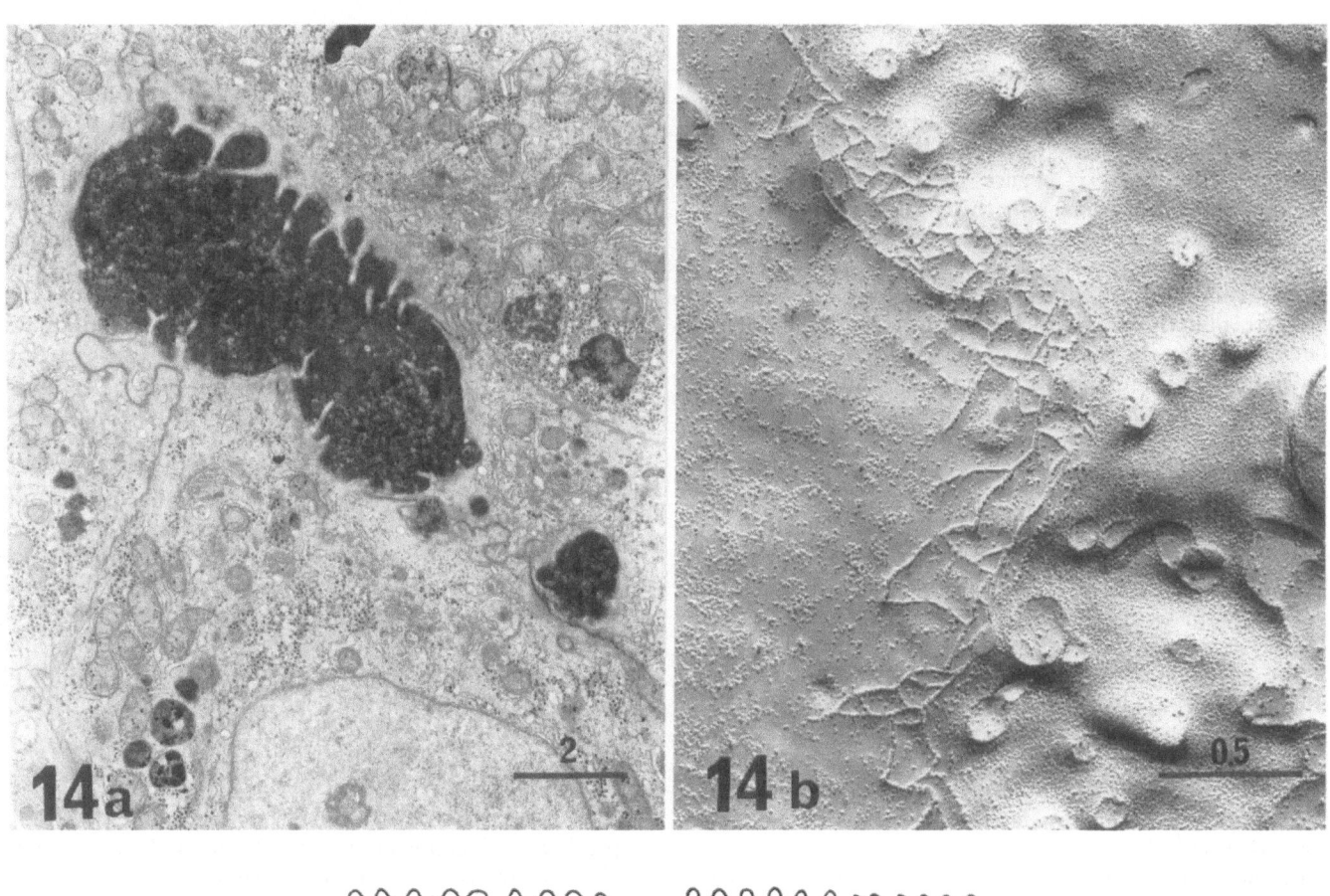

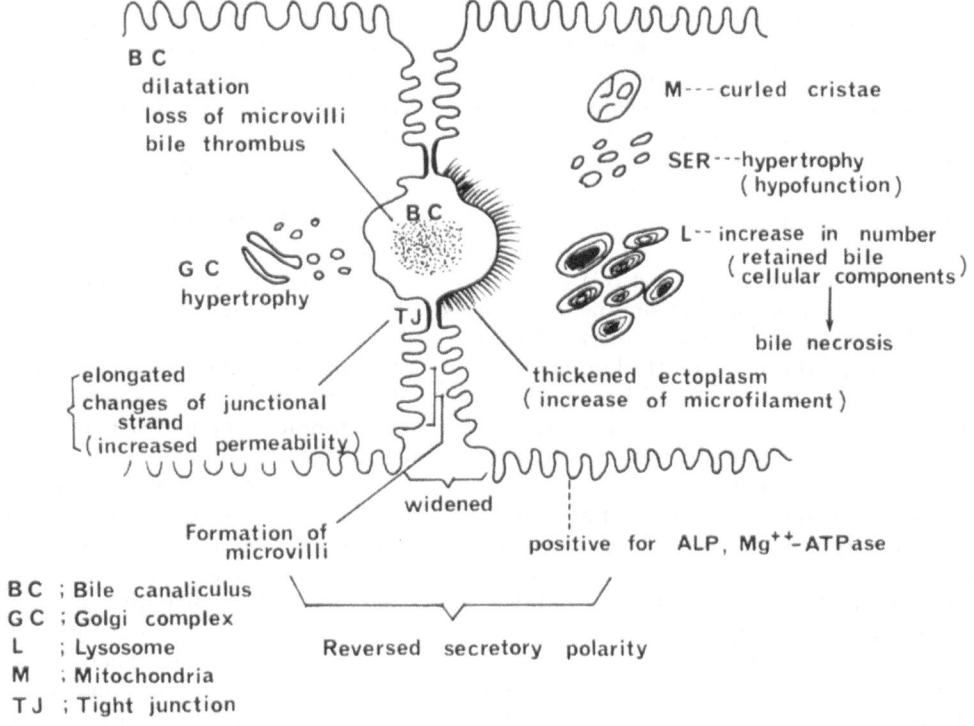

Figure 14 Changes in the bile canaliculus in intrahepatic cholestasis. The bile canaliculus appears dilated, showing loss of microvilli, and the canalicular lumen is filled by a bile thrombus with widened pericanalicular ectoplasm (12a). A freeze-cleave replica study shows junctional strands of the tight junction to be irregularly arranged and partly disrupted (arrow) (12b)
Figure 15 Schematic representation of fine structural changes in the hepatocyte seen in cholestasis

estasis, however, it is due mainly to dysfunction of the microfilaments surrounding the canaliculus, resulting in its paralysis[33,34].

Changes in the canalicular membrane are the most prominent events occurring at this level and are thought to represent primary events of lithocholate-induced intrahepatic cholestasis[35]. In this pathological state, an increased cholesterol content is noted in the canalicular membrane[36]. However, in cytochalasin B- or norethandrolone-induced intrahepatic cholestasis, decreased cholesterol in the canalicular membrane has been noted[37]. The changes in the P/C ratio in the canalicular membrane may affect enzyme activity, membrane fluidity and permeability in this region, resulting in disturbances of bile excretion and cholestasis. In addition, the disappearance of the canalicular membrane glycocalyx is also noted in cholestasis[38].

In long-standing cholestasis, the hepatocytes surrounding the dilated bile canaliculus are often observed in a tubular arrangement. This is probably an adaptive phenomenon to marked cholestasis[39] and may be considered a primitive manifestation. The thrombi found in the canalicular lumen generally appear as granular, fibrillar or lamellar electron-dense materials having various shapes. Such thrombi are sometimes continuous with canalicular membranes, suggesting a partly membranous composition. However, it is not clear whether these materials in bile thrombi have particular fine structural aspects.

In cholestasis, the hepatocyte also contains numerous electron-dense materials, most of which are seen in lysosomes. These materials are probably composed of stagnated bile components and degenerated organelles and membranes produced by the cholestatic condition. Given their detergent properties, stagnant bile acids within the hepatocyte may be one of the most important factors in damage occurring to subcellular components.

The Golgi apparatus has been known to be associated with vesicular transport, not only to the basolateral surface of the hepatocyte, but also to the bile canaliculus[40,41]. Thus, a possible role of this organelle in the pathogenesis of cholestasis has been considered. Unfortunately, however, very little is currently known about it. In fact, in cholestasis, the Golgi complex appears to be hypertrophic and the pericanalicular vesicles are more numerous; in long-standing cholestasis, however, these organelles prove fewer in number[42].

Recently, the cytoskeletal system of the hepatocyte has been studied extensively in relation to the pathogenesis of cholestasis. It has been well established that the microfilaments surrounding the bile canaliculus play a pivotal role in bile flow through the canalicular lumen[43]. In fact, in cholestasis, the pericanalicular ectoplasm appears to be thickened and to contain an increased number of microfilaments. However, whether this is a primary alteration or a secondary event in cholestasis remains to be clarified.

The junctional complexes are generally elongated in cholestasis, and freeze-cleave replica studies indicate increased permeability of the tight junction. Moreover, the junctional strands are irregularly arranged, discontinuous and lose parallelism (Figure 14b), all of which is suggestive of increased permeability of this paracellular pathway in human intrahepatic cholestasis[44]. In exper-

imental cholestasis, an increase in the permeability of tracers, such as horseradish peroxidase, lanthanum, etc., has been shown. In long-standing cholestasis, rupture of the tight junction has been noted[45], but this seems to be a late event. These changes observed in cholestasis are partly primary, but mostly secondary, and it is currently difficult to differentiate the former from the latter. Nevertheless, these changes complement one another in the promotion of cholestasis. Fine structural changes seen in the hepatocyte in cholestasis are schematically presented in Figure 15. It has generally been accepted that the principal cause of intrahepatic cholestasis rests at the level of the hepatocyte. However, in the cholestatic kind of acute Type A hepatitis, electron microscopy shows prominent bile ductal changes in the portal tract, associated with considerable lymphocyte infiltration.

In primary biliary cirrhosis, ductal changes in the portal tract are remarkable and are described together as a chronic, non-suppurative, destructive cholangitis[46]. Electron microscopy reveals shrunken ductal cells possessing an electron-dense cytoplasm containing markedly altered mitochondria, and lymphocytes intimately associated with these cells, suggesting involvement of cytotoxic processes in this disease[47].

FIBROSIS AND CIRRHOSIS

It is assumed that all cell types have the potential to produce collagenous materials. In normal liver, however, electron microscopy indicates that production of fibre within the portal tract, space of Disse and the vicinity of the central vein is accomplished, respectively, by fibroblasts, fat-storing cells and myofibroblasts[48]. These three types of cells, which have been well described ultrastructurally, always seem to be more or less surrounded by connective tissue fibres. Collagen Types I, II and IV have been identified in the liver and are all increased several-fold in the fibrotic liver. Under the electron microscope, thick fibrils of Type I collagen, having a diameter of 25–100 nm and a periodicity of 660 Å, thinner fibrils of Type III collagen, 20–40 nm in diameter, and amorphous substances are observed in the extracellular matrix. The basement membrane, composed mainly of collagen Types IV and V, is also clearly demonstrable. During the development of fibrosis, Type III collagen increases before Type I does.

In the fibrous septa of the fibrotic liver, numerous bundles of collagen appear intermingled with some fibroblasts. Newly formed small vessels, which probably act as shunts, are found within the septa but do not pass through the hepatic parenchyma[50]. In areas of focal hepatocellular necrosis, considerable numbers of fat-storing cells are found. Such cells have dilated RER cisternae containing amorphous materials, which seems to indicate that these cells are involved in active procollagen production[50]. In necrotic areas, only amorphous materials and fine fibrils are seen in the extracellular matrix.

The fat-storing cells are also well preserved in wider areas of necrosis, as is the case in the zonal or massive necrosis of fulminant hepatitis. This morphological evidence seems to indicate that the fat-storing cells play an important role in fibrogenesis following hepatocellular necrosis.

In the portal fibrosis associated with chronic hepatitis,

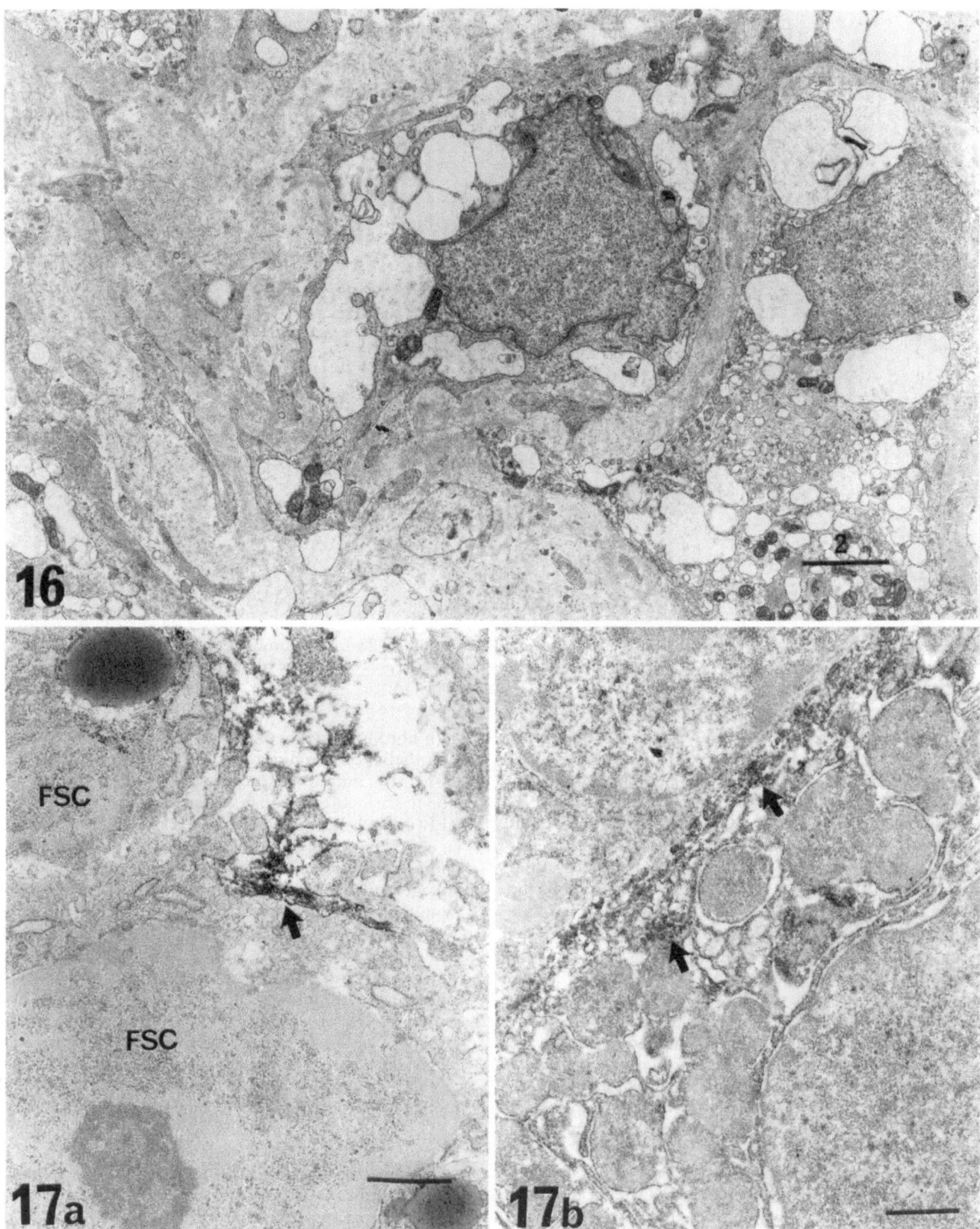

Figure 16 Fat-storing cell in chronic hepatitis. A fat-storing cell, surrounded by fibrous tissue, shows remarkably dilated RER and a few fat droplets in the cytoplasm

Figure 17 Ultrastructural demonstration of collagen-producing cells. Staining reactions to monoclonal antibody against type III collagen (arrow) are noted in the RER of a fat-storing cell (FSC) in chronic hepatitis (**17a**). Staining reactions to monoclonal antibody against type III collagen (arrows) are also noted in the RER of the hepatocyte (**17b**) in cirrhosis

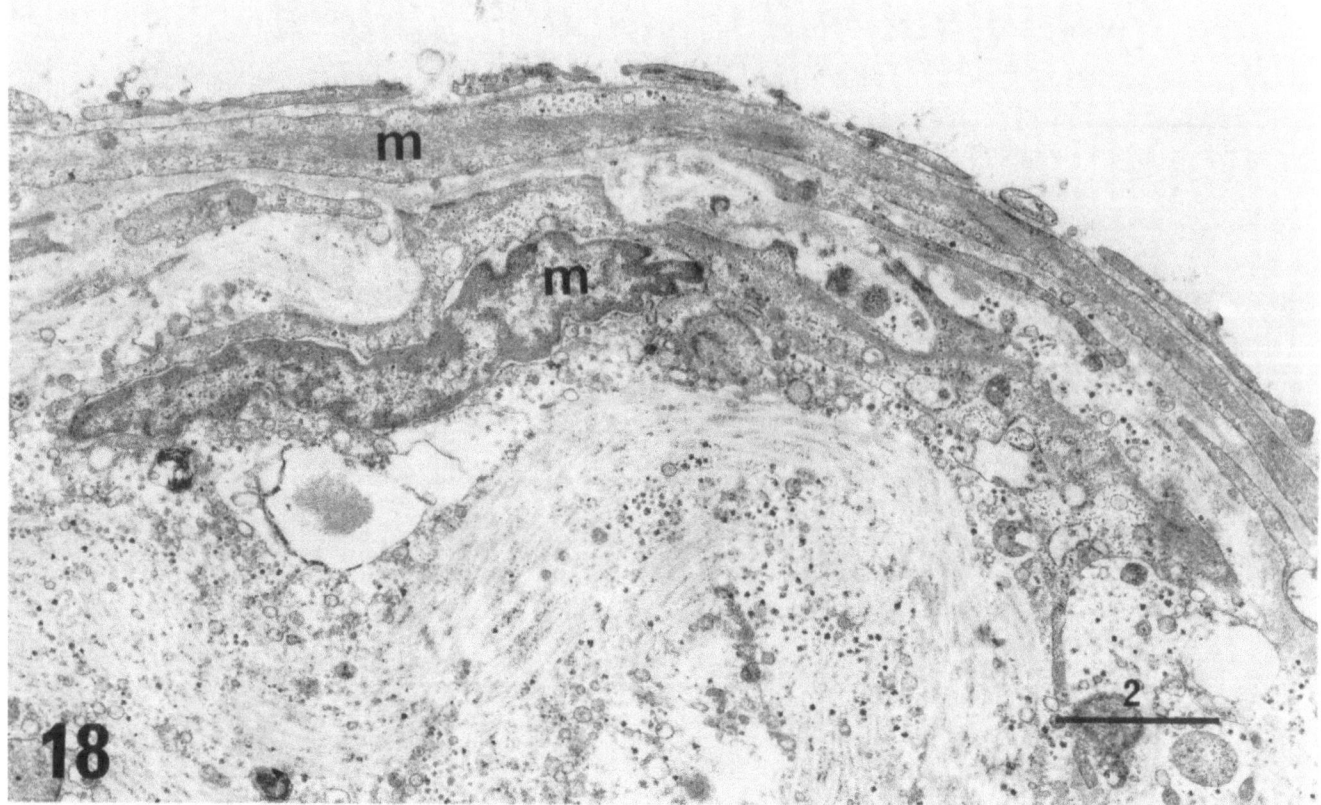

Figure 18 Myofibroblasts in the centrolobular area in alcoholic liver injury. Two myofibroblasts (m) are located in the area of perivenular fibrosis. The myofibroblasts have long microfilaments with dense areas along the plasma membrane

the number of fat-storing cells increases as fibrous tissue increases. Compared with the typical fat-storing cells observed in normal liver, the cells encountered in this pathological condition have a more prominent RER, more numerous mitochondria, fewer lipid droplets and an elongated indented nucleus (Figure 16). In fact, immunohistochemical studies, using monoclonal antibodies against Type III collagen, show positive reactions in the RER of fat-storing cells in such areas[51] (Figure 17a). These cells are probably in a transitional phase between the resting and active stages of collagen synthesis.

Proliferation of the bile ductules in or near the portal tract is usually found in chronic liver injuries and in cholestasis. Although it is not clear what factors are involved in such proliferation, ductular proliferation accompanies fibrosis. Under the electron microscope, few fibroblasts appear in these proliferative regions; thus, to some extent, the bile ductules appear to be responsible for collagen synthesis. It is also noteworthy that small hepatocytes are often intermingled with ductular cells in such areas of ductular proliferation[52]. Pericellular fibrosis, usually seen in the centrolobular zone, is characteristic of alcoholic liver injuries and non-alcoholic fatty liver-associated fibrosis. By electron microscopy, fibrous bundles are noted around the hepatocytes and fat-storing cells, suggesting that both cells may be responsible for fibrogenesis in this type of fibrosis. Poor oxygen supply, noted in the centrolobular zone, may be one of the factors which stimulate hepatocytes or fat-storing cells to produce collagen in alcoholic liver injuries or in non-alcoholic fatty liver-associated fibrosis.

In fibrous tissue, hepatocytes are often not covered by endothelial cells and are therefore exposed to connective tissue. By immunohistochemical studies using monoclonal antibodies against collagen Types I and III, the RER of such hepatocytes is often positive for these collagens (Figure 17b). This evidence indicates that, in pathological states, the hepatocytes actively synthesize collagen proteins which may serve to protect these cells from their noxious environment.

In the areas of central sclerosis characteristically seen in alcoholic liver injuries and in non-alcoholic fatty liver-associated fibrosis, increased numbers of myofibroblasts and greater amounts of fibrous tissue are seen in the region of the central vein (Figure 18), which is often narrowed and occasionally obliterated. Thus, myofibroblasts seem to participate in this type of fibrosis. Some of these cells possess small lipid droplets and probably represent a transitional form of the fat-storing cell[48].

The basement membrane, composed mainly of collagen Types IV and V, laminin and fibronectin, can be easily recognized by electron microscopy by its electron-dense membranous structure. In normal liver, the basement membrane is found around the portal vein, hepatic artery, bile duct or ductule, large lymphatics and nerve endings in the portal tract. The basement membrane is also seen beneath the endothelial cells of the central vein and, in part, around the myofibroblast[53]. However, the membrane is not detectable in the space of Disse. From fine structural observations, it has been suggested that, in normal liver, the basement membrane is produced by the endothelial cells of the arteries and veins and by the epithelial cells of bile ducts and ductules. It has further been suggested that the basement membrane, not only contributes to the regulation of exchanges of materials occurring between the cell and its surroundings, but that it also acts as an anchor for morphogenesis[48].

In hepatic cirrhosis, the basement membrane is often detected beneath the endothelial cells of the sinusoid. A marked decrease in the number of endothelial cell fenestrations can also be seen by electron microscopy. In this state, exchanges of substances between the hepatocytes and sinusoidal lumen are inhibited, resulting in poor oxygen and nutrient supply to the hepatocyte; this has been called 'capillarization of the hepatic sinusoid'[54].

Under the electron microscope, the basement membrane is demonstrated on the surface of the hepatocytes directly facing the connective tissue. This finding indicates that the hepatocyte produce not only Types I or III collagen, but also Type IV in some pathological conditions[51]. Formed membranes seem to control the uptake and secretion of materials in the hepatocytes, protecting them from their surroundings since the hepatocytes are not covered by endothelial cells as they are in normal liver.

These fine structural observations of fibrous tissue in the liver seem to support the concept by which the fat-storing cells transform into fibroblasts or myofibroblasts, depending on their location in the lobule or the particular pathological state, and by which they play an important role in fibrogenesis, especially following hepatocellular necrosis. The myofibroblast is probably responsible for central sclerosis. The hepatocyte also seems to synthesize Types I and III collagen, and, in certain pathological states, even basement membrane proteins which probably serve a protective role.

METABOLIC DISORDERS AND STORAGE DISEASES

Since the liver constitutes the body's centre of metabolism, metabolic disorders or storage diseases are reflected by more or less extensive morphological changes at the hepatic level. Among such diseases, haemochromatosis and Wilson's disease are relatively frequently encountered.

In haemochromatosis, numerous haemosiderin granules, which contain fine ferritin particles and are surrounded by a membrane, are observed in the hepatocyte and in the Kupffer cell. In Wilson's disease, liver histology is characterized by numerous copper granules within the hepatocyte. By electron microscopy, dense granules, together with several electron-lucid globules of similar size are distributed throughout the cytoplasm[55]. Electron microscopic analysis demonstrates that these granules have a high content of copper[56]. However, in the subclinical stage of Wilson's disease, mitochondrial alterations, such as increased matrix density, widened spaces between the inner and outer membranes or loss of mitochondrial granules, are prominent[57,58].

In storage diseases of various aetiologies, substance deposits often show a characteristic fine structure[59-61]. Thus, in such diseases, electron microscopy is often diagnostic.

HEPATIC MALIGNANCIES

Hepatocellular carcinoma is the most common primary hepatic malignancy and has recently shown a rise in prevalence.

There are notable fine structural differences between the well-differentiated and poorly differentiated forms of this malignant disease[62,63]. In well-differentiated hepatocellular carcinoma, the malignant cell appears to contain structures similar to those seen in the normal hepatocyte. Alpha-type glycogen particles and small fat droplets are often seen in the cytoplasm, and bile canalicular formation is noted between two adjacent malignant cells. By contrast, poorly differentiated hepatocellular carcinoma cells show fine structures quite different from those noted in normal hepatocytes. However, bile canaliculus-like structures are occasionally detected even in the poorly differentiated form. Thus, the detection of such structures is one of the important clues for the ultrastructural diagnosis of hepatocellular carcinoma.

Fine structural observations of the areas constituting the border between malignant cells and surrounding non-malignant tissue have been incomplete. We have been paying especially close attention to these zones in small hepatocellular carcinomas. Fortunately, recent ultrasonographic techniques have rendered possible the detection of tumours less than 2 cm in diameter, as well as the removal of such small tumours by liver biopsy. In the future, the interactions between malignant cells and surrounding tissue, and, subsequently, the various modes of malignant invasion should be at least partially clarified by electron microscopy.

References

1. Setoyama, H., Sata, M., Benninger, R. P., Matsumoto, H., Ueda, H., Yoshida, H., Ikejiri, N., Kawaguchi, M., Abe, H., Tanikawa, K. and Shimizu, Y. K. (1981). Hepatitis A virus-like particles in human liver tissue. *J. Clin. Electron Microsc.*, 14, 5

2. Shimizu, K. Y., Shikata, T., Benninger, R. P., Sata, M., Setoyama, H., Abe, H. and Tanikawa, K. (1982). Detection of hepatitis A antigen in human liver. *Infect. Immun.* 36, 320

3. Tanikawa, K., Sata, M., Setoyama, H. and Abe, H. (1986). Changes of the Kupffer cell and clinical manifestations in acute hepatitis Type A. In Kirn, A., Knook, D. L. and Wisse, E. (eds.) *Cell of the Hepatic Sinusoid*, Vol. I, p. 371. (HV Rijswijk, The Netherlands: Kupffer Cell Foundation)

4. Tanikawa, K. and Sata, M. (1986). Hepatitis virus and tissue reaction in the liver. *Proceedings of XIth International Congress on Electron Microscopy*, pp. 2133. (Kyoto, Japan)

5. Gudat, F., Bianchi, L., Sonnabend, W., Thiel, G., Aenishaenslin, W. and Stalder, G. A. (1975). Pattern of core and surface expression in liver tissue reflects state of specific immune response in heptitis B. *Lab. Invest.*, 32, 1

6. Huang, S-N. and Neurath, A. R. (1979). Immunohistologic demonstration of hepatitis B viral antigens in liver, with reference to its significance in liver injury. *Lab. Invest.*, 40, 1

7. Kamimura, T., Yoshikawa, A., Ichida, F. and Sasaki, H. (1981). Electron microscopic studies of Dane particles in hepatocytes, with special reference to intracellular develop-

ment of Dane particles and their relationship with HBeAg in serum. *Hepatology*, 1, 392

8. Huang, S. N., Groh, V., Beaudoin, J. G., Dauphinee, W. D., Guttmann, R. D., Morehouse, D. D., Aronoff, A. and Gault, H. (1974). A study of the relationship of virus-like particles and Australia antigen in liver. *Hum. Pathol.*, 5, 209

9. DeVos, R., Vanstapel, M. J., Desmyter, J., DeWolf-Peeter, C., DeGroote, G., Colaert, J., Mortelmans, J., Degroore, J., Fevery, J. and Desmet, V. (1983). Are nuclear particles specific for non-A, non-B hepatitis? *Hepatology*, 3, 532

10. Shimizu, Y. K., Feinstone, S. M., Purcell, R. H., Alter, H. J. and London, W. (1979). Non-A, non-B hepatitis: Ultra-structural evidence for two agents in experimentally infected chimpanzees. *Science*, 205, 197

11. Schaffner, F. (1985). Epstein-Barr virus in chronic hepatitis. In Bianchi, L., Gerok, W. and Popper, H. (eds.) *Trends in Hepatology*, p. 209. (Lancaster: MTP Press)

12. Matsuda, Y. K., Baraona, E., Salaspuro, M. and Liever, C. S. (1979). Effects of ethanol on liver microtubules and Golgi apparatus. *Lab. Invest.*, 41, 455

13. Tandler, B., Erlandson, R. A. and Wynder, E. L. (1975) Riboflavin and mouse hepatic cell structure and function. I. Ultrastructural alterations in simple deficiency. *Am. J. Pathol.*, 52, 69

14. Tanikawa, K. and Miyakoda, U. (1973). Étude au microscope electronique des mecanismes de depot et de disparition des lipides hépatiques dans la steatose ethylique. *Ann. Gastroenterol. Hepatol.*, 9, 411

15. Yokoo, H., Minick, O., Batti, F. and Kent, G. (1972). Morphologic variants of alcoholic hyalin. *Am. J. Pathol.*, 69, 25

16. Bhatal, P. S. (1972). Presence of modified fibroblasts in cirrhotic livers in man. *Pathology*, 4, 139

17. Nakano, M., Worner, T. M. and Lieber, C. S. (1982). Perivenular fibrosis in alcoholic liver injury: ultrastructure and histologic progression. *Gastroenterology*, 83, 777

18. Kawahara, T., Sakisaka, S., Yamauchi, K., Abe, H. and Tanikawa, K. (1986). Effect of alcohol on cultured Kupffer cells. In Kirn, A., Knook, D. L. and Wisse, E. (eds.) *Cell of the Hepatic Sinusoid*, Vol. 1, p. 323. (HV Rijswijk, The Netherlands: Kupffer Cell Foundation)

19. Tanikawa, K. (1986). Effects of alcohol and bile acids on the endocytosis of the Kupffer cell. *Proceedings of XIth International Congress on Electron Microscopy*, pp. 1957. (Kyoto, Japan)

20. Trump, B. F. and Arstila, A. U. (1971). Cellular and subcellular reactions of cells to injury. In LaVia, N. and Hill, R. (eds.) *Principles of Pathobiology*, p. 9. (New York: Oxford University Press)

21. Arstila, A. U., Smith, M. and Trump, B. F. (1972). Microsomal lipid peroxidation; morphological characterization. *Science*, 175, 530

22. Trump, B. F., Dess, J. H. and Sherburne, J. S. (1973). The ultrastructure of the human liver cell and its common patterns of reaction to injury. In Gall, E. A. and Mostofi, F. K. (eds.) *The Liver*, pp. 80. (Baltimore: Williams & Wilkins)

23. Franklin, M., Schaffmer, F. and Popper, H. (1969). Hepatitis after exposure to halothane. *Ann. Intern. Med.*, 71, 467

24. Oda, T., Shikata, T. and Suzuki, H. (1969). Phospholipidosis of the liver cell: A report of three cases with a new type of fatty liver. *Acta Hepatol. Jpn.*, 10, 530

25. De La Iglesia, F. A., Feuer, G. and Takada, A. (1974). Morphologic studies on secondary phospholipidosis in human liver. *Lab. Invest.*, 30, 539

26. Elias, E. and Boyer, J. L. (1979). Mechanisms of intrahepatic cholestasis. In Popper, H. and Shaffner, F. (eds.) *Progress in Liver Diseases*, Vol. VI, p. 457. (New York: Grune & Stratton)

27. Desmet, V. J. (1972). Morphologic and histochemical aspects of cholestasis. In Popper, H. and Shaffner, F. (eds.) *Progress in Liver Diseases*, Vol. IV, p. 97. (New York: Grune & Stratton)

28. Toda, G., Kato, M., Oka, H., Oda, T. and Ikeda, Y. (1978). Uneven distribution of enzymatic alterations on the liver cell surface in experimental extrahepatic cholestasis of rat. *Exp. Mol. Pathol.*, 28, 10

29. Sternlieb, I. (1979). Electron microscopy of mitochondria and peroxisomes of human hepatocytes. In Popper, H. and Shaffner, F. (eds.) *Progress in Liver Diseases*, Vol. IV, p. 81. (New York: Grune & Stratton)

30. Mathis, R. K., Watkins, J. B., Szczepanik-Van Leeuwen, P. and Lott, I. T. (1980). Liver in the cerebro-hepatorenal syndrome: defective bile acid synthesis and abnormal mitochondria. *Gastroenterology*, 79, 1311

31. Jones, A. L. and Schmucker, D. L. (1977). Current concepts of liver structure as related to function. *Gastroenterology*, 73, 833

32. Yamauchi, H., Koyama, K., Matsuo, Y., Kashimura, S., Takagi, Y., Muto, I., Owada, Y., Otowa, T., Ouchi, K., Anezaki, T. and Itoh, K. (1975). Morphometric studies on the rat liver in biliary obstruction. *Jpn. J. Gastroenterol.*, 72, 392

33. Fisher, M. M. and Phillips, M. J. (1979). Cytoskeleton of the hepatocyte. In Popper, H. and Shaffner, F. (eds.) *Progress in Liver Diseases*, Vol. VI, p. 105. (New York: Grune & Stratton)

34. Phillips, M. J., Oda, M. and Funatsu, K. (1979). Reactions of the liver to injury. Cholestasis, its ultrastructural aspects. In Farber, E. and Fisher, M. M. (eds.) *Toxic Injury of the Liver*, Part A, p. 333. (New York: Dekker)

35. Fisher, M. M. (1979). Biochemical basis for toxic injury. Lithocholate hepatotoxicity. In Farber, E. and Fisher, M. M. (eds.) *Toxic Injury of the Liver*, Part A, p. 155. (New York: Dekker)

36. Kakis, G., Philips, M. J. and Yousef, I. M. (1980). The respective roles of membrane cholesterol and of sodium potassium adenosine triphosphatase in the pathogenesis of lithocholate-induced cholestasis. *Lab. Invest*, 43, 73

37. Phillips, M. J., Yousef, I. M., Kakis, G., Oda, M. and Funatsu, K. (1979). Biochemical pathology of canalicular membrane in intrahepatic cholestasis. In Rreisig, R. and Bircher, J. (eds.) *The Liver. Quantitative Aspects of Structure and Function*, p. 185. (Berne: Editio Cantor Aulendorf)

38. Loosli, H., Gardiol, D. and Gautier, A. (1981). Experimental intrahepatic cholestasis. *Virchows Arch. (Cell Pathol.)*, 35, 213

39. Desmet, V. J. and De Vos, R. (1982). Tight junctions in the liver. In Popper, H. and Shaffner, F. (eds.) *Progress in Liver Diseases*, Vol. VII, p. 31. (New York: Grune & Stratton)

40. Bianchi, L., Ott, R. and Rohr, H. P. (1971). Ultrastrukturell-morphometrische untersuchungen an der liberparenchym-zelle der ratte nach cholereticagabe. *Acta Hepatosplenol.*, 18, 305

41. Boyer, J. L., Itabashi, M. and Hruban, Z. (1979). Formation of pericanalicular vacuoles during sodium dehydrocholate

Rreisig, R. and Bircher, J. (eds.) *The Liver. Quantitative Aspects of Structure and Function*, p. 163. (Berne: Editio Cantor Aulendorf)

42. Jones, A. L., Schmucker, D. L., Renston, R. H. and Murakami, Y. (1980). The architecture of bile secretion. A morphological perspective of physiology. *Dig. Dis. Sci.*, **25**, 609

43. Oshio, C. and Phillips, M. J. (1981). Contractility of bile canaliculi: implications for liver function. *Science*, **212**, 1041

44. Matsumoto, H., Ikejiri, N., Eguchi, T., Abe, H. and Tanikawa, K. (1979). Ultrastructural changes of tight junction in cholestatic human liver. *J. Clin. Electron Microsc.*, **12**, 5

45. Tanikawa, K. (1980). Pathology of jaundice and cholestasis at the ultrastructural level. In *Pathology of Cell Membranes II*, p. 381. (New York: Academic Press)

46. Rubin, E., Schaffner, F. and Popper, H. (1965). Primary biliary cirrhosis. Chronic non-suppurative destructive cholangitis. *Am. J. Pathol.*, **46**, 387

47. Tanikawa, K., Sakisaka, S. and Kojima, M. (1983). Fine structural characteristics of chronic, non-suppurative, destructive cholangitis (in Japanese). *Kan Tan Sui.* **7**, 207

48. Tanikawa, K. and Ueno, T. (1985). Fine structural features and roles of fat-storing cell and basement membrane in hepatic fibrosis. In Hirayama, C. and Kivirikko, K. I. (eds.) *Pathobiology of Hepatic Fibrosis*, p. 3. (Amsterdam: Excerpta Medica)

49. Fleischmajer, R., Olsen, B. R., Timple, R., Perlish, J. S. and Lovelace, O. (1983). Collagen fibril formation during embryogenesis. *Proc. Natl. Acad. Sci.*, **80**, 3354

50. Tanikawa, K. (1975). Ultrastructure of hepatic fibrosis and fat-storing cells. In Popper, H. and Becker, K. (eds.) *Collagen Metabolism in the Liver*, p. 93. (New York: Stratton Intercontinental Medical Book)

51. Clement, B., Grimaud, J-A., Campion, J-P., Deugnier, Y. and Guillouzo, A. (1986). Cell types involved in collagen and fibronectin production in normal and fibrotic human liver. *Hepatology*, **6**, 225

52. Phillips, P. A. and Purcell, S. (1981). Modern aspects of the morphology of viral hepatitis. *Hum. Pathol.*, **12**, 1060

53. Tanikawa, K., Ueno, T. and Sakisaka, S. (1985). Basement membrane in the liver and its changes. In Shibata, S. (ed.) *Basement Membrane*, p. 453. (Amsterdam: Elsevier Science Publishers)

54. Schaffner, F. and Popper, H. (1963). Capillarization of hepatic sinusoids in man. *Gastroenterology*, **44**, 239

55. Tanikawa, K. (1968). *Ultrastructural Aspects of the Liver and its Disorders*, p. 218, (Berlin: Springer-Verlag)

56. Tanikawa, K., Abe, H. and Miyakada, U. (1973). Electron microscopic observation and X-ray analysis of deposit granules in the hepatocyte. *J. Clin. Electron Microsc.*, **6**, 332

57. Sternlieb, I. (1968). Mitochondrial and fatty changes in hepatocytes of patients with Wilson's disease. *Gastroenterology*, **55**, 354

58. Sternlieb, I. (1972). Evolution of the hepatic lesion in Wilson's disease (hepatolenticular degeneration). In Popper, H. and Schaffer, F. (eds.) *Progress in Liver Diseases*, Vol IV, p. 511. (New York: Grune & Stratton)

59. Hers, H. G. and Van Hoof, F. (1970). The genetic pathology of lysosomes. In Popper, H. and Schaffner, F. (eds.) *Progress in Liver Diseases*, Vol III, p. 185. (New York: Grune & Stratton)

60. Volk, B. H., Wellmann, K. F. and Wallace, B. J. (1970). Hepatic changes in various lipidoses: electron microscopic and histochemical studies. In Popper, H. and Schaffner, F. (eds.) *Progress in Liver Diseases*, Vol III, p. 206. (New York: Grune & Stratton)

61. Hug, G. (1973). Non-bilirubin genetic disorders of the liver. In Gall, E. A. and Mostofi, F. K. (eds.) *The Liver*, p. 21. (Baltimore: Williams & Wilkins)

62. Tanikawa, K. (1979). *Ultrastructural Aspects of the Liver and its Disorders*, 2nd Edn., p. 338. (Tokyo, Igaku-shoin)

63. Isomura, T. and Nakashima, T. (1980). Ultrastructure of human hepatocellular carcinoma. *Acta Pathol. Jpn.*, **30**, 713

11

Normal and pathological liver cells as studied in freeze-fracture replicas

J. METZ and H. ROBENEK

INTRODUCTION

The freeze-fracture technique has become a routine procedure for the preparation of biological specimens for electron microscopic analysis within the last 25 years. The methodological development, practical aspects as well as innovations of the procedure, have been reviewed by several authors[1-4]. In practice, rapidly frozen tissue is fractured in vacuum and the exposed surface is shadowed with carbon–platinum to give a replica which yields a three-dimensional image of the ultrastructure when studied in the transmission electron microscope. Cells are fractured either in a crosswise manner, revealing cytoplasm and cell organelles, or the fracture level runs intramembranously, principally following the central hydrophobic plane of the lipid bilayer, exposing the inner faces of the membrane. According to the nomenclature that was established in 1975, the exposed part of the bilayer, which is directed to the extracellular space, is called the E-face, while the P-face is the exposed part adjacent to the cytoplasm[5].

The major advantage of the freeze-fracture method is to give more information on the ultrastructural details of intra- and extracellular membranes and their specializations, such as intercellular junctions. Freeze-fracturing and standard thin section methods, in combination with tracer experiments and biochemical analyses, offer additional information on the functional geometry, e.g. of the membrane specializations[6-8].

NORMAL LIVER

The liver was among the first organs to be ultrastructurally analysed using the freeze-fracture method[9]. Misinterpretations, which were made soon after the introduction of this method and primarily concerned the fracture levels within the hepatocellular plasmalemma, have been ruled out in the meantime[9-13].

Sinus endothelial cell

The sinusoids constitute an abundant vascular network within the liver lobules that converges from the lobular periphery towards the central veins. The sinusoidal endo-thelial cells delineate with their inner surfaces the blood space, while their outer circumference faces the perisinusoid space of Disse. In human and most mammals, endothelial cells form a continuous wall that displays sieve areas, where numerous openings (fenestrations) of various sizes are arranged[14] (Figure 1). The diameter of the fenestrations seems to be influenced by various parameters[15,16]. Blood cells down to the level of thrombocytes appear to be restricted from passage, as well as chylomicrons[15].

Kupffer cell

The Kupffer cells are situated within the lumen of the sinusoids. In freeze-fracture images, they differ from the endothelial cells by their irregular surface structure (Figure 2). Numerous membrane-enclosed vesicles, which are mainly lysosomes, are present within these cells.

Hepatocyte

Plasmalemma

A functional polarization of the hepatocytes is indicated, not only by the arrangement of the organelles within the cytoplasm, but can also be derived from structural variations of the plasmalemma and its specializations. Distinct membrane areas (domains) on the cell surface can be differentiated depending on the location of the hepatocyte within the lobule:

(a) Plasmalemmal areas facing the perisinusoidal Disse's space (basal or perisinusoidal hepatocyte plasmalemmal domain),

(b) Plasmalemmal areas on the transition from the perisinusoidal to the interhepatocellular space (basolateral or juxtasinusoidal hepatocyte plasmalemmal domain),

(c) Plasmalemmal surfaces between the hepatocytes (lateral hepatocyte plasmalemmal domain) which exhibit the membrane specializations of the interhepatocellular contacts (nexus, zonulae occludentes, desmosomes),

(d) Plasmalemmal surfaces that limit the bile canaliculi (bile canalicular hepatocyte plasmalemmal domain).

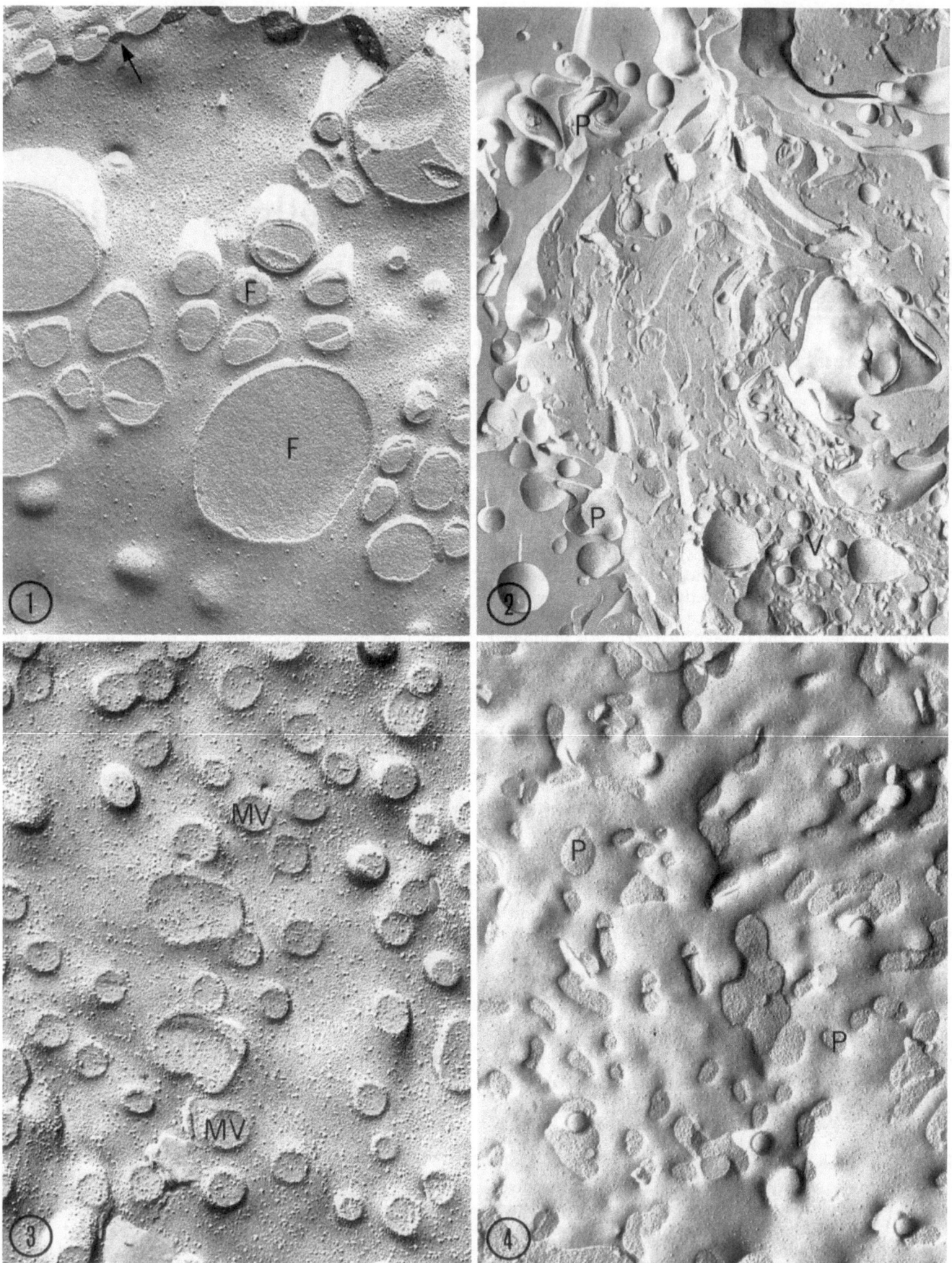

Figure 1 Freeze-fracture of a sinusoidal endothelial cell: fenestrations (F) of different size suggest a size-dependent permeability between the lumen of the sinus and the Disse space. Crosswise fractures (arrows) through the cytoplasm show the small diameter of the endothelial wall. × 48 000

Figure 2 Kupffer cell fractured crosswise: the surface exhibits frequent protrusions and processes (P). Numerous vesicular structures (V), which probably represent lysosomes, are seen in the cytoplasm. × 12 000

Figure 3 P-face of an intramembranous fracture of the perisinusoidal domain of a hepatocyte: numerous microvillous structures (MV) are fractured crosswise. × 57 600

Figure 4 Freeze-fracture of the basolateral hepatocellular domain: cytoplasmic protrusions (P), larger in size than the microvillous structures on the perisinusoidal domain, are fractured crosswise. × 38 400

Additional plasmalemmal areas are found in only a limited number of cells, for example, those cells which contact portal connective tissue or the central veins.

Basal (perisinusoidal) plasmalemmal domain: The surface area of the hepatocyte facing the perisinusoidal (Disse) space exhibits numerous microvillous and irregularly shaped cytoplasmic protrusions (Figure 3). A few collagen bundles and nerve fibres, which often possess varicosities adjacent to the hepatocyte, are located within the perisinusoidal space.

Basolateral (juxtasinusoidal) plasmalemmal domain: In comparison with the basal plasmalemmal domain, larger and more irregular protrusions are typical of the basolateral hepatocyte surface (Figure 4). This transitional area between the basal and the lateral membrane compartments, however, is variable and may change under pathological conditions.

Lateral plasmalemmal domain: The interhepatocellular plasmalemma is smooth in the region between two adjacent hepatocytes and exhibits interdigitations on the transition where three hepatocytes abut. Numerous membrane-associated particles, which range in size from 6 to 120 nm, are randomly distributed on the P-face of the membrane. Fewer particles are generally found on the E-face. The unequal distribution of particles suggests membrane asymmetry. Experimental evidence indicates that the particles are mainly protein components, while the smooth areas between the particles represent lipid molecules. Gap junctions (nexus) and desmosomes (maculae adherentes) are observed in mediolateral and juxtabiliary areas. Tight junctions demarcate the border of the bile canalicular membrane.

Gap junction (nexus, macula communicans): Gap junctions are identified in freeze-fracture replicas as irregularly formed macular arrays of particle aggregations on the P-face and corresponding pits on the E-face of the plasmalemma[12–18] (Figures 5 and 6). They have been detected in all species examined, including human. Particle aggregations situated within juxtabiliary plasmalemmal regions are often closely associated with tight-junctional strands. The number and size of these particle aggregations vary between species and are dependent on the physiological and pathological stage of the hepatocytes[6,19,20]. In human liver, gap junctions occupy about 1% of the hepatocellular plasmalemma[21,22]. In rat and mice particle aggregations are larger and account about 1.5% of the total hepatocyte surface or 2.9–3.6% of the lateral plasmalemmal domain[6,19].

The formation of gap junctions between cells was investigated in embryonic tissue[21,23] and in cell cultures[24]. According to these studies, 'large' precursor particles appear within formation plaques on the plasmalemma. They assemble in progressively enlarging polygonal arrangements of junctional particles, which seem to be smaller than the precursor particles. Similar results were obtained in hepatectomized[20] and cholestatic[25] animals where disappearance and reconstitution of gap junctions were studied.

Gap junctions are specialized membrane regions of intercellular contact that serve as the pathway for cell-to-cell communication[26–29]. Experimentally, the intercellular

passage of substances between cells via gap junctions has been demonstrated[30]. Intercellular communication has also been shown electrophysiologically. Thus, communicating hepatocytes may be referred to as electronically or metabolically coupled. However, it is not possible to predict, on the basis of routine freeze-fracture studies, to what degree particle aggregations are in a coupled state, since gap junctions uncouple during aldehyde fixation[31].

Tight junction (zonula occludens): The tight junctional complex is a specialized area at the border between the bile canaliculus and the lateral hepatocytic plasmalemma. In thin sections, the zonula occludens forms a continuous zone of intimate contacts between the plasma membranes of neighbouring liver cells. In freeze-fracture replicas, the junctional structure is confined to narrow belt-like arrays, which, in aldehyde-fixed tissue, usually consists of 3–5 continuous strands on the P-face of the membrane[32] (Figure 7). The lumen is lined by an uninterrupted strand, from which anastomoses extend laterally to other parallelly running strands. Perpendicularly arranged strands of varying length extend frequently towards the lateral hepatocellular plasmalemma. Aggregations of particles are occasionally intercalated at places where the strands intersect. On the E-face of the membrane, complementary grooves or pits correspond to the strands or to the particle aggregations on the P-face (Figures 7 and 8). On blind originations or on outpocketings of bile canaliculi, strands are more numerous. At points where the edges of three hepatocytes abut, the tight junctional meshwork exhibits a lateral extension with a structurally different pattern compared with the juxtabiliary network. On the P-face, parallel (horizontally) to the course of the bile canaliculus, arranged strands extend at various levels from a thick perpendicularly running strand and connect in a ladder-like fashion other vertical elements (Figure 9). The formation of tight junctions in the liver is similar to that in other organs. In embryonic liver, tight-junctional structures grow around newly developing bile canaliculi by aligning particles within the presumptive pericanalicular region of the plasmalemma[23,33]. After subsequent fusion into beaded ridges, they transform into smooth unbroken lines which are often arranged in discontinuous networks. Small clusters of tightly packed particles which probably represent developing or mature gap junctions are characteristically associated with these tight junctional structures.

Functionally, tight junctions around the bile canaliculi appear to build a permeability barrier between the biliary and interhepatocytic compartments, restricting paracellular transfer. This is shown in studies where electron-dense tracers are applied via the blood circulation[6,34–37]. Functional conclusions, based solely on the freeze-fracture image of the tight junctional arrangement, can be made only with reservation, since the nature of the intercellular sealing is still unsolved.

Difficulty in identification arises where junctional structures within the juxtabiliary plasmalemma of adult hepatocytes are mixed, e.g. when particle aggregations are intercalated between strands. They are either considered as part of a pool of unorganized structural subunits of the tight junctional strands, or regarded as gap junctions. Experimental data indicate that particle aggre-

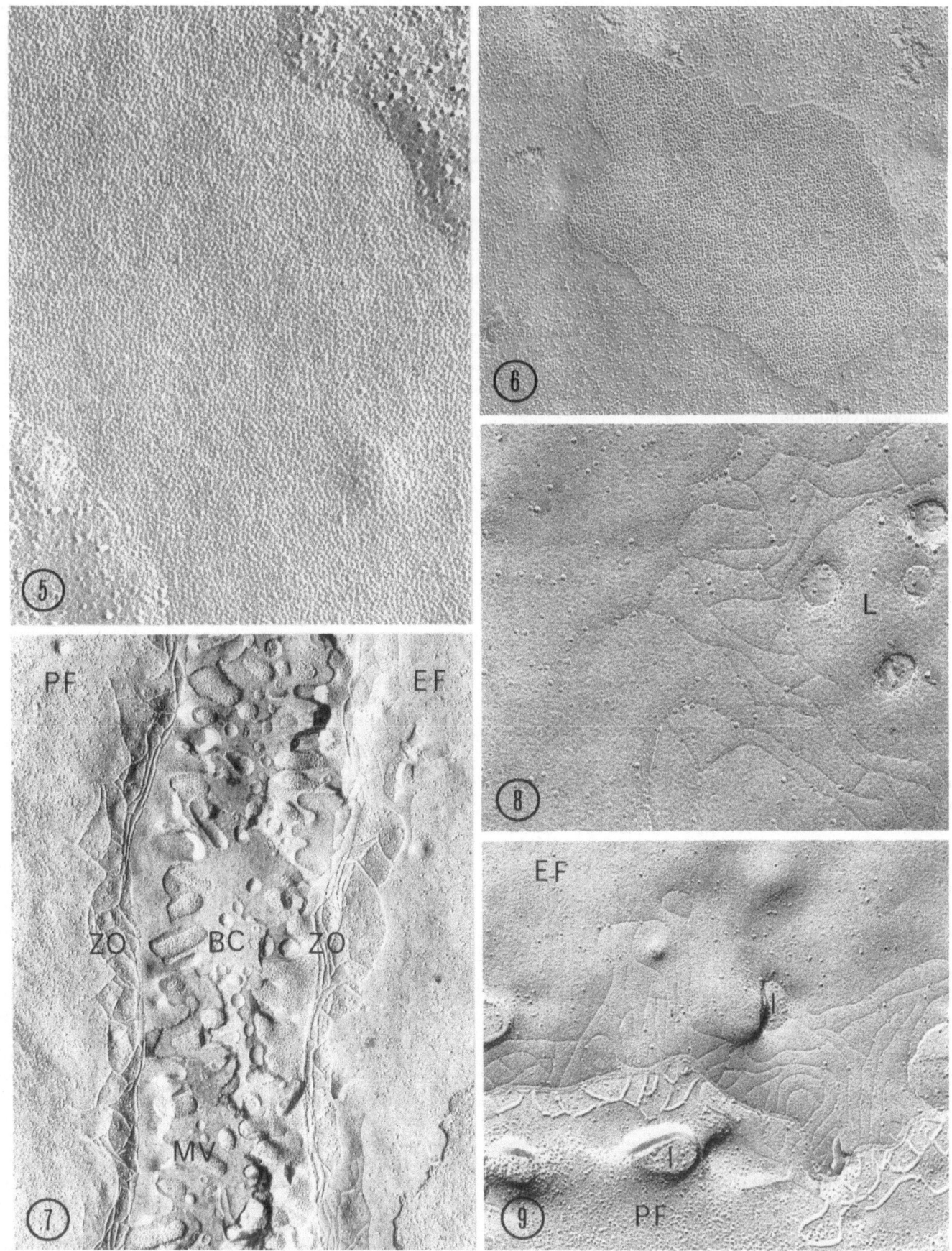

Figure 5 E-face of a gap junction on the lateral hepatocellular plasmalemma: characteristically, pits are seen in contrast to surrounding plasmalemma, where randomly distributed particles are scattered. × 106 000

Figure 6 P-face of the lateral plasmalemmal domain: the gap-junctional area is identified by the densely packed particle aggregation. × 53 000

Figure 7 Arrangement of a bile canaliculus (BC) and the demarcating zonula occludens (ZO) of a human hepatocyte: the canalicular lumen exhibits numerous microvilli (MV). P-Face (PF); E-Face (EF) of the hepatocyte plasma membrane. × 48 000

Figure 8 E-Face of the juxtabiliary plasmalemmal area: a network of grooves represents the zonula occludens. Lumen of the bile canaliculus (L). × 96 000

Figure 9 Freeze-fracture of a contact area of three hepatocytes: the lateral extension of the zonula occludens is fractured on the E-Face (EF) and P-Face (PF) of the plasmalemma. Interdigitations (I) are fractured crosswide. × 62 400

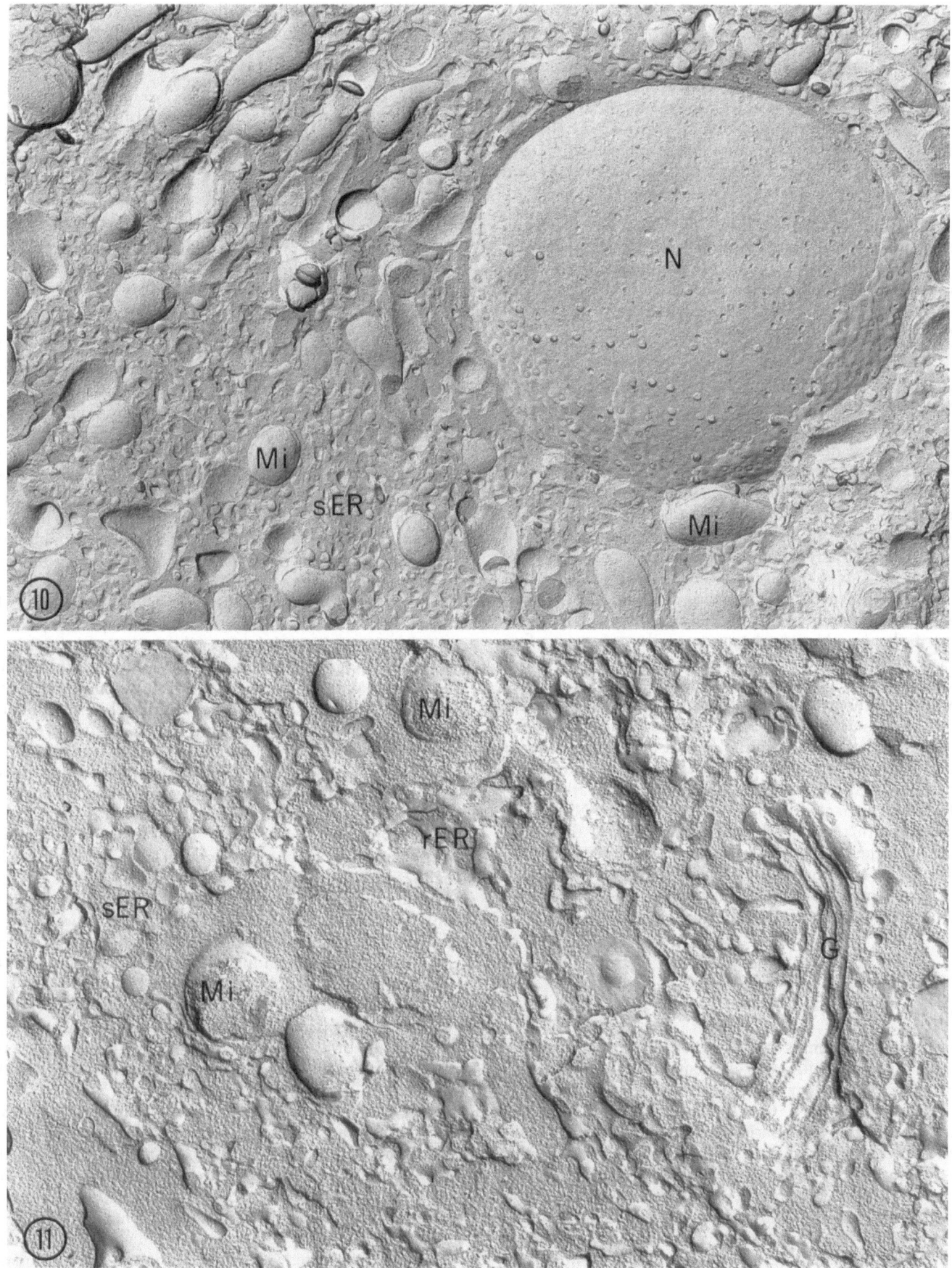

Figure 10 Crosswise-fracture through the cytoplasm of a human hepatocyte: the nuclear envelope (N), which exhibits numerous pores, is fractured along the E-face and P-face. The larger vesicular structures correspond mainly to mitochondria (Mi). The smooth endoplasmic reticulum (sER) exhibits an intricate system of small vesicular structures. × 22 000

Figure 11 Freeze-fracture through a normal human hepatocyte: membrane faces of the Golgi apparatus (G), mitochondria (Mi), rough (rER) and smooth endoplasmic reticulum (sER) are seen. × 59 500

gations arise more frequently in the juxtabiliary region under certain pathological conditions[6,25].

Desmosome (macula adherens): Desmosomes are found in variable numbers at the lateral hepatocytic plasmalemma of several species. In men, they are predominantly located in the proximal regions near the bile canaliculi[21]. The freeze-fracture image exhibits numerous granules and short segments of filaments on the E- and P-faces.

Bile canalicular plasmalemma: The canaliculi are small bile spaces which arise as blind branches between the hepatocytes in the centre of the lobules and continue finally into larger canalicular structures in the periportal regions. Microvilli and larger protrusions project from the wall into the lumen which has a diameter of 0.5–1.5 μm (Figure 7).

Cytoplasm: Within the cytoplasm of the large polyhedral hepatocytes, generally one or two round nuclei are centrally located. Nuclear pores between the outer and inner membranes are distributed randomly and comprise about 8% of the surface[21] (Figure 10). The inner membrane exhibits numerous associated particles, whereas the outer membrane of the nuclear envelope is smooth. Fractures running along the external membrane of the mitochondria reveal larger numbers of particles on the P-face than on the E-face (Figure 10). The interior arrangement of crosswise-fractured mitochondria is clearly distinguishable only in deeply etched specimens. The cisternae of the rough endoplasmic reticulum appear often as parallel lamellae which exhibit typical fenestrations (Figure 11). In smooth endoplasmic reticulum, anastomosing tubular and caveolar structures are prominent in building an irregular intricate network (Figure 10). The Golgi complex is found in the area of the bile canalicular membrane (Figure 11). This cell organelle consists of closely packed membranous structures which form parallel lamellae that exhibit lateral enlargements. Numerous vesicular structures are found at the faces of the membranes, suggesting a rather dynamic status. Numerous corpuscular structures, in the range of 0.2–2.0 μm, which represent lysosomes, fat droplets or vacuoles, are distributed throughout the cytoplasm.

PATHOLOGICAL LIVER CELLS

Cholestasis

Cholestasis in animals can be experimentally induced by obstructing the bile duct system (extrahepatic cholestasis)[6,25,35,38-46] or by administering drugs (intrahepatic cholestasis)[13-32,36,47-65]. One hypothesis to explain the pathway of bile regurgitation into the blood during cholestasis is the free passage of bile from the bile canaliculus to the sinusoid. Structural alterations of the canaliculosinusoidal barrier (=tight junctions) following cholestasis provide a possible pathway for bile regurgitation. In recent studies using the freeze-fracture technique in combination with tracer experiments, altered geometrical arrangement and focal disruptions of the zonula occludens were correlated with increased permeability properties of the canaliculo-sinusoidal barrier after bile duct ligation in rats[6,25]. In a few studies, similar alterations in

the plasmalemmal specializations have been shown during extrahepatic cholestasis in man[22,66,67].

Extrahepatic cholestasis

The freeze-fracture technique, in combination with morphometric methods, was employed to evaluate normal morphology and assess quantitative changes in the intercellular junctions in the human liver following extrahepatic cholestasis.

Fracture images of the bile canaliculi reveal that the diameter of the canalicular lumen within cholestatic livers is not quite as uniform as in control specimens (Figure 12). Dilatation of the canalicular space and loss of the microvilli are the prominent changes observed. The margins of the canaliculi are irregular, and outpouchings, side branches and large extensions are frequent. The branching pattern and the number of strands of the zonulae occludentes are altered. Various degrees of response to cholestasis are found, varying from approximately unmodifed junctions to completely destroyed contacts, and the wide range of variations seems to be randomly distributed in the tissue of a given patient. Most of the zonulae occludentes lose the typical arrangement of their strands (Figures 12–14). The primarily more or less parallelly arranged luminal strands become less ordered, forming a network of frequently anastomosing ridges. Tight junctional strands are no longer just associated with the bile canaliculus, but also appear on the lateral plasmalemmal domain. Partly they are scattered all over the surface of the lateral domain without a preferential topography. Quantitative analysis reveals that both normal and cholestatic livers show great variability in the length of tight junctions per μm of bile canaliculus; the values range from 4 to 14 μm (mean 7.4 μm) in normal livers and from 2 to 20 μm (mean 6.5 μm = −12%) in cholestatic livers. The same phenomenon applies to the width and number of tight junctional strands. The mean width of the zonula occludens in 0.32 μm in the normal liver, consisting on average of 5.4 strands. Zonulae occludentes in the cholestatic livers have a mean width of 0.25 μm (= −19%) and 4.4 strands (−19%). Tight junctions in cholestatic livers are frequently reduced to only one strand. Most importantly, interruptions within the zonulae occludentes suggest that no junctional seals may exist in these regions, resulting in a leakage of the canaliculo-sinusoidal barrier (Figure 14).

Claude and Goodenough[68] correlated the permeability of various epithelia with the freeze-fracture morphology of tight junctions in these tissues. They proposed a classification, based on the width of the tight junctions and the number of strands, ranging from 'very leaky' to 'very tight'. Using these criteria, the permeability characteristics of the tight junctions of normal human liver might fall in the range of 'leaky' to 'tight'. However, the general applicability of these findings has been debated[69,70]. In our opinion, average values do not provide reliable information about actual permeability characteristics along the course of the bile canaliculi. The zonulae occludentes in normal human liver occasionally consist of only one strand; however, interruptions are never found. The assumption that one strand is sufficient to restrict the passage of bile into the blood circulation is confirmed by the clinical aspect and by tracer exper-

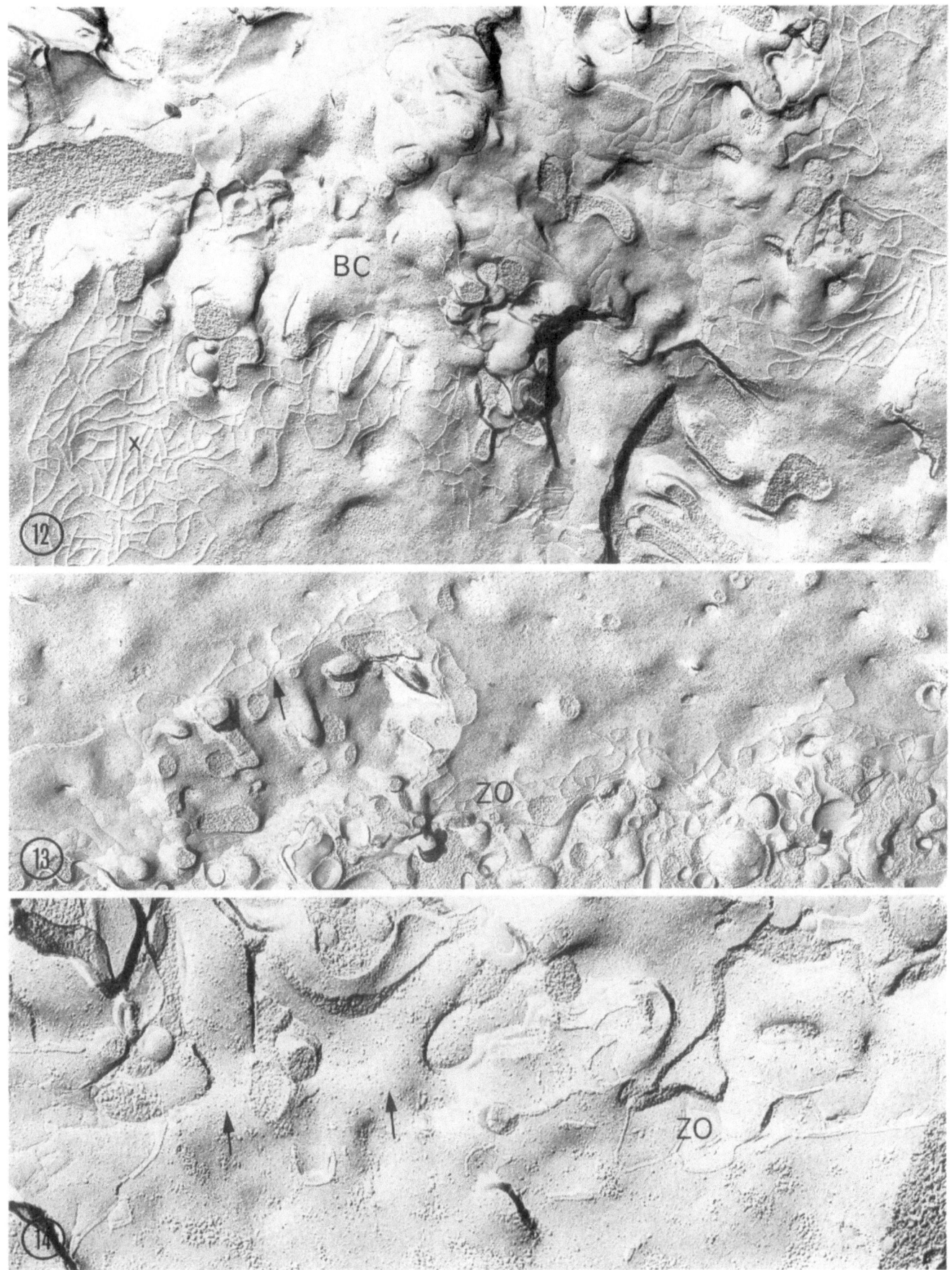

Figure 12 Human cholestatic liver: the bile canaliculus (BC) is enlarged and exhibits an irregular course. The zonula occludens reaches in restricted regions (*) the depth of about 1.5–2.0 μm and covers broad areas of plasma membrane around the bile canaliculus. × 33 000

Figure 13 Human cholestatic liver: regional disorganization of the zonula occludens (ZO). The tight-junctional strands are loosened, and their number is sometimes reduced to one or two strands (arrow). × 21 000

Figure 14 Human cholestatic liver: a broad interruption (arrows) of the zonula occludens (ZO) is seen. × 57 600

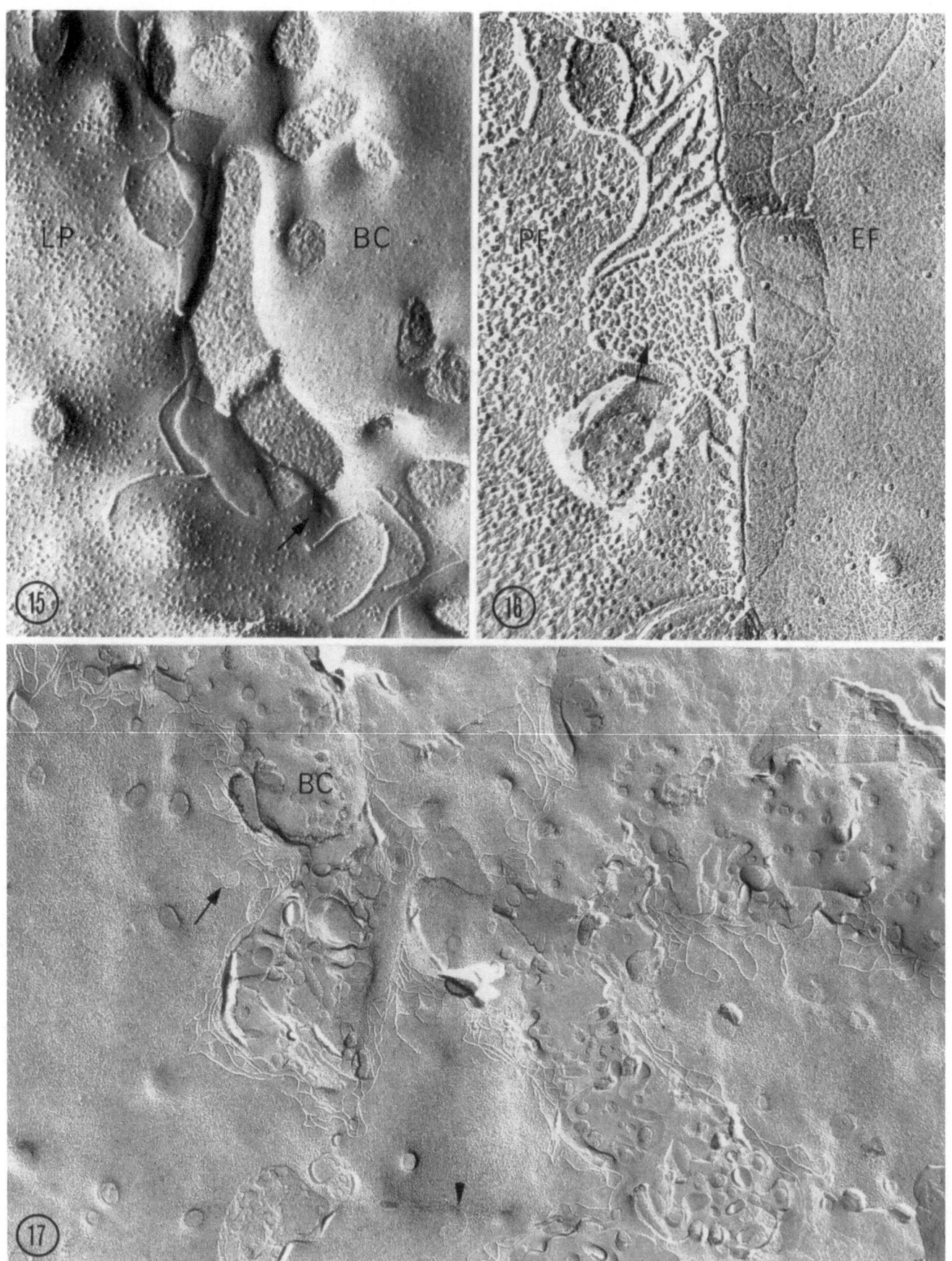

Figure 15 Rat cholestatic liver: disorganization of the zonula occludens, and a diminution of the number and interruptions of the strands (arrow) are seen. E-face of the bile canalicular plasmalemma (BC); P-face of the lateral hepatocellular plasmalemma (LP). × 125 000

Figure 16 Regeneration experiment: 24 hours after recanalization of the common bile duct particle aggregation (arrow) is found intercalated in the tight-junctional network. P-Face and E-Face of the membrane. × 86 400

Figure 17 Regeneration experiment: at low magnification, the irregular course of the bile canaliculi (BC), disorganization of the tight-junctional network and strand-associated particle aggregations (arrow) are seen. A small gap junction (arrowhead) is located on the lateral plasmalemmal domain. × 29 000

iments in animals. In rats, lanthanum and peroxidase do not pass across tight junctions under normal conditions, while in cholestasis an increase in permeability is seen[6,11,36,37,71-73]. If, on the other hand, the data for cholestatic livers are considered, the assumption can be made that it is not the reduction in number, but rather actual interruptions, of tight-junctional strands, which are responsible for the escape of bile into the blood[6]. The general reduction and disorganization of the zonulae occludentes may be interpreted as a consequence and adaptation of the liver to increased bile canalicular pressure; however, probably without any effect on the permeability characteristics. Gap junctions in the normal human liver occupy approximately 1% of the hepatocyte plasma membrane. In the cholestatic liver, the gap-junction area is drastically diminished to 0.3% (−60%), whereas the number of gap junctions is reduced by 14%. As far as particle packing is concerned, an increase in spacing is often observed between individual particles. Gap junctions, however, partially exhibit particles clustered into tighter and more ordered arrays than in controls. Metabolic co-operation between hepatocytes in the cholestatic liver is judged to be drastically reduced as a consequence of the considerable loss of gap-junctional area[6]. The extent to which the suspected reduction in metabolic communication may be the source of imbalances in metabolic activity, or of a more individual behaviour of adjacent hepatocytes, requires further investigation.

Regeneration after extrahepatic cholestasis: Regeneration of liver cells has been investigated following experimental extrahepatic cholestasis in rats[25] and guinea pigs[45]. In rats, forty-eight hours after common bile duct ligation, the ligature was released, and, after successful recanalization, which was biochemically judged, ultrastructural studies of the liver were performed[25].

Reformation of tight-junctional structures in the juxtabiliary area of the hepatocytes is observed even 45 min after release of the ligature. The strands, which, similar to the alterations in human cholestatic liver, exhibit interruptions in their continuity, irregularities in their pattern, as well as diminished numbers (Figure 15), now become continuous, regularly arranged, and their number increases. Small clusters of particles intercalated more frequently within the strands appear to contribute to their reconstitution (Figure 16). Although bilirubin values return to normal within 24 h after recanalization, the configuration and geometry, compared with controls, is reestablished only after 72-96 h (Figure 17).

The first stages of gap-junctional reformation are characterized by aggregations of single particles, which progressively assemble into clusters and groups. Since these structures appear within the tight-junctional network, in the juxtabiliary region as well as in the area of the lateral hepatocellular plasmalemma, it is probable that reformation of gap junctions occurs at more than one site (Figure 17)[25]. Gap junctions appear in excess, at least temporarily, in the juxtacanalicular area, suggesting that they form predominantly in this region. After 72-96 h, however, the distribution and appearance of gap junctions on the lateral hepatocellular plasmalemma is similar to that of controls again. The regeneration of junctional structures after recanalization experiments in rats[25] and

guinea pigs[45] was similar to that after partial hepatectomy in rats[19,20].

Intrahepatic cholestasis

Oestradiol valerate: Oestrogens have long been recognized as agents capable of producing intrahepatic cholestasis with jaundice[64], the pathogenesis of which is controversially discussed. Limited secretion of bile components has been proposed[74], while other investigators favour diffusion via the tight junctions as a decisive factor[75,76].

Morphological alterations in bile canaliculi and extensive alterations in the tight-junctional pattern were induced by long-term administration of œstradiol valerate (1.5 mg (kg body weight)$^{-1}$ week^{-1}) – a distinctly lower dosage than that used by other authors[48] in order not to exceed the clinical dose range in an unrealistic manner and to eliminate secondary alterations caused by very pronounced cholestasis which might overshadow the original pathogenetic factors – over a period of 20 weeks to male Wistar rats[36,50]. Most of the zonulae occludentes lose the typical arrangement of their strands. The luminal strands, usually more or less parallel, become less orderly and form a network of frequently anastomosing ridges. In restricted areas, the zonulae occludentes increase in width, indicating localized proliferation. Compared with controls, there appear to be many simplified junctions. Although the number of strands in general is diminished and very narrow junctions, consisting of only one or two strands, are present, morphological interruptions in the tight-junctional strands are never observed. Our morphological interpretation that tight junctions, both in controls and in oestrogen-treated animals, are impermeable to medium-sized molecules, such as bile acids, is supported by perfusion studies which show that the barrier is tight, at least with respect to colloidal lanthanum. Noticeable intramembranous particle aggregations on the P face of the lateral plasmalemma, which correspond to a random arrangement of particles on the P face of the bile canaliculus, might be a further indication of the integrity of an additional tight-junctional function (Figure 18). The conception that zonulae occludentes may prevent mixing of the components between various zones of a continuous membrane is also supported by other studies[77].

Long-term treatment with oestradiol valerate also induces distinct alterations in gap junctions with a noteworthy temporal pattern. The variations involve the spacing and regularity of packing of the membrane particles on the P face and the complementary pits on the E face, as well as changes in the number, size and shape of the junctional domains. Three remarkable results are established in the oestrogen-treated animals:

(1) The average size of gap junctions decreases.

(2) The number of gap junctions per unit area of lateral plasma membrane increases.

(3) Alterations in the gap junctions vary over the 20 weeks experimental period and exhibit a clear-cut time dependence.

Bile salts: Taurolithocholate: Taurolithocholate is known to cause severe intrahepatic cholestasis in rats and

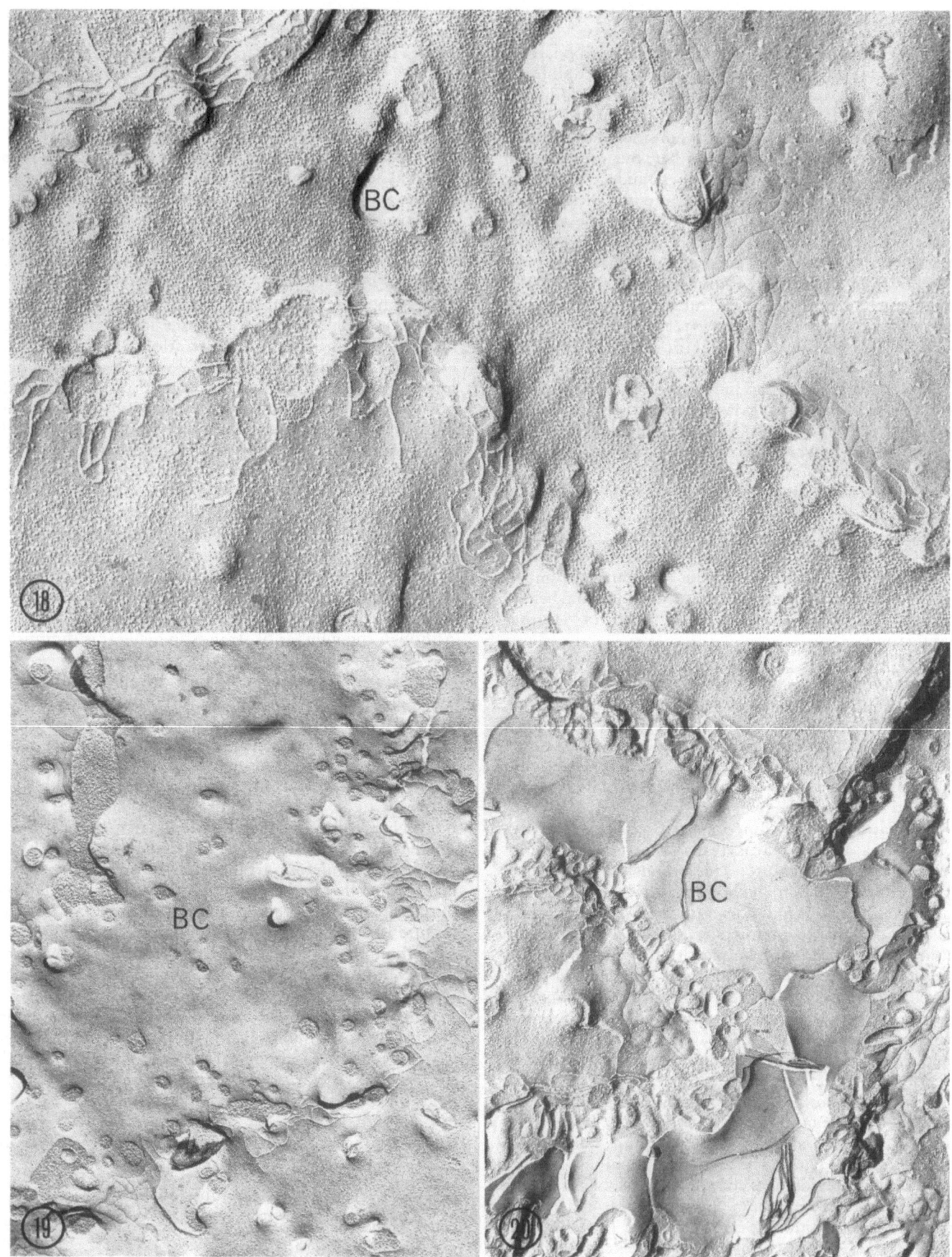

Figure 18 Oestradiol valerate: fracture faces of the bile canalicular (BC) and lateral plasmalemmal domain after 16 weeks of treatment with oestradiol valerate. The P-face of the plasma membrane displays aggregations of intramembranous particles, whereas the P-face of the bile canalicular membrane maintains the normal random distribution of particles found in controls. Note the loss of microvilli. × 53 800

Figure 19 Taurolithocholate: dilated canaliculus (BC) showing a loss of microvilli after treatment with sodium taurolithocholate for 24 h. × 37 400

Figure 20 Taurolithocholate (24 h): bizarre transformation of canaliculus (BC) showing fractured lamellar membranes. Note the absence of intramembranous particles. × 27 400

hamsters[51,55,65,78]. In this type of acute cholestasis, specific ultrastructural changes in the bile canalicular membrane and in the pericanalicular region can be demonstrated by transmission and scanning electron microscopy[56,58-60,79].

Freeze-fracture studies show that administration of a single dose (100 mg (kg body weight)$^{-1}$) of sodium taurolithocholate to male Wistar rats results in characteristic ultrastructural changes located primarily within the bile canaliculi, whereas intracellular organelles are hardly affected. A few dilated bile canaliculi with partial or total loss of microvilli can be detected as early as 4 h after treatment and are most prominent after 12 to 24 h when only a few canaliculi remain virtually unaffected (Figure 19). Frequently, bizarre transformations of the canalicular membrane, consisting of multiple projections and a diverticulation of the canalicular wall, are observed (Figure 20). As is obvious from freeze-fracture replicas, intramembranous particles are almost completely absent from the wide and thin lamellae, whereas membrane areas maintaining their normal configuration are studded with these particles. In addition to changes in the canalicular membrane, extensive alterations in the tight-junctional pattern occur. The strands show a highly irregular pattern and fragmentation. It seems possible that the fragments detach from the pericanalicular complex and move abluminally, where they become dispersed on the lateral plane of the plasma membrane, forming small macular tight junctions. Recently, we have shown that primary monolayer cultures of rat hepatocytes are a suitable experimental system to study 'de novo' synthesis of bile canaliculi and that they may serve as an appropriate model of taurolithocholate-induced cholestasis[52,80,81]. Exposure of cultured hepatocytes to sodium taurolithocholate resulted in severe ultrastructural changes, similar to those observed in rat livers in vivo[59,60] as well as in isolated perfused livers[58]. Localization of cholesterol in plasma membranes of taurolithocholate-affected hepatocytes by the use of filipin[82] revealed extensive accumulation of cholesterol in membranes of dilated canaliculi and also in outpouchings of the contiguous membrane in the immediate vicinity. Furthermore, a pronounced secretion of cholesterol-rich membrane material into the lumen of dilated canaliculi and into enlargements of the intercellular space could be observed. In contrast, a total absence of cholesterol was noted in the lamellar projections of the bizarre transformed canaliculi[52].

Experimental intoxication

Despite the volume of literature pertaining to the zonula occludens, our knowledge, so far, about their chemical composition and relationship to the other components of the plasmalemma is still limited and fragmentary[83]. To study the development and function of tight junctions in more detail, it is important that their modulation can be induced at will. Recently, it is becoming increasingly clear that modulation of the tight-junctional organization is a relatively common reaction to a number of different kinds of physiological stimuli. Thus, the production of experimental changes in the organization of tight junctions in the liver has provided model systems suitable for ultrastructural research on their derivation, formation and function[21,84-86].

Galactosamine

After administration of the amino sugar, D-galactosamine, to rats, a dose-dependent diffuse hepatocellular injury develops, with focal necrosis and an inflammatory infiltration of the periportal regions[87]. Secondary lesions, resulting from an inhibition of uracil-nucleotide-dependent synthesis of macromolecules, occur and structural disturbances of cell organelles, particularly nucleoli, endoplasmic reticulum and plasmalemma, are evident[88].

24 h after administration of 500 mg (kg body weight)$^{-1}$ galactosamine, freeze-fracture replicas reveal that the number of gap junctions is focally reduced and the tight-junctional network becomes disarranged[21]. The number of strands is often reduced and their continuity is interrupted. Often, a particulate substructure of strands is obvious. Perpendicularly running strands appear in a direction toward the lateral plasmalemma and also toward the bile canalicular compartment. After application of 1500 mg (kg body weight)$^{-1}$, however, severely necrotic areas with disintegration of parenchymal cell groups are observed. Gap junctions and zonulae occludentes diminish and are often absent from their typical location (Figures 21 and 22). Separated and dislocated fragments of zonulae occludentes are seen scattered over the lateral hepatocyte membrane.

Several cell organelles are affected besides the hepatocellular plasmalemma and its specializations. The number of nuclear pores is reduced and they are frequently aggregated in groups within the nuclear envelope, suggesting a large disturbance of the nuclear metabolism (Figure 23). Lamellar structures that consist of whorled membranes are particularly conspicuous in the cytoplasm of parenchymal cells in freeze-fracture replicas (Figure 24). Cisternae of rough endoplasmic reticulum are frequently continuous with the lamellar structures. Many fat droplets are observed in the altered hepatocytes (Figure 25). Although the lesions of the hepatocytes caused by galactosamine appear to be an expression of a multifactorial process, the alterations in the extra- and intracellular membranes and in the intercellular junctions could be primarily evoked by disturbances of cellular calcium metabolism[89].

N-Nitrosomorpholine (NNM)

The administration of NNM offers a model for investigation of proliferation and evolution of tight junctions in the rat liver. After 2 to 10 weeks of chronic administration of N-nitrosomorpholine[84], extensive dilatation of the canaliculi and a wide variety of responses of tight junctions are observed using the freeze-fracture technique. A loosening of the abluminal meshwork of the zonulae occludentes is seen after two weeks of treatment. The predominantly long strands oriented parallel to the bile canaliculus seem to remain unaffected. After chronic administration of NNM for 5 weeks, striking changes in the overall orientation of the tight-junctional network occurs, when compared with control rats. Their meshwork is progressively loosened and disarranged. After 7 and 10 weeks of treatment, the tight-junctional strands extend abluminally in highly irregular patterns, frequently covering broad areas of the membrane faces around the bile canaliculi. Large macular tight junctions,

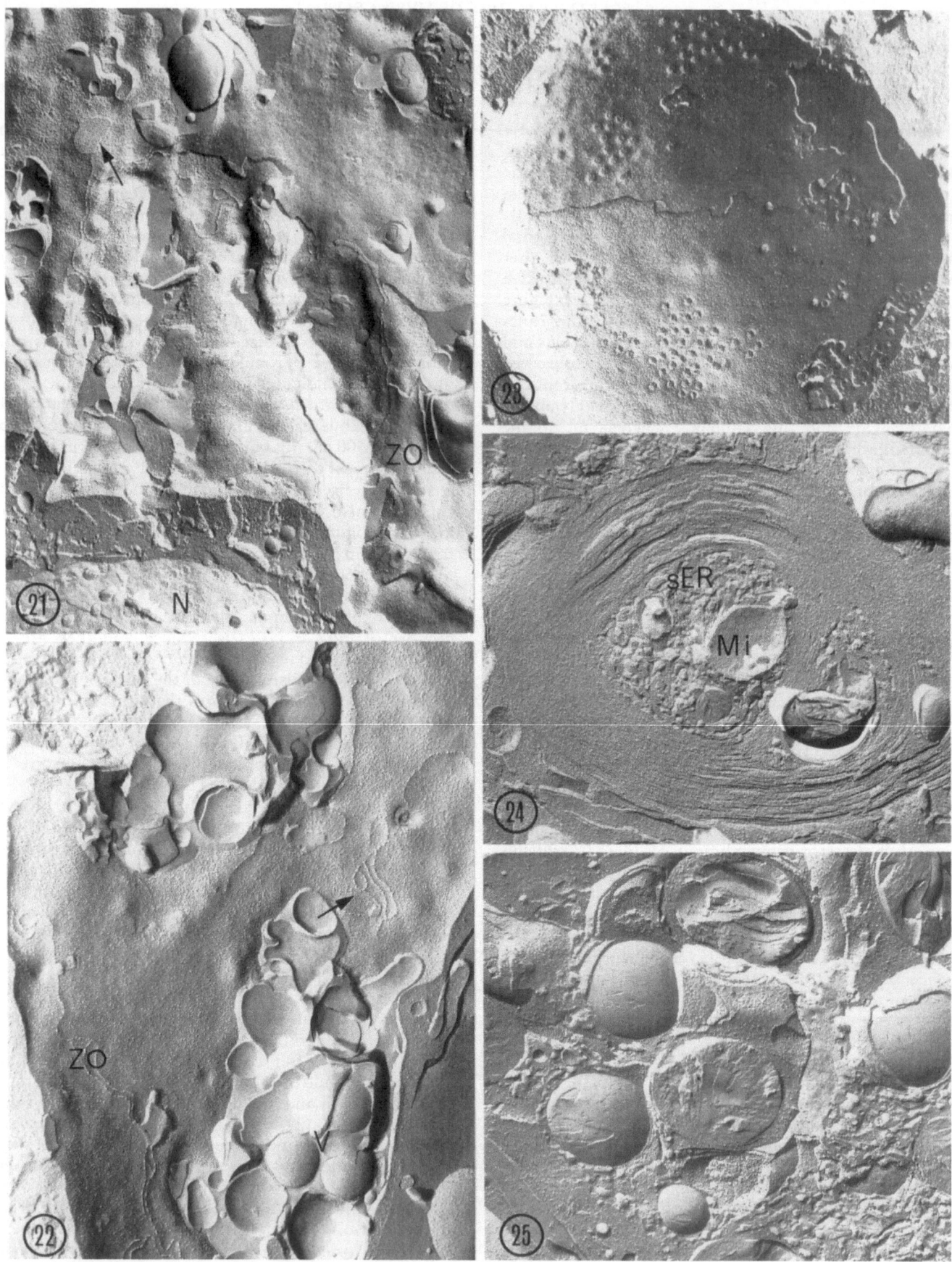

Figure 21   Galactosamine: a disorganized and interrupted zonula occludens (ZO) delineates a dilated bile canalicular membrane. No microvilli are seen; gap junction (arrow); nucleus (N). × 24 000

Figure 22   Galactosamine: on the P-face of the lateral hepatocellular plasmalemma fragmentations of tight-junctional strands (arrow) are seen detached from the zonula occludens (ZO). Vesicular structures (V) are seen within the cytoplasm. × 29 000

Figure 23   Galactosamine: the pores of the nuclear envelope are aggregated into groups. × 29 000

Figure 24   Galactosamine: crossfracture of a whorl body. The densely packed membranes encircle smooth endoplasmic reticulum (sER) and mitochondria (Mi). × 19 000

Figure 25   Galactosamine: the cytoplasm contains numerous fat droplets. × 38 400

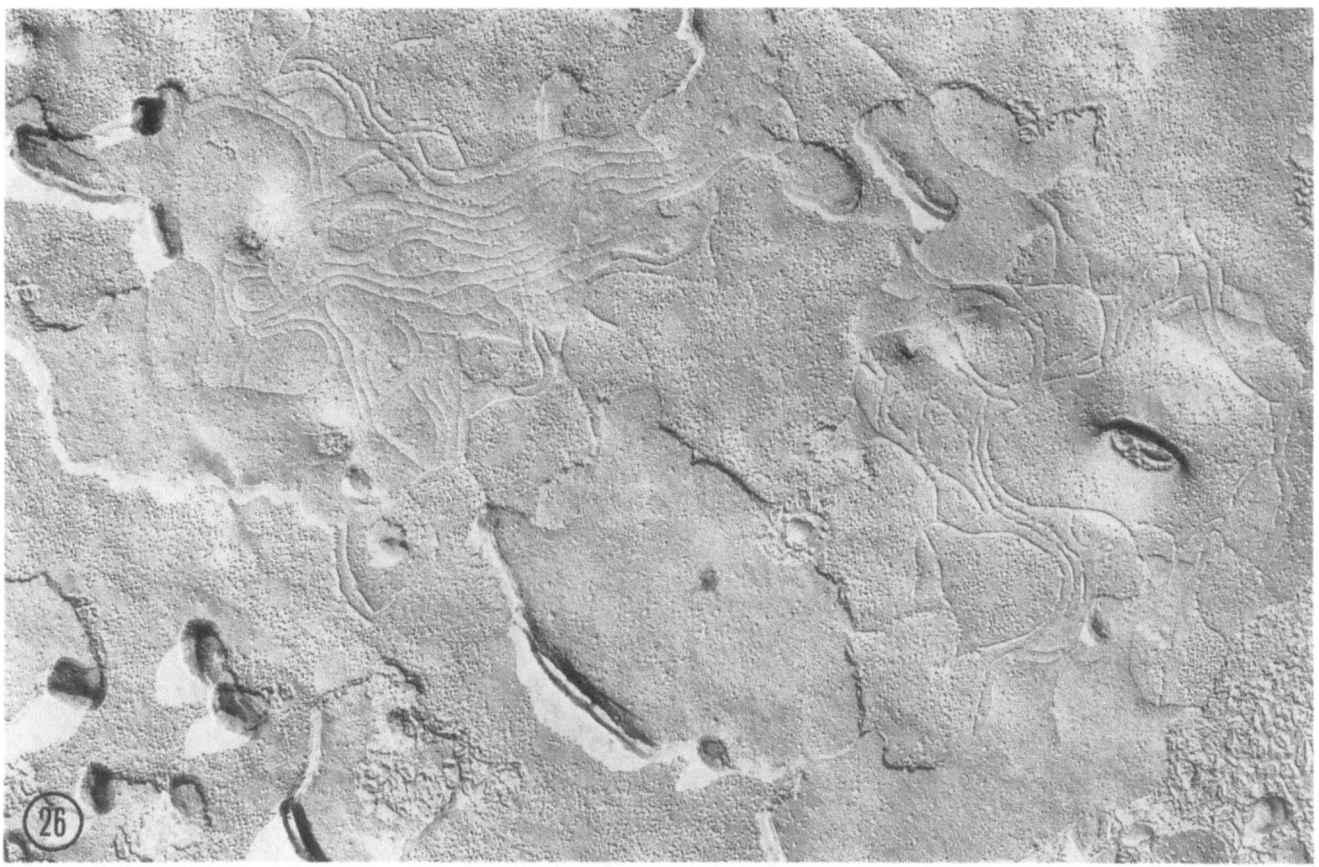

Figure 26 *N*-nitrosomorpholine (NNM): macular tight junction on the lateral plasmalemma located apart from its usual pericanalicular position in rats treated with NNM for 10 weeks. × 44 000

consisting of a network of numerous anastomosing junctional ridges, are observed in the lateral region of the plasmalemma (Figure 26). Gap junctions are sometimes intercalated within the meshwork, or in close association with these structures. The changes within the rat liver are similar to those described for other experimental systems[90–92].

In most cases, the mechanisms responsible for the alteration in tight junctions and the functional consequences are not understood. Although a progression in the proliferation of tight junctions, during the different stages of our experiments, is observed, there is great variability in the response of tight junctions to the drug used. Even after 10 weeks of treatment, more or less unchanged tight junctions are found. At present, we cannot provide any evidence concerning the origin of the newly formed tight junctions. However, some of our observations about the formation of tight junctions during progressive proliferation seem to be in agreement with the models of other development systems[23,93,94].

Cytoskeleton-affecting drugs

According to the Singer–Nicolson membrane model[95], most membrane components seem to be capable of lateral movement. However, movement has to be controlled in order to maintain the orderly arrangement of surface structures[96,97]. Nicolson[98] proposed that motility of membrane proteins is restricted, to some extent, by the cyto-

skeleton (microfilaments and microtubules). In view of the fact that the protein particles of gap and tight junctions exist in specific arrays within a certain domain of the plasma membrane, it seems appropriate to explore the relationship between junctions and the cytoskeleton.

It was the aim of our studies to address this problem more closely and to seek further evidence for the possible involvement of microfilaments and microtubules in the formation of tight and gap junctions in the liver. These studies encompassed investigations on the effects of the drugs, vincristine[72], colchicine[73], vincamine[99] and vinblastine[37,81], known to destroy microtubules, and cytochalasin B[100], known to disrupt microfilaments, both in *in vivo* and *in vitro* experiments on mice and rat liver cells. We found severe alterations in the morphology of bile canaliculi, and tight and gap junctions following treatment with these cytoskeleton-destroying drugs. The bile canaliculi dilate (Figure 27), and both a reduced number as well as extensive proliferation of canalicular tight-junctional strands occur. In accordance with other studies, we found increased permeability of the tight-junctional network to lanthanum hydroxide. The observation that vinblastine changes the bile canaliculi and associated tight junctions in liver cells *in vivo* fits well with similar alterations caused by this drug *in vitro*[81]. This is particularly valid with respect to tight junctional complexes, whereas no comparable alterations in the number and size of gap junctions were found. Proliferation and expansion in size of gap junctions, which

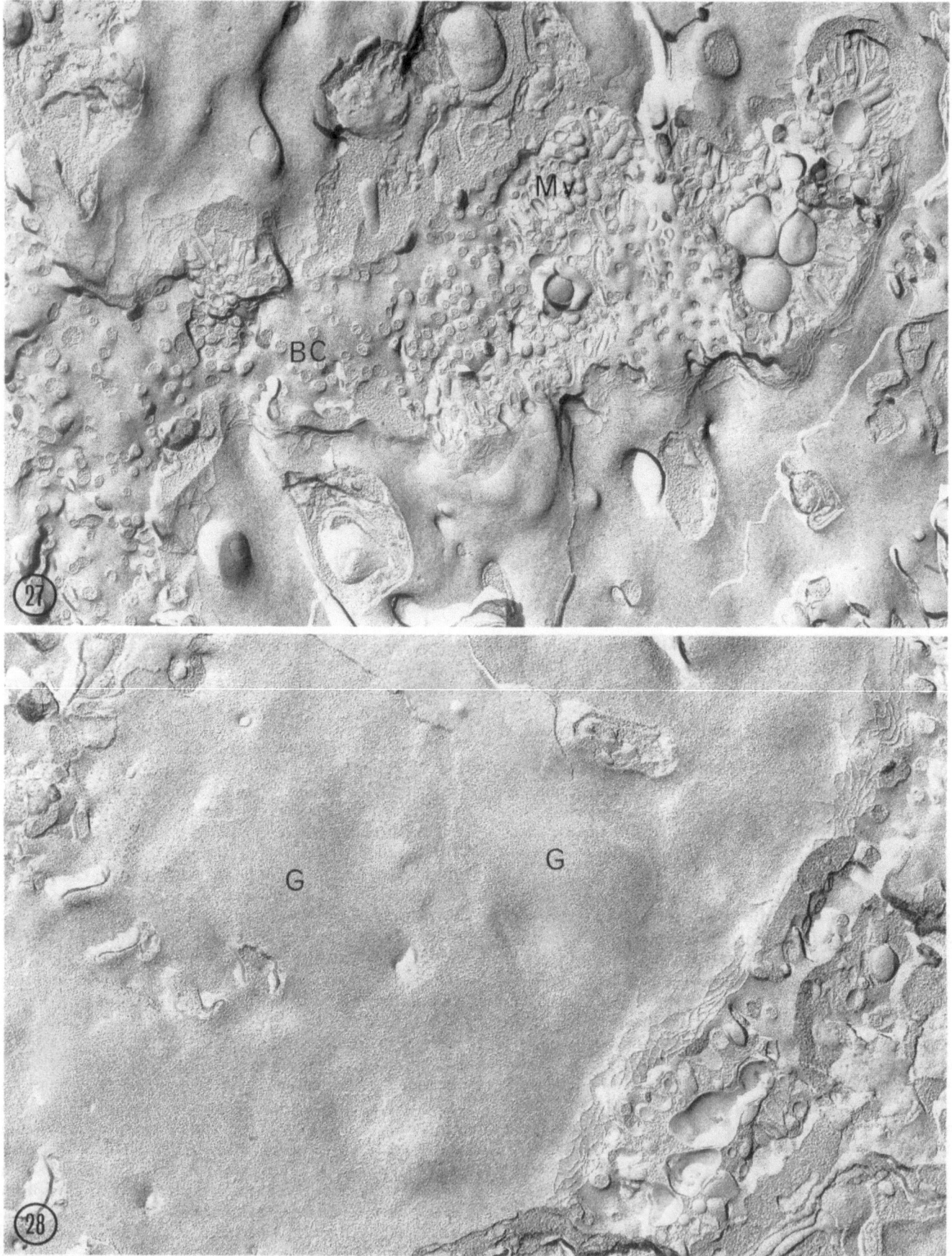

Figure 27   Vinblastine: the bile canaliculus (BC) exhibits an irregular course; the diameter of the lumen is enlarged and outpouchings are frequent 16 h after vinblastine sulphate application. Microvilli (MV). × 17 800

Figure 28   Colchicine: several very large gap junctions (G) on the plasma membrane of a mouse hepatocyte 8 h after colchicine administration. × 25 400

is most dramatic in colchicine-treated animals, are observed as well (Figure 28). The size of gap junctions is four times that of controls. The effect of colchicine on the gap junction attained a maximum after only 1 h and continued unattenuated for 8 h.

From similar results obtained with vinblastine, vincamine and colchicine, and the ineffectiveness of lumicolchicine[101], it appears quite certain that the effects of these drugs are mediated by disruption of the microtubular network. Obviously, this breaks down the structural fixation of the junctional complexes encircling the bile canaliculi. The participation of microfilaments in the maintenance of bile-canalicular and gap-junctional structures becomes obvious from the dramatic alterations caused by cytochalasin B or phalloidin[62,71,72,102]. A number of authors have recently found evidence for the involvement of microfilaments in the formation of tight junctions[103–105] and gap junctions[106] in other systems. Although the nature of participation of cytoskeletal elements in junction formation and development of bile canaliculi remains to be characterized in molecular terms, some involvement of microfilaments and microtubules – in the latter perhaps via hypothetical crossbridges to microfilaments – in the formation of gap and tight junctions in the liver cells might be suspected.

CONCLUSION

The freeze-fracture method is used to analyse the ultrastructure of the liver under normal and experimental conditions. This procedure is especially advantageous for the investigation of membranes and associated processes. Different domains of the plasmalemma of liver cells can be characterized, e.g. perisinusoidal, lateral or bile canalicular hepatocytic plasmalemmal regions. Among the various intercellular junctions, species variations particularly concern the desmosomes (macula adherens) and the gap junctions (nexus), while the tight junctions (zonula occludens) exhibit a regular arrangement around the bile canaliculi. In crossfractures through the interior of liver cells, principal information is obtained from fractures along membranes of cell organelles, i.e. about nuclear pores or fenestrations of the rough endoplasmic reticulum, membranous organization of the Golgi complex.

Significant changes within the individual membrane domains and especially the intercellular connections occur under experimental and pathological conditions. Degenerative processes, as well as regeneration after extra- and intrahepatic cholestasis, liver intoxication, and cytoskeleton-affecting drugs, are characterized by specific alterations. The freeze-fracture images provide the morphological substrate for the interpretation of functional consequences that occur within intracellular as well as intercellular compartments. The freeze-fracture method in combination with other morphological and functional analytical methods is an important tool with which to gain further information on normal hepatocellular functioning as well as on the pathogenesis of liver diseases.

Acknowledgments

The authors are indebted to Ms J. Kölb for preparing the manuscript.

References

1. Benedetti, E. L. and Favard, P. (eds.) (1973). *Freeze-etching Techniques and Applications*. (Paris: Société Francaise de Microscope Elektronique)
2. Koehler, J. K. (ed.) (1973). *Advanced Technique in Biological Electron Microscopy*. (Berlin: Springer)
3. Rash, J. E. and Hudson, C. S. (eds.) (1979). *Freeze Fracture Methods, Artefacts and Interpretations*. (New York: Raven)
4. Heuser, J. E., Reese, T. S., Dennis, M. J., Yan, Y., Yan, L. and Evans, L. (1979). Synaptic vesicle exocytosis captured by quick freezing and correlated with quantal transmitter release. *J. Cell. Biol.*, **81**, 275–300
5. Branton, D., Bullivant, S., Gilula, N. B., Karnovsky, M. J., Moor, H., Mühlethaler, K., Northcote, D. H., Packer, L., Satir, B., Satir, P., Speth, V., Staehelin, L. A., Steere, R. L. and Weinstein, R. S. (1975). Freeze-etching nomenclature. *Science*, **190**, 54–56
6. Metz, J., Aoki, A., Merlo, M. and Forssmann, W. G. (1977). Morphological alterations and functional changes of interhepatocellular junctions induced by bile duct ligation. *Cell. Tiss. Res.*, **182**, 299–310
7. Krell, H., Höke, H. and Pfaff, E. (1982). Development of intrahepatic cholestasis by alpha-naphthylisothiocyanate in rats. *Gastroenterology*, **82**, 507–514
8. Krell, H., Metz, J., Jäschke, H., Höke, H. and Pfaff, E. (1987). Drug-induced intrahepatic cholestasis: characterization of different pathomechanisms. *Arch. Toxicol.*, **60**, 124–130
9. Kreutziger, G. (1968). Freeze-etching of intercellular junctions of mouse liver. *Proc. Electron Microsc. Soc. Am.*, **2**, 234–235
10. Spycher, M. A. (1970). Intercellular adhesions. An electron microscope study on freeze-etched rat hepatocytes. *Z. Zellforsch.*, **111**, 64–74
11. Goodenough, D. R. and Revel, J. P. (1970). A fine structural analysis of intercellular junctions in the mouse liver. *J. Cell. Biol.*, **45**, 272–290
12. Chalcroft, J. P. and Bullivant, S. (1970). An interpretation of liver cell membrane and junction structure based on observation of freeze-fracture replicas of both sides of the fracture. *J. Cell. Biol.*, **47**, 49–60
13. Pinto da Silva, P. and Branton, D. (1970). Membrane splitting in freeze-etching. *J. Cell. Biol.*, **598–605**
14. Montesano, R. and Nikolescu, P. (1978). Fenestrations in endothelium of rat liver sinusoids revisited by freeze-fracture. *Anat. Rec.*, **190**, 861–870
15. Wisse, E. and Knook, D. L. (1979). The investigation of sinusoidal cells, a new approach to the study of liver function. In Popper, H. and Schaffner, F. (eds.) *Progress in Liver Diseases*, Vol. 6, pp. 151–171. (New York: Grune and Stratton)
16. Meirs, S., Nimmrich, H., Weihe, E., Metz, J. and Forssmann, W. G. (1979). Scanning electron microscopy for the study of vascular endothelia. (Abstr.) *5th European Anatomical Congress Prague*, p. 451
17. Friend, D. and Gilula, N. (1972). Variations in tight and gap junctions in mammalian tissues. *J. Cell. Biol.*, **53**, 757–776
18. Revel, J. and Karnovsky, J. (1967). Hexagonal array of subunits in intercellular junctions of the mouse heart and liver. *J. Cell. Biol.*, **57**, 7–12
19. Yancey, S. B., Easter, D. and Revel, J. P. (1979). Cyto-

logical changes in gap junctions during liver regeneration. *J. Ultrastruct. Res., 67,* 229–242

20. Yee, A. G. and Revel, J. H. (1978). Loss and reappearance of gap junction in regenerating liver. *J. Cell. Biol., 78,* 554–564

21. Metz, J. (1982). Freeze-fracture of hepatic fine structure under normal and pathological conditions. In Motta, P. M. and DiDio, L. J. A. (eds.). *Basic and Clinical Hepatology,* pp. 51–68. (Hague/Boston/London: M. Nijhoff Publishers)

22. Robenek, H., Rassat, J. and Themann, H. (1981). A quantitative freeze-fracture analysis of gap and tight junctions in the normal and cholestatic human liver. *Virchows Arch. (Cell. Pathol.),* **38,** 39–56

23. Montesano, R., Friend, D. S., Perrelet, A. and Orci, L. (1975). In vivo assembly of tight junctions in fetal rat liver. *J. Cell. Biol., 57,* 310–319

24. Johnson, R., Hammer, M., Sheridan, J. and Revel, J. (1974). Gap junction formation between reaggregated Novikoff hepatoma cells. *Proc. Natl. Acad. Sci. USA,* **71,** 4536–4540

25. Metz, J. and Bressler, D. (1979). Reformation of gap and tight junctions in regenerating liver after cholestasis. *Cell Tiss. Res., 199,* 257–270

26. Payton, B. W., Bennet, M. V. L. and Pappas, G. D. (1969). Permeability and structure of junctional membranes at an electronic synapse. *Science, 166,* 1641–1643

27. Dewey, M. M. and Barr, L. (1962) Intercellular connections between smooth muscle cells: the nexus. *Science,* **137,** 670–672

28. Dreifuss, J. J., Giradier, L. and Forssmann, W. G. (1966). Etude de la propagation de l'excitation dans le ventricule du rat au moyen de solutions hypertonique. *Pfluegers Arch.,* **292,** 15–33

29. Gilula, N., Reeves, O. and Steinbach, A. (1972). Metabolic coupling, ionic coupling and cell contacts. *Nature (London),* **235,** 262–265

30. Loewenstein, W. (1977). Permeability of the junctional membrane channel. In Brinkley, B. R. and Porter, K. (eds.) *International Cell Biology,* pp. 70–82. (New York: Rockefeller University Press)

31. Bennett, M. V. L. (1973). Function of electronic junctions in embryonic and adult tissues. *Fed. Proc.,* **32,** 65–75

32. Van Deurs, B. and Luft, J. H. (1979). Effects of glutaraldehyde fixation on the structure of tight junctions. A quantitative freeze-fracture analysis. *J. Ultrastruct. Res.,* **68,** 160–172

33. Montesano, R., Mira-Moser, F., Stefan, Y., Perrelet, A. and Orci, L. (1978) Tight junctions in fetal rat liver explants grown in vitro. *J. Ultrastruct. Res.,* **64,** 182–190

34. Matter, A., Orci, L. and Rouiller, C. (1969). A study on the permeability barriers between Disse space and the bile canaliculus. *J. Ultrastruct. Res. (Suppl.),* **11**

35. Koga, A. and Todo, S. (1978). Morphological and functional changes in the tight junctions of the bile canaliculi induced by bile duct ligation. *Cell Tiss. Res., 195,* 267–276

36. Robenek, H., Rassat, J., Grosser, V. and Themann, H. (1982). Ultrastructural study of cholestasis induced by longterm treatment with estradiol valerate. I. Tight junctional analysis and tracer experiments. *Virchows Arch. (Cell. Pathol.),* **40,** 201–215

37. Rassat, J., Robenek and Themann, H. (1981). Ultra-

structural changes in mouse hepatocytes exposed to vinblastine sulfate with special reference to the intercellular junctions. *Eur. J. Cell. Biol.,* **24,** 203–210

38. Aronson, K. F. (1961). Liver function studies during and after complete extra-hepatic biliary obstruction in the dog. *Acta Chir. Scand. (Suppl.),* **275,** 1–114

39. Compagno, J. and Grisham, W. (1974). Scanning electron microscopy of extrahepatic biliary obstruction. *Arch. Pathol., 97,* 48–51

40. Carpino, F., Gaudio, E., Marinozzi, G., Melis, M. and Motta, P. M. (1981). A scanning transmission electron microscopic study of experimental extrahepatic cholestasis in the rat. *J. Submicrosc. Cytol., 13,* 581–598

41. De Vos, R., De Wolf-Peeter, C., Desmet, V., Bianchi, L. and Rohr, H. P. (1975). Significance of liver canalicular changes after experimental bile duct ligation. *Exp. Mol. Pathol., 23,* 12–34

42. De Vos, R. and Desmet, V. J. (1978). Morphologic changes of the junctional complex of the hepatocytes in rat liver after bile duct ligation. *Br. J. Exp. Pathol., 59,* 220–227

43. Jones, A. L., Schmucker, D. L., Mooney, J. S., Adler, R. D. and Ockner, R. K. (1976). Morphometric analysis of rat hepatocytes after total biliary obstruction. *Gastroenterology, 71,* 1050–1060

44. Lee, E., Ross, D. B. and Haines, J. R. (1972). The effect of experimental bile duct obstruction on critical biosynthetic functions of the liver. *Br. J. Surg., 59,* 564–568

45. Mutoh, H. (1981). Freeze replica observations on the junction structures in the guinea pig liver after bile duct ligation and recanalization. *Arch. Histol. Jpn., 44,* 345–367

46. Nishi, M. (1978). Scanning electron microscope study on the mechanism of obstructive jaundice in rats. *Arch. Histol. Jpn., 41,* 411–426

47. Bonvicini, F., Gautier, A., Gardiol, D. and Borel, G. A. (1978). Cholesterol in acute cholestasis induced by taurolithocholic acid. A cytochemical study in transmission and scanning electron microscopy. *Lab. Invest., 38,* 487–495

48. De Vos, R. and Desmet, V. (1981). Morphology of liver tight junctions in ethinyl estradiol induced cholestasis. *Pathol. Res. Pract., 171,* 381–388

49. Dubin, M., Maurice, M., Feldmann, G. and Erlinger, S. (1978). Phalloidin-induced cholestasis in the rat: relation to changes in microfilaments. *Gastroenterology, 75,* 450–455

50. Grosser, V., Robenek, H., Rassat, J. and Themann, H. (1982). Ultrastructural study of cholestasis induced by longterm treatment with estradiol valerate. I. Gap junctional analysis. *Virchows Arch. (Cell. Pathol.),* **40,** 365–378

51. Javitt, N. B. (1966). Cholestasis in rats induced by taurolithocholate. *Nature (London),* **210,** 1262–1263

52. Jung, W., Gebhardt, R. and Robenek, H. (1982). Primary cultures of rat hepatocytes as a model system of canalicular development, biliary secretion and intrahepatic cholestasis. II. Taurolithocholate-induced alterations of canalicular morphology and of the distribution of filipin-cholesterol complexes. *Eur. J. Cell. Biol., 29,* 77–82

53. Kakis, G. and Yousef, J. M. (1978). Pathogenesis of lithocholate- and taurolithocholate-induced intrahepatic cholestasis in rats. *Gastroenterology, 75,* 595–607

54. Kakis, G., Phillips, M. J. and Yousef, J. M. (1980). The respective roles of membrane cholesterol and of sodium potassium adenosine triphosphatase in the pathogenesis

of lithocholate induced cholestasis. *Lab. Invest.*, **43**, 73–81

55. King, J. E. and Schoenfield, L. (1971). Cholestasis induced by sodium taurolithocholate in isolated hamster liver. *J. Clin. Invest.*, **50**, 2305–2312

56. Layden, T. J., Schwarz, J. and Boyer, J. L. (1975). Scanning electron microscopy of the rat liver. Studies of the effect of taurolithocholate and other models of cholestasis. *Gastroenterology*, **69**, 724–738

57. Loosley, H., Gardiol, D. and Gautier, A. (1981). Experimental intrahepatic cholestasis. A comparative physiopathological, ultrastructural, and cytochemical study of different types. *Virchows Arch. (Cell. Pathol.)*, **35**, 213–228

58. Miyai, K., Price, V. M. and Fisher, M. M. (1971). Bile acid metabolism in mammals: Ultrastructural studies on the intrahepatic cholestasis induced by lithocholic and chenodeoxycholic acids in the rat. *Lab. Invest.*, **24**, 292–301

59. Miyai, K., Mayr, W. W. and Richardson, A. L. (1975). Acute cholestasis induced by lithocholic acid in the rat – a freeze-fracture replica and thin section study. *Lab. Invest.*, **32**, 527–535

60. Miyai, K., Richardson, A. L., Mayr, W. and Javitt, N. B. (1977). Subcellular pathology of rat liver in cholestasis and choleresis induced by bile salts. 1. Effects of lithocholic, 3β-hydroxy-15-cholenoic, cholic and dehydrocholic acids. *Lab. Invest.*, **36**, 249–258

61. Nemchausky, B. A., Layden, T. J. and Boyer, J. L. (1977). Effects of chronic choleretic infusions of bile acid on the membrane of the bile canaliculus: a biochemical and morphological study. *Lab. Invest.*, **36**, 259–267

62. Phillips, M. J., Oda, M., Mak, M., Fisher, M. M. and Jeejeebho, K. N. (1975). Microfilament dysfunction as a possible cause of intrahepatic cholestasis. *Gastroenterology*, **69**, 48–58

63. Phillips, M. J., Oda, M. and Funatsu, K. (1978). Evidence for microfilament involvement in norethandrolone-induced intrahepatic cholestasis. *Am. J. Pathol.*, **93**, 729–744

64. Plaa, G. L. and Priestley, B. G. (1977). Intrahepatic cholestasis induced by drugs and chemicals. *Pharmacol. Rev.*, **28**, 207–273

65. Schaffner, F. and Javitt, N. B. (1966). Morphological changes in hamster liver during intrahepatic cholestasis induced by taurolithocholate. *Lab. Invest.*, **15**, 1783–1792

66. Robenek, H., Herwig, J. and Themann, H. (1980). The morphologic characteristics of intercellular junctions between normal human liver cells and cells from patients with extrahepatic cholestasis. *Am. J. Pathol.*, **100**, 93–114

67. Robenek, H. (1983). Freeze-fracture study of the liver. In Popper, H., Köttgen, E., Reutter, W. and Gudat, F. (eds.) *Structural Carbohydrates in the Liver*, pp. 121–146. (Lancaster: MTP Press)

68. Claude, P. and Goodenough, D. A. (1973). Fracture faces of zonulae occludentes from 'tight' and 'leaky' epithelia. *J. Cell. Biol.*, **58**, 390–400

69. Martinez-Palomo, A. and Erlij, D. (1975). Structure of tight junctions in epithelia with different permeability. *Proc. Natl. Acad. Sci. USA*, **72**, 4487–4491

70. Mollgard, K., Malinowska, D. H. and Saunders, N. R. (1976). Lack of correlation between tight junction morphology and permeability properties in developing choroid plexus. *Nature (London)*, **264**, 293–294

71. Staehelin, L. (1974). Structure and function of intercellular junctions. *Int. Rev. Cytol.*, **39**, 191–283

72. Rassat, J., Robenek, H. and Themann, H. (1981). Ultrastructural alterations in the mouse liver following vincristine administration. *J. Submicrosc. Cytol.*, **13**, 321–335

73. Rassat, J., Robenek, H. and Themann, H. (1982). Alterations of tight and gap junctions in mouse hepatocytes following administration of colchicine. *Cell. Tiss. Res.*, **223**, 187–200

74. Gumucio, J. J. C. and Valdivieso, V. C. (1971). Studies on the mechanism of the ethynyl estradiol impairment of bile flow and bile salt excretion in the rat. *Gastroenterology*, **61**, 339–344

75. Forker, E. L. (1969) The effect of estrogen on bile formation in the rat. *J. Clin. Invest.*, **48**, 654–663

76. Berk, P. D. and Javitt, N. B. (1978). Hyperbilirubinemia and cholestasis. *Am. J. Med.*, **64**, 311–326

77. Hoi-Sang, Ü, Sauer, M. H., Ellisman, J. R. and Ellisman, M. H. (1980). Tight junction formation is closely linked to the polar redistribution of intramembranous particles in aggregating MDCK epithelia. *Exp. Cell. Res.*, **122**, 384–391

78. Javitt, N. B. and Emerman, S. (1968). Effect of sodium taurolithocholate on bile flow and bile acid secretion. *J. Clin. Invest.*, **47**, 1002–1014

79. Priestley, B. G., Cote, M. G. and Plaa, G. L. (1971). Biochemical and morphological parameters of taurolithocholate-induced cholestasis. *Can. J. Physiol. Pharmacol.*, **49**, 1078–1091

80. Gebhardt, R., Jung, W. and Robenek, H. (1982). Primary cultures of rat hepatocytes as a model of canalicular development, biliary secretion and intrahepatic cholestasis. I. Distribution of filipin-cholesterol complexes during de novo formation of bile canaliculi. *Eur. J. Cell. Biol.*, **29**, 68–76

81. Robenek, H. and Gebhardt, R. (1983). Primary cultures of rat hepatocytes as a model of canalicular development, biliary secretion and intrahepatic cholestasis. IV. Disintegration of bile canaliculi and disturbance of tight junction formation caused by vinblastine. *Eur. J. Cell. Biol.*, **31**, 283–289

82. Severs, N. J. and Robenek, H. (1983). Detection of microdomains in biomembranes. An appraisal of recent developments in freeze-fracture cytochemistry. *Biochem. Biophys. Acta*, **737**, 373–408

83. Robenek, H., Jung, W. and Gebhardt, R. (1982). The topography of filipin-cholesterol complexes in the plasma membrane of cultured hepatocytes and their relation to cell junction formation. *J. Ultrastruct. Res.*, **78**, 95–106

84. Robenek, H., Döldissen, M. and Themann, H. (1980). Morphological changes of tight junctions in the rat liver after chronic administration of N-nitrosomorpholine (NNM) as revealed by freeze-fracturing. *J. Ultrastruct. Res.*, **70**, 82–91

85. Robenek, H., Themann, H. and Ott, K. (1979). Carbon tetrachloridide-induced proliferation of tight junctions in the rat liver as revealed by freeze-fracturing. *Eur. J. Cell. Biol.*, **20**, 62–70

86. Robenek, H. and Themann, H. (1979). Effects of chronic administration of Thioacetamide (TAA) on the structure of bile canaliculi and tight junctions in the rat liver as revealed by freeze-fracturing. *Virchows Arch. (Cell. Pathol.)*, **32**, 57–67

87. Decker, K. and Keppler, D. (1974). Galactosamine hepatitis: key role of the nucleotide deficiency period in the pathogenesis of cell injury and cell death. *Rev. Physiol. Biochem. Pharmacol.*, **71**, 77–106

88. El Mofty, S. K., Scrutton, M. C., Serroni, A., Nicolini, C. and Farber, J. L. (1975). Early reversible plasma membrane injury in galactosamine induced liver cell death. *Am. J. Pathol.*, **79**, 579–595

89. Schanne, F., Kane, A., Young, E. and Farber, J. (1979). Calcium dependence of toxic cell death: A final common pathway. *Science*, **206**, 700–702

90. Orci, L., Amherdt, M., Henquin, J. C., Lambert, A. E., Unger, R. H. and Renold, A. E. (1973). Pronase effect on pancreatic beta cell secretion and morphology. *Science*, **180**, 647–649

91. Elias, P. M. and Friend, D. S. (1976). Vitamin-A-induced mucous metaplasia: an in vitro system for modulating tight and gap junction differentiation. *J. Cell. Biol.*, **68**, 173–188

92. Meldolesi, J., Castiglioni, G., Parma, R., Nassivera, N. and De Camilli, P. (1978). Ca^{++}-dependent disassembly and reassembly of occluding junctions in guinea pig pancreatic acinar cell. Effect of drugs. *J. Cell. Biol.*, **79**, 159–172

93. Montesano, R., Gabbiani, G., Perrelet, A. and Orci, L. (1976). In vivo induction of tight junction proliferation in rat liver. *J. Cell. Biol.*, **68**, 793–798

94. Porvaznik, U. (1979). Tight junction disruption and recovery after sublethal gamma-irradiation. *Pediatr. Res.*, **78**, 233–250

95. Singer, S. J. and Nicolson, G. L. (1972). The fluid mosaic model of the structure of cell membranes. *Science*, **175**, 720–731

96. Robenek, H. and Schmitz, G. (1985). Receptor domains in the plasma membrane of cultured mouse peritoneal macrophages. *Eur. J. Cell. Biol.*, **39**, 77–85

97. Robenek, H. (1987). Distribution and mobility of receptors in the plasma membrane. In S. W. Hui (ed.), *Freeze–Fracture Studies of Membrane Structure*. CRC Press

98. Nicolson, G. L. (1976). Transmembrane control of the receptors on normal and tumor cells. 1. Cytoplasmic influence over cell surface components. *Biochim. Biophys. Acta*, **457**, 57–108

99. Rassat, J., Robenek, H. and Themann, H. (1982). Changes in mouse hepatocytes caused by vincamin. A thin-sectioning and freeze-fracture study. *Naunyn-Schmiedebergs Arch. Pharmacol.*, **318**, 349–357

100. Rassat, H., Robenek, H. and Themann, H. (1981). Cytochalasin B affects the gap and tight junctions of mouse hepatocytes in vivo. *J. Submicrosc. Cytol.*, **14**, 427–439

101. Gebhardt, R. (1983). Disappearance of visible bile canaliculi caused by vinblastine in primary cultures of rat hepatocytes. *Exp. Cell Res.*, **144**, 218–223

102. Elias, E., Hruban, Z., Wade, J. B. and Boyer, J. L. (1980). Phalloidin-induced cholestasis: a microfilament mediated change in junctional complex permeability. *Proc. Natl. Acad. Sci. USA*, **77**, 2229–2233

103. Bentzel, C. J., Hainau, B., Edelmann, A., Anagnostopoulos, T. and Benedetti, E. L. (1976). Effect of plant cytokinins on microfilaments and tight junctions permeability. *Nature (London)*, **264**, 666–668

104. Bentzel, C. J., Hainau, B., Ho, S., Hui, W., Edelmann, A., Anagnostopoulos, T. and Benedetti, E. L. (1980). Cytoplasmic regulation of tight junction permeability: Effect of plant cytokinins. *Am. J. Physiol.*, **239**, C 75–C 89

105. Saxon, M. E., Popov, V. J., Kirkin, A. H. and Allakhverdov, B. L. (1978). De novo formation of tight-like junctions induced with phalloidin between mouse lymphocytes. *Naturwissenschaften*, **65**, 62–63

106. Larsen, W. J., Tung, H. N., Murray, S. A. and Swenson, C. A. (1979). Evidence for the participation of actin microfilaments and bristle coats in the internalization of gap junction membranes. *J. Cell. Biol.*, **83**, 576–587

12

Ultrastructure of hepatic tumours in teleosts

J. A. HAMPTON, J. E. KLAUNIG and P. J. GOLDBLATT

INTRODUCTION

Teleosts provide sensitive animal models for use in carcinogenesis studies[1-4]. The Mt. Shasta strain of rainbow trout (*Salmo gairdneri*) is the most sensitive animal model used to study the tumorigenic effects of aflatoxin[4]. The brown bullhead (*Ictalurus nebulosus*) has emerged as a freshwater teleost species which is sensitive to induction of tumours by chemical carcinogen exposure, both experimentally in the laboratory and in the environment[5-10]. The brown bullhead, as well as other teleost species, may serve as sentinel organisms for the detection of biohazardous material in the environment[2-6]. We report for the first time the light- and electron-microscopic features of experimentally induced hepatic tumours 9 months after 28-day exposure to an aqueous solution (100 ppm) of diethylnitrosamine (DENA) in 1 y old male and female brown bullheads. Lesions in the bullhead liver will be described in terms derived from the study of mammalian (rodent) hepatocarcinogenesis. Microscopic features of experimentally induced hepatic tumours will be compared with hepatic tumours found in feral brown bullheads previously sampled from the Black River, Lorain, Ohio. However, before descriptions and interpretations of the pattern and progression of lesions seen in bullhead liver during carcinogenesis can be made, knowledge of the normal architecture and component cell types is necessary.

Normal hepatic morphology

Teleost liver is qualitatively similar to mammalian liver in component cell types (hepatocytes, endothelial, fat-storing, exocrine pancreatic, circulating blood cells, and fixed macrophages); however, significant differences exist in a number of cells present and in the hepatic architectural arrangement[3,11-17]. Not normally seen in mammalian liver, the association of exocrine pancreatic tissue within the walls and periadventitia of hepatic portal veins has led to the use of the term 'hepatopancreas' to describe this co-occurrence[14,15]. Reviewed by early workers as tubular glands[11] and, more recently, as laminar or composed of interconnecting walls penetrated by sinusoids, all vertebrate liver was thought to be similarly organized[18]. However, findings of tubular arrangement in liver of teleosts examined with high-resolution light microscopy[19,20], especially following perfusion fixation of the hepatic vascular bed[16,21], have been reported. Hepatic tubules have been described as composed of hepatocytes whose apices are directed towards a central biliary element and bases directed towards a sinusoid[16]. Well described in the teleost[14,21], fenestrated endothelial cells line sinusoids. In some teleost species, fenestrae have been reported to be organized into sieve plates[21]. Formed by processes of endothelial cells and hepatocytes, and containing hepatocyte microvillus-like projections, the space of Disse appears as well developed in teleosts as in mammals[14]. Residing within the space of Disse, perisinusoidal fat-storing cells have been reported in at least 50 species of bony and cartilaginous fishes[14-17,19,21]. Apparently absent in salmonids[16,17], phagocytic Kupffer cells have been reported in a variety of other teleost species[14,15]. The exact architectural arrangement and cellular components of the bullhead liver have not been fully reported (Figure 1). Most portal and hepatic venous tributaries can be distinguished by the presence of exocrine pancreatic tissue associated with the former (Figure 1).

Ultrastructurally, hepatocytes contain a centrally placed irregularly shaped nucleus, sparse perinuclear granular endoplasmic reticulum (GER) in parallel array, few mitochondria, fibrillar lysosomes, dispersed glycogen and smooth (agranular) endoplasmic reticulum (SER) associated with glycogen deposits (Figure 2). Bile canaliculi can be observed between hepatocytes. Lacking a separating basal lamina, small bile preductular and ductular epithelial cells are intimately associated with adjacent hepatocytes (Figure 3). In teleost liver in general, and bullhead liver in particular, lobules and portal regions as defined in mammals are either poorly defined or absent[3,13-16,22].

Hepatic tumour pathology

Histological progression of hepatic neoplasia in teleosts has not been studied as extensively as in rodents[22-28]. In rodent liver, three distinct hepatocyte lesions have been

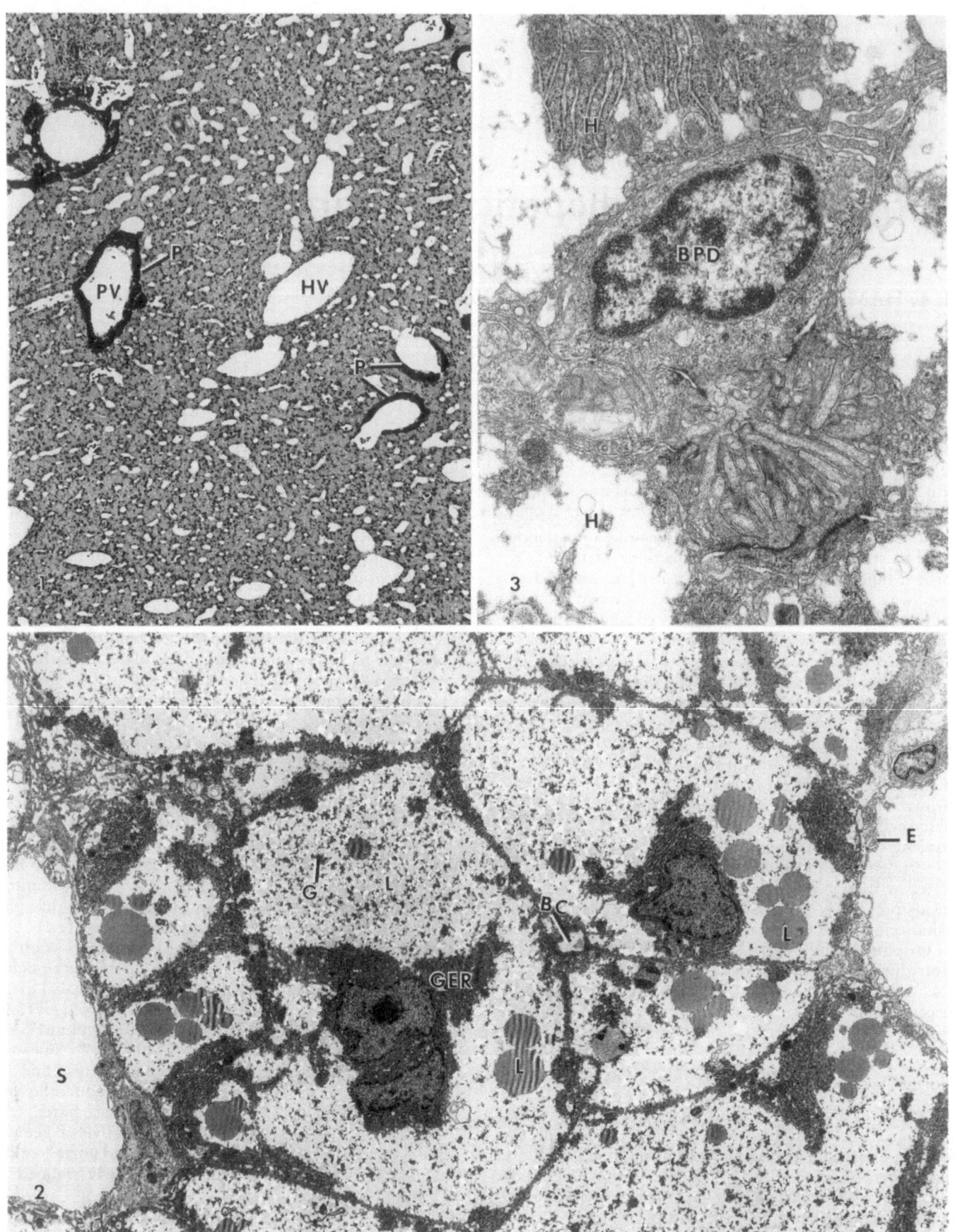

Figure 1 Low-magnification view of normal bullhead liver. Portal (PV) and hepatic (HV) venous tributaries can be distinguished by the presence of exocrine pancreatic (P) tissue with the former. H + E stained paraffin section (4 μm). × 68

Figure 2 Low-magnification transmission electron micrograph (TEM) of normal bullhead hepatic parenchyma. Hepatocytes contain a centrally placed nucleus, sparse granular endoplasmic reticulum (GER), few mitochondria, abundant lipid deposits (L) of different electron density, and dispersed glycogen (G). A bile canaliculus (BC) can be seen between 3 adjacent hepatocytes. S = sinusoids; E = sinusoidal endothelium. Uranyl acetate and lead citrate. × 4000

Figure 3 TEM of a bile preductule in the normal bullhead liver. A preductule is a biliary channel which at its origin is bounded by one or more hepatocytes (H) and by a bile preductular epithelial cell (BPD) with both cell types contributing microvilli to the biliary lumen. Uranyl acetate and lead citrate. × 19 500

described associated with chronic exposure to hepatocarcinogens. These include:

(1) Focal areas of cellular alteration (commonly referred to as foci);
(2) Neoplastic nodules or adenomas (also sometimes referred to as hyperplastic nodules); and
(3) Hepatocellular carcinomas[29].

In addition to these preneoplastic and neoplastic lesions arising from hepatocytes, other hepatic histological elements (biliary epithelium and sinusoidal lining cells) have been shown to be the target of cellular transformation. Thus, cholangiomas and cholangiocarcinomas (biliary epithelium), as well as haemangiomas and haemangiosarcomas, may be induced by chemical carcinogens[29].

Foci

In rodents, following exposure to most hepatocarcinogens, the primary cell target of neoplastic transformation is the hepatocyte. The three hepatocellular lesions (foci, adenomas and carcinomas) arising from these cells are classified on the basis of both morphology and oncogenic behaviour. Focal areas of cellular alteration (foci) are usually the earliest lesions seen in the liver following exposure to hepatocarcinogens. These lesions are thought to be preneoplastic and can either regress to apparently normal cells or progress to adenomas and/or carcinomas. Morphologically, rodent foci are small aggregates of hepatocytes (usually less than a lobule in size) distinguished from the surrounding 'normal' hepatocytes by differences in staining with haematoxylin and eosin (H + E), In rodents, four types of foci have been described, based upon their H + E staining properties: basophilic; acidophilic; clear cell; or mixed (combination of two of the three). In addition to the particular H + E staining characteristics, these foci have also demonstrated increased staining for glucose-6-phosphate dehydrogenase, γ-glutamyl transpeptidase and glycogen; decreased staining for glucose-6-phosphatase (G-6-Pase), adenosine triphosphatase (ATPase); and inability to store iron when made sideriotic. In teleosts, only decreased staining for G-6-Pase and ATPase have shown consistent results in carcinogen-induced hepatic lesions[4,30]. In mammalian, as well as teleost, hepatocarcinogenesis, it remains controversial how the staining characteristics of these focal lesions bear on the future biological behaviour of these lesions, i.e. regression or progression[4,22,29]. In addition, foci do not display invasive or expansive properties.

Since teleost liver lacks lobular organization, a more arbitrary definition of hepatic lesions is necessary. In the bullhead liver, following carcinogen exposure, we have defined foci as focal areas of cellular alteration less than 0.5 mm in diameter which usually exhibit tinctorial differences (increased basophilia, acidophilia, clear cell) from the surrounding normal hepatic cells[4] (Figures 4–6). Not compressing surrounding normal tissue, basophilic (Figure 4) and acidophilic (Figure 5) foci are composed of cells which exhibit enlarged nuclei with a mitotic index greater than surrounding normal liver. In mammalian and teleost foci, basophilia is imparted by an abundance of free ribosomes or GER with dilated cisternae while

acidophilia is indicative of proliferated dilated SER[12,31]. Frequently, flocculent material is present within dilated cisternae[12]. In the trout[4] and bullhead liver, clear cell foci appear as empty cells with small, dark nuclei (Figure 6). Although the biological significance of clear cell lesions in mammalian and teleost carcinogenesis is unknown, they result from excessive glycogen or lipid storage and subsequent loss during histological processing[22].

Adenoma

Rodent hepatic adenomas are usually larger than a lobule in size with component cells displaying similar histological and histochemical characteristics seen in hepatocellular foci and are similarly classified (basophilic, acidophilic, mixed or clear cell)[25,29]. Adenomas, also referred to as hyperplastic and/or preneoplastic nodules, exhibit expansile growth which results in compression of surrounding normal hepatic parenchyma. Compression of normal parenchyma results in a pseudocapsule-like appearance of the adenoma. In the rainbow trout liver, it has been suggested that basophilic lesions larger than 0.5 mm in diameter progress to malignant tumours[4]. Based on this finding, basophilic lesions larger than 0.5 mm were termed 'carcinomas'[4]. Little is known about the biology of hepatic neoplasia in the bullhead; therefore, we are reluctant to classify lesions solely upon size and prefer to classify adenomas and carcinomas on their biological behaviour.

Rarely used to describe teleost hepatic lesions[12,32–34] and used in mammalian research interchangeably with the terms neoplastic or hyperplastic nodule, we feel the term 'adenoma' is appropriate in labelling indeterminant (i.e. regress or progress) lesions of the bullhead liver that exhibit expansile growth. In the rainbow trout, an adenoma can be: acidophilic; basophilic; clear cell type; or mixed[12]. These lesions are larger than a focus and frequently produce raised protrusions of the capsule when seen near the surface of the liver[12]. Additionally, adenomas in rainbow trout liver may or may not be surrounded by fibrous connective tissue[12]. In acidophilic adenomas in the bullhead liver, hepatocytes appear as thickened laminae with frequent mitotic figures (Figure 7). In the rainbow trout, hepatocytes composing adenomas are ultrastructurally characterized by round, dense bodies which contain whorled membranes, extensive GER, numerous mitochondria and a prominent Golgi[12]. We have seen similar basophilic and acidophilic lesions in the bullhead liver. In trout, acidophilic and clear cell lesions larger than 0.5 mm are rare and are not believed to be neoplastic in nature, and, when observed, these larger lesions have been termed 'nodules'[4]. In the bullhead liver, large clear cell lesions have also been termed nodules[10].

Other lesions

Large cyst-like spaces have been observed in the liver of the Japanese medaka (*Oryzias latipes*) following exposure to an aqueous solution of methylazoxymethanol acetate (MAM)[33,35]. Similar lesions have been observed in the sheepshead minnow (*Cyprinodon variegatus*) following exposure to DENA[36]. Similar to

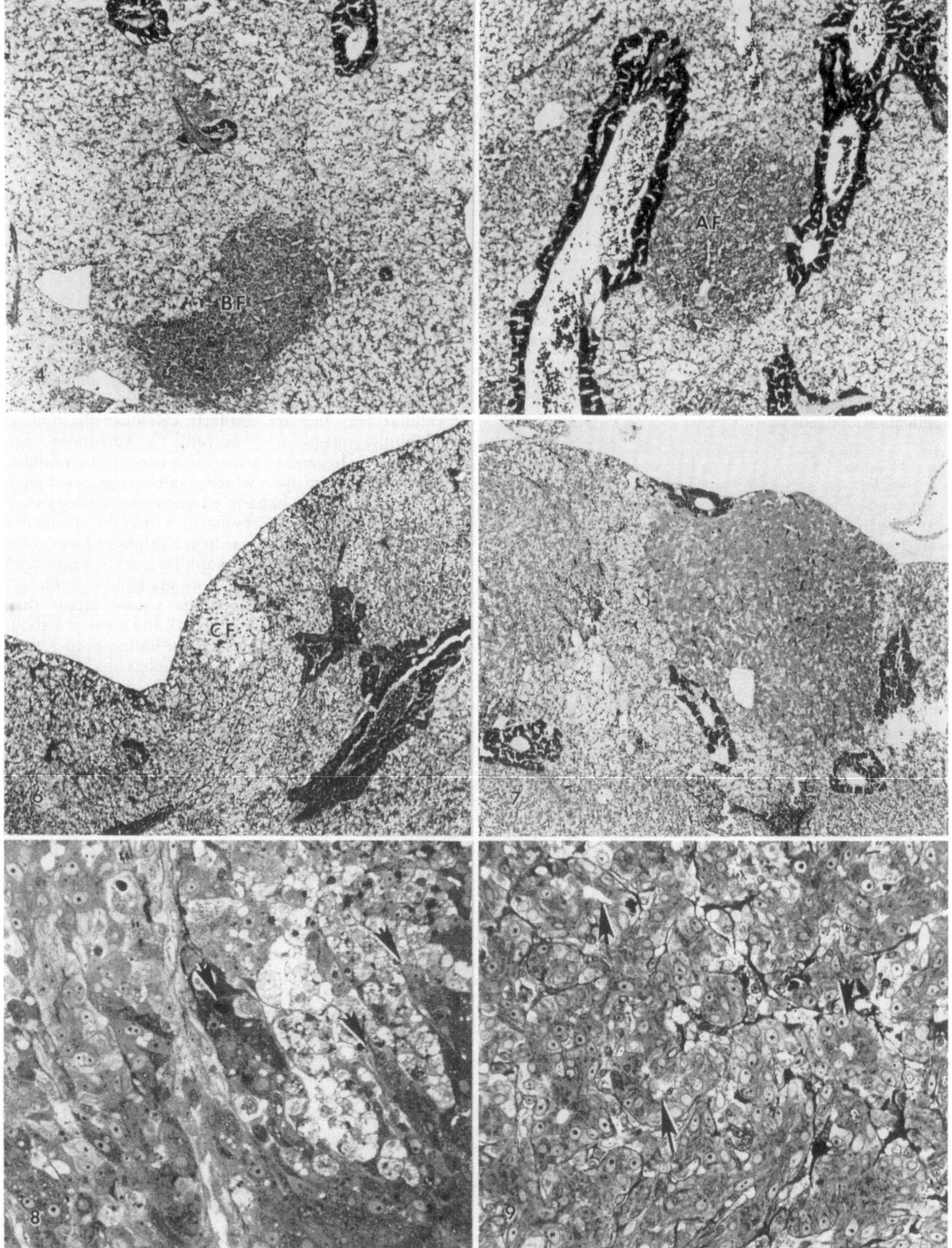

Figure 4 Low-magnification light micrograph of a basophilic focus (BF) within the bullhead liver 9 months following a 28-day exposure to 100 ppm DENA. Focus is less than 0.5 mm in diameter. H + E stained paraffin section (4 μm). × 66

Figure 5 Low-magnification light micrograph of an acidophilic focus (AF) within the bullhead liver. Compression of surrounding tissue is not evident. Sampling and staining procedures are identical to those described in Figure 4. × 66

Figure 6 Low-magnification light micrograph of a clear cell focus (CF) within the bullhead liver. Sampling and staining procedures are identical to those described in Figure 4. × 66

Figure 7 Low-magnification light micrograph of an acidophilic adenoma from the bullhead liver. Visible grossly on the surface of the liver and greater than 0.5 mm in diameter, the adenoma is unencapsulated and compression of surrounding tissue is not evident. Sampling and staining procedures are identical to those described in Figure 4. × 56

Figure 8 Light micrograph of darkly stained trabecular hepatocellular carcinoma cells (arrows). Toluidine blue stained epoxy section (0.5–1.0 μm). × 412

Figure 9 Centrally within trabecular tumours and with little supporting connective tissue, bile duct or duct-like (arrows) structures are observed in both cross- and longitudinal section. Toluidine blue stained epoxy section (0.5–1.0 μm). × 412

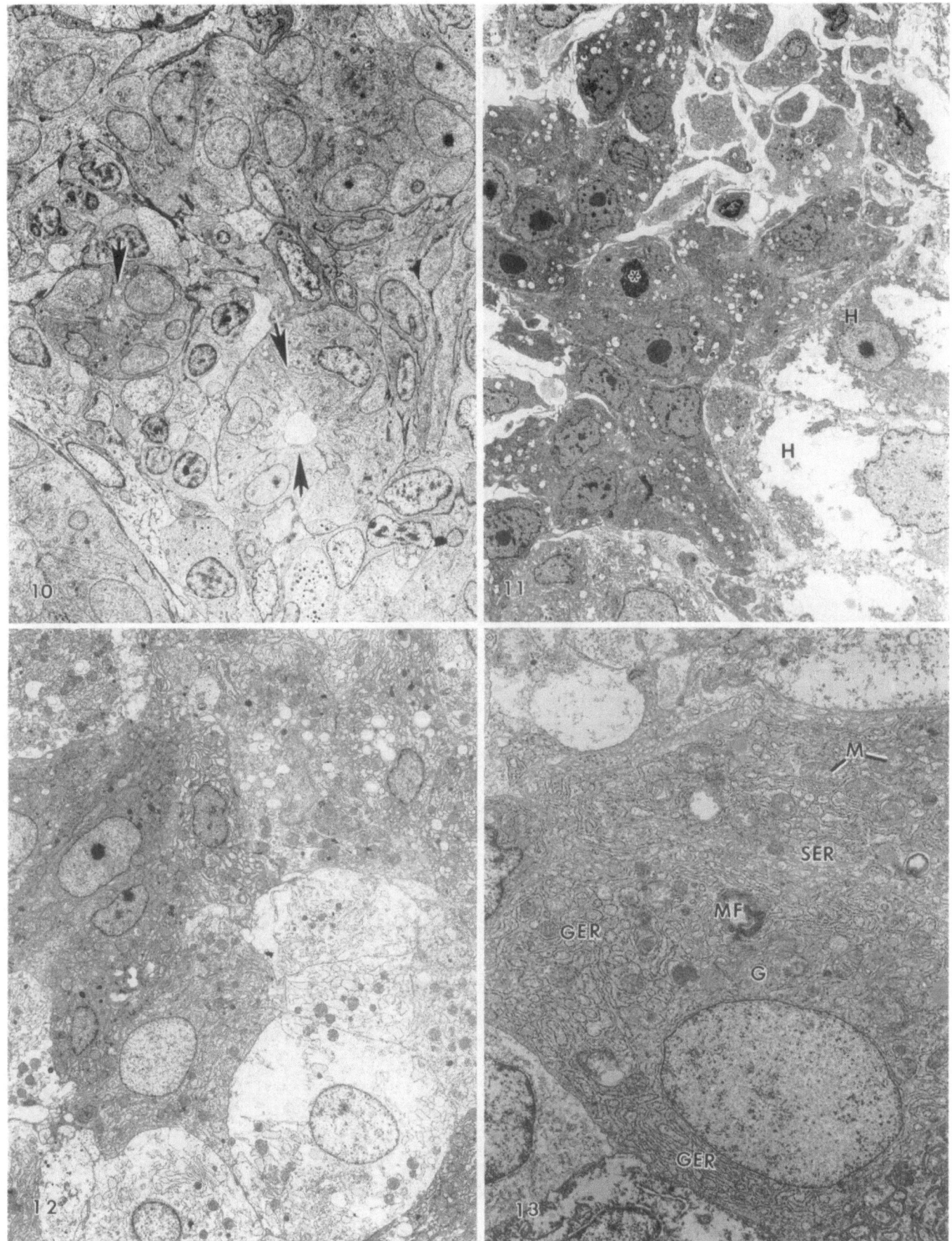

Figure 10 Containing little supporting connective tissue, bile duct or duct-like structures (arrows) are observed centrally within trabecular tumours. Uranyl acetate and lead citrate. × 1800

Figure 11 Low-magnification TEM of darkly stained peripheral trabecular carcinoma cells. Injured, as well as more normal appearing, hepatocytes (H) are seen adjacent to carcinoma cells. Few canalicular structures are seen and cellular borders are difficult to distinguish. Asterisk indicates an early metaphase nucleus. Uranyl acetate and lead citrate. × 2025

Figure 12 Higher magnification view of darkly stained peripheral carcinoma cells illustrates reduced nuclear and cytoplasmic volumes. Uranyl acetate and lead citrate. × 2200

Figure 13 Cytoplasmically, transformed hepatocytes exhibit loss of lipid, proliferation and dilation of GER and SER, free ribosomes, well-developed Golgi (G), absence of cytoplasmic filaments, electron-dense lysosomes, myelin figures (MF) and numerous mitochondria (M). Uranyl acetate and lead citrate. × 6050

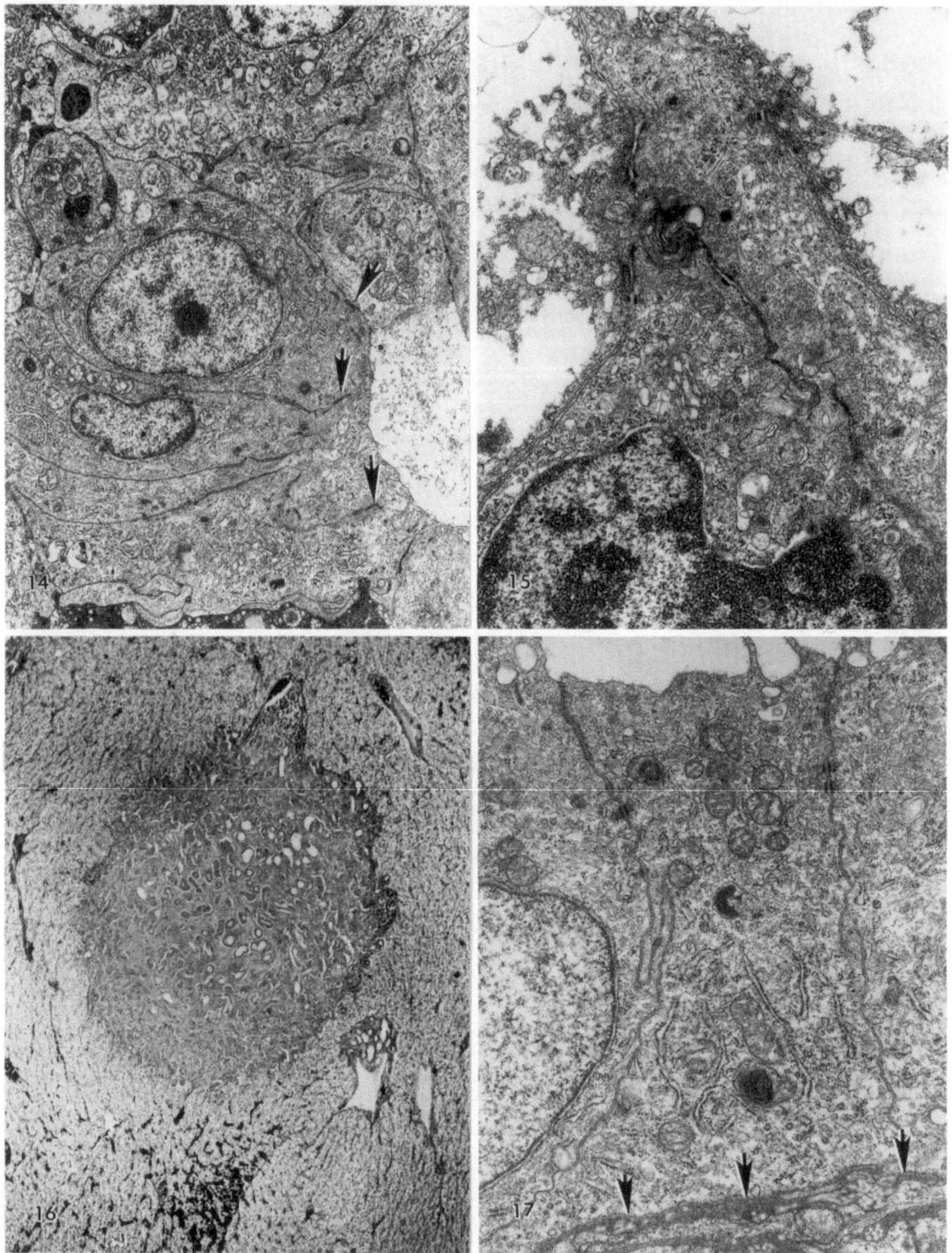

Figure 14 Centrally within trabecular tumours, electron-dense cells forming duct-like structures resemble normal biliary cells within the bullhead liver. Cells contain sparse amounts of GER, numerous free ribosomes, few mitochondria, well-developed SER and Golgi with numerous smooth vesicles, and abundant intermediate filaments. Apically tight junctions and desmosomes are observed (arrows). A basal lamina separating ductal and surrounding cells is absent. Uranyl acetate and lead citrate. × 6050

Figure 15 Although considerably smaller, normal bile preductular cells are ultrastructurally similar to cells forming small duct-like structures seen within trabecular tumours. In the normal bullhead liver, a basal lamina between bile preductular cells and hepatocytes is absent. Uranyl acetate and lead citrate. × 19 250

Figure 16 Light micrograph of a cholangioma from a feral brown bullhead sampled from the Black River, Lorain, Ohio. Lesion is composed entirely of ductal cells and supporting connective tissue. H + E stained paraffin section (4 μm). × 75

Figure 17 Transmission electron micrograph of a cholangioma from a bullhead exposed to DENA. Lesion is composed of cuboidal to columnar epithelial cells with a basally located nucleus. A basal lamina (arrows) is present. Ductal cells contain numerous intermediate filaments, sparse GER, well-developed SER and Golgi, numerous smooth vesicles, and few mitochondria. Numerous interdigitations and junctional complexes join adjacent cells. Uranyl acetate and lead citrate. × 15 700

lesions in the rat termed 'spongiosis hepatis'[37], lesions in the medaka and sheepshead minnow involve cells rich in intermediate filaments identified as empty perisinusoidal fat-storing (Ito) liver cells. Presence of this lesion in the brown bullhead and other teleost species is unknown.

Hepatocellular carcinoma

In rodents, hepatocellular carcinomas occur either 'spontaneously' late in life (in some strains) and/or following chronic administration of chemical carcinogens[29]. Usually only one or two carcinomas are found per liver. These lesions are characterized by their invasive growth pattern, large size (usually greater than 1–2 mm in diameter) and histological appearance[29]. Frequently, an area of central necrosis within the carcinoma is seen. Histologically, most rodent hepatocellular carcinomas present in a trabecular pattern displaying cords of two or more hepatocytes in thickness[29].

Hendricks *et al.*[4] described similar tumours in the rainbow trout exposed to various carcinogens as 'hepatocellular (trabecular) and adenocarcinomas'. As previously described[4], a trabecular carcinoma is characterized by broad discontinuous laminae of hepatocytes (3–10 cells thick) which alternate with sinusoids. Similar lesions are observed in the bullhead liver following exposure to chemical carcinogens (Figure 8). These laminae are usually slightly basophilic and exhibit numerous mitotic figures. Reported previously in the rainbow trout[4] and observed in the bullhead liver, bile ducts or duct-like structures and sparse supporting connective tissue are seen centrally within trabecular lesions (Figures 9 and 10). Both dead and dying hepatocytes, as well as more normal appearing hepatocytes, are observed in surrounding tissue adjacent to trabecular carcinoma cells (Figure 11). Additionally, nuclear and cytoplasmic volumes appear to be reduced in peripheral trabecular carcinoma cells (Figure 12). Few canalicular structures are observed and cellular borders are difficult to distinguish (Figure 12). Cytoplasmically, transformed hepatocytes exhibited a loss of lipid and glycogen, proliferated and dilated GER and SER free ribosomes, well-developed Golgi, absence of cytoplasmic filaments and numerous mitochondria (Figures 12 and 13). Centrally within trabecular tumours, duct or duct-like structures with little supporting connective tissue are observed (Figures 10 and 14). Cytoplasmically similar to normal biliary epithelium, these duct-like cells possess sparse amounts of GER, numerous free ribosomes, few mitochondria, well-developed Golgi with numerous vesicles, and abundant intermediate filaments (Figure 14). Near the apical border of cells forming duct-like structures, numerous tight junctions and desmosomes are observed (Figure 14). Similar to bile preductular (Figures 3 and 15) and ductular epithelium in the normal bullhead liver, a basal lamina is absent between cells forming small duct-like structures and surrounding cells within trabecular tumours (Figures 10 and 14). Associated with large bile ducts in the normal liver, basement membrane-like material is only associated with large duct-like structures within trabecular tumours. Whether bile duct proliferation results from transformed hepatocytes, enveloped portal regions by an expanding trabeculat carcinoma[4], or from hyperplasia and hypertrophy of bile preductular cells is unknown.

Adenocarcinoma

Less frequently observed in teleost liver, lesions which possess a glandular or acinar appearance have been described[1,4,32]. Termed 'adenocarcinoma', due to the presence within such lesions of duct-like structures with supporting connective tissue elements and solid nests of cells recognized as hepatocytes, controversy exists, even in mammalian research, over whether biliary epithelium or hepatocytes give rise to these lesions[22]. Although not observed in the bullhead liver, cells which compose this lesion are usually slightly basophilic and exhibit numerous mitotic figures[4]. Closely resembling neoplastic bile ducts, the term 'hepatocholangiocarcinoma' has been proposed as appropriately describing this lesion in the teleost liver[4,36].

Bile duct tumours

Benign (cholangiomas) and malignant (cholangiocarcinomas) tumours arising from ductal epithelium have been described in rodent liver[22,29]. In particular, chronic treatment with nitrosamine carcinogens has been very effective in the production of cholangiomas and cholangiocarcinomas[29].

In the feral bullhead liver, the term cholangioma has been used to describe tumours which are composed exclusively of bile ductular epithelial cells and supporting connective tissue[5,9] (Figure 16). These lesions consist of proliferated ductal structures with a dilated lumen surrounded by a flattened cuboidal to columnar epithelium. Epithelial cells have a round to oval nucleus with a dispersed chromatin pattern (Figure 16). The nucleus occupies the entire width of the cytoplasm of the cells, and most have a small rim of cytoplasm extending in the circumferential axis of the duct. At high magnification, the lumenal border contains hair-like processes consistent with cilia. Cross-sections of these ducts show an irregular outline with frequent interdigitations and outpouchings. The ductal structures are surrounded by a small number of proliferated young fibroblastic appearing cells and a few lymphocytes which infiltrate the stroma. The outline of these areas is irregular, and there does not appear to be overt compression of the surrounding liver parenchyma. At times, periductular fibrous tissue is much more sclerotic and the ducts are compressed by the proliferation of fibrous tissue. A designation of 'cholangiofibroma' may be appropriate for this area (Figure 16).

In feral bullheads as well as those exposed to DENA, bile ductular tumours were identical. Ducts were separated from surrounding connective tissue by a basal lamina (Figure 17). Ductal cells contained a basally located nucleus, numerous intermediate filaments, well-developed Golgi with numerous smooth vesicles, well-developed SER, sparse GER, and few mitochondria (Figure 17). Numerous interdigitations and junctional complexes joined adjacent cells.

In the rat, disparate synonyms reflect confusion about origin, nature and eventual fate of bile preductular and ductular epithelial cells[38]. Following chronic exposure to hepatocarcinogens, hyperplasia of bile preductular cells are thought to give rise to so called 'oval cells'. Termed oval cells due to their light-microscopic morphology, their appearance occurs early, preceding the development of other proliferative lesions[22,39-45]. When Grisham[45] attempted long-term culture of rat liver cells, only cells which resembled bile preductular cells remained viable, indicating that bile preductular cells may act as hepatocyte stem cells. Yaswen *et al.*[41] showed that oval cells isolated from rats fed a choline-deficient diet were: γ-glutamyl transpeptidase positive; either biliary epithelial cells or small transitional hepatocytes; and positive for albumin and α-fetoprotein as demonstrated immunocytochemically. Additionally, in the rat, bile preductular cells have been shown to: activate carcinogens directly; be susceptible to direct or indirect effects of metabolites activated by hepatocytes; influence hepatocyte conversion to malignancy; or develop into hepatomas directly[39]. Examination of the role(s) of bile preductular and ductular epithelium in teleost carcinogenesis warrants further study.

Interestingly, studies of fish liver carcinogenesis induced by chemical carcinogens showed co-existence of cholangio- and hepatocellular carcinoma[1,33,35,46-49]. This finding may be due to the intimate association of hepatocytes and biliary elements, especially bile preductules and ductular cells[16,17,21,33]. Therefore, the role of these cells in carcinogenesis in the teleost liver deserves further study. Since evidence exists that bile preductular cells may serve as stem cells from which hepatocytes, exocrine pancreatic, intestinal epithelial and hepatocellular carcinoma cells arise in rodents[39,42,44,45], teleost liver in general and the brown bullhead liver in particular may serve as an excellent model for the study of the role(s) of bile preductular cells in carcinogenesis.

References

1. Stanton, M. F. (1965). Diethylnitrosamine-induced hepatic degeneration and neoplasia in the aquarium fish, *Brachydanio rerio*. *J. Natl. Cancer Inst.*, 34, 117–130
2. Ishikawa, T. and Takayama, S. (1979). Importance of hepatic neoplasms in lower vertebrate animals as a tool in cancer research. *J. Toxicol. Environ. Health*, 5, 537–550
3. Gingerich, W. H. (1982). Hepatic toxicology of fishes. In Weber, L. J. (ed.) *Aquatic Toxicology*, pp. 55–105. (New York: Raven Press)
4. Hendricks, J. D., Meyers, T. R. and Shelton, D. W. (1984). Histological progression of hepatic neoplasia in rainbow trout (*Salmo gairdneri*). *Natl. Cancer Inst. Monogr.*, 65, 321–336
5. Dawe, C. J., Stanton, M. F. and Schwartz, F. J. (1964). Hepatic neoplasms in native bottom-feeding fish of Deep Creek Lake, Maryland. *Cancer Res.*, 24, 1194–1201
6. Wellings, S. R. (1969). Neoplasia and primitive vertebrate phylogeny: echinoderms, prevertebrates, and fishes. A review. *Natl. Cancer Inst. Monogr.*, 31, 59–128
7. Brown, E. R., Hazdra, J. J., Keith, L., Greenspan, I., Kwapinski, J. B. G. and Beamer, P. (1973). Frequency of fish tumors found in a polluted watershed and compared to nonpolluted Canadian waters. *Cancer Res.*, 33, 189–198
8. Black, J. J. (1983). Field and laboratory studies of environmental carcinogenesis in Niagara River fish. *J. Great Lakes Res.*, 9, 326–334
9. Klaunig, J. E., Ruch, R., Krall, C., Hamlett, W. C., Morse, D. and Goldblatt, P. J. (1984). Morphology of liver tumors in brown bullhead catfish (*Ictalurus nebulosus*) from the Black River in Ohio. *Mics. Micros. Acta*, 15, 111–112
10. Black, J., Fox, H., Black, P. and Bock, F. (1985). Carcinogenic effects of river sediment extracts in fish and mice. In Jolley, R. L., Bull, R. J., Davis, W. P., Katz, S., Roberts, M. H. and Jacobs, V. A. (eds.) *Water Chlorination Chemistry, Environmental Impact and Health Effects*, pp. 415–427. (Chelsea, Michigan: Lewis Publishers, Inc.)
11. Shore, T. W. and Jones, H. L. (1889). On the structure of the vertebrate liver. *J. Physiol. (London)*, 10, 408–428
12. Scarpelli, D. G., Greider, M. H. and Frajola, W. J. (1963). Observations on hepatic cell hyperplasia, adenoma, and hepatoma of rainbow trout (*Salmo gairdnerii*). *Cancer Res.*, 23, 848–857
13. Simon, R. C., Dollar, A. M. and Smuckler, E. A. (1967). Descriptive classification on normal and altered histology of trout livers. In Halver, J. E. and Mitchell, I. A. (eds.) *Trout Hepatoma Research Conference Papers*, pp. 18–28. (Washington: U.S. Fish and Wildlife Service)
14. Hinton, D. E. and Pool, C. R. (1976). Ultrastructure of the liver in channel catfish *Ictalurus punctatus* (Rafinesque). *J. Fish Biol.*, 8, 209–219
15. Hinton, D. E., Walker, E. R., Pinkstaff, C. A. and Zuchelkowski, E. M. (1984). Morphological survey of teleost organs important in carcinogenesis with attention to fixation. *Natl. Cancer Inst. Monogr.*, 65, 291–320
16. Hampton, J. A., McCuskey, P. A., McCuskey, R. S. and Hinton, D. E. (1985). Functional units in rainbow trout (*Salmo gairdneri*, Richardson) liver. I. Histochemical properties and arrangement of hepatocytes. *Anat. Rec.*, 213, 166–175
17. Hampton, J. A., Lantz, R. C. and Hinton, D. E. (1988). Functional units in rainbow trout (*Salmo gairdneri*, Richardson) liver. III. Morphometric analysis of parenchyma, stroma and component cell types. *Am. J. Anat.* (In press)
18. Elias, H. and Bengelsdorf, H. (1952). The structure of the liver of vertebrates. *Acta Anat.*, 14, 297–337
19. Ito, T., Watanabe, A. and Takahashi, Y. (1962). Histologische und cytologische utersuchungen der leber bei fisch und cyclostomata, nebst bemerkungen die fettsspeicherungszellen. *Arch. Histol. Jpn.*, 22, 429–463
20. Elias, H. and Sherrick, J. C. (1969). *Morphology of the Liver*. (New York: Academic Press)
21. Tanuma, Y., Ohata, M. and Ito, T. (1982). Electron microscopic study on the sinusoidal wall of the liver in the flatfish, *Kareius bicoloratus*: demonstration of numerous desmosomes along the sinusoidal wall. *Arch. Histol. Jpn.*, 45, 453–472
22. Stewart, H. L., Williams, G., Keysser, C. H., Lombard, L. S. and Montali, R. J. (1980). Histologic typing of liver tumors of the rat. *J. Natl. Cancer Inst.*, 64, 179–206
23. Lipsky, M. M., Hinton, D. E., Klaunig, J. E. and Trump, B. F. (1981). Biology of hepatocellular neoplasia in the mouse. I. Histogenesis of safrole-induced hepatocellular carcinoma. *J. Natl. Cancer Inst.*, 67, 365–376
24. Lipsky, M. M., Hinton, D. E., Klaunig, J. E., Goldblatt, P. J. and Trump, B. F. (1981). Biology of hepatocellular neoplasia in the mouse. II. Sequential enzyme histochemical analysis of BALB/c mouse liver during safrole-induced carcinogenesis. *J. Natl. Cancer Inst.*, 67, 377–392
25. Lipsky, M. M., Hinton, D. E., Klaunig, J. E. and Trump, B. F. (1981). Biology of hepatocellular neoplasia in the mouse. III. Electron microscopy of safrole-induced hepatocellular adenomas and hepatocellular carcinomas. *J. Natl. Cancer Inst.*, 67, 393–405

26. Farber, E. (1984). The multistep nature of cancer development. *Cancer Res.*, **44**, 4217–4223

27. Farber, E. (1984). Precancerous steps in carcinogenesis: their physiological and adaptive nature. *Biochem. Biophys. Acta*, **738**, 171–180

28. Schulte-Hermann, R. (1985). Tumor promotion in the liver. *Arch. Toxicol.*, **57**, 147–158

29. Frith, C. H. and Ward, J. M. (1980). A morphologic classification of proliferative and neoplastic hepatic lesions in mice. *J. Environ. Pathol. Toxicol.*, **3**, 329–351

30. Nakazawa, T., Hamaguchi, S. and Kyono-Hamaguchi, Y. (1985). Histochemistry of liver tumors induced by diethylnitrosamine and differential sex susceptibility to carcinogenesis in *Oryzias latipes*. *J. Natl. Cancer Inst.*, **75**, 567–573

31. Klaunig, J. E., Lipsky, M. M., Trump, B. F. and Hinton, D. E. (1979). Biochemical and ultrastructural changes in teleost liver following subacute exposure to PCB. *J. Environ. Pathol. Toxicol.*, **2**, 953–963

32. Pliss, G. B. and Khudoley, V. V. (1975). Tumor induction by carcinogenic agents in aquarium fish. *J. Natl. Cancer Inst.*, **55**, 129–136

33. Hinton, D. E., Lantz, R. C. and Hampton, J. A. (1984). Effects of age and exposure to a carcinogen on the structure of the medaka liver: a morphometric study. *Natl. Cancer Inst. Monogr.*, **65**, 239–249

34. Murchelano, R. A. and Wolke, R. E. (1985). Epizootic carcinoma in the winter flounder, *Pseudopleuronectes americanus*. *Science*, **228**, 587–589

35. Hinton, D. E., Hampton, J. A. and McCuskey, P. A. (1985). The Japanese medaka (*Oryzias latipes*) liver tumor model: Review of literature and new findings. In Jolley, R. L., Bull, R. J., Davis, W. P., Katz, S., Roberts, M. H. and Jacobs, V. A. (eds.) *Water Chlorination Chemistry, Environmental Impact and Health Effects*, pp. 439–450. (Chelsea, Michigan: Lewis Publishers, Inc.)

36. Couch, J. A. and Courtney, L. A. (1985). Attempts to abbreviate time to endpoint in fish hepatocarcinogenesis assays. In Jolley, R. L., Bull, R. J., Davis, W. P., Katz, S., Roberts, M. H. and Jacobs, V. A. (eds.) *Water Chlorination Chemistry, Environmental Impact and Health Effects*, pp. 377–398. (Chelsea, Michigan: Lewis Publishers, Inc.)

37. Bannasch, P., Bloch, M. and Zerban, H. (1981). Spongiosis hepatis. *Lab. Invest.*, **44**, 252–264

38. Steiner, J. W. and Carruthers, J. S. (1961). Studies on the fine structure of the terminal branches of the biliary tree. *Am. J. Pathol.*, **38**, 639–661

39. Sell, S. and Leffert, H. L. (1982). An evaluation of cellular lineages in the pathogenesis of experimental hepatocellular carcinoma. *Hepatology*, **2**, 77–86

40. Lombardi, B. (1982). On the nature, properties and significance of oval cells. *Recent Trends Chem. Carcinogen.*, **1**, 37–56

41. Yaswen, P., Hayner, N. T. and Fausto, N. (1984). Isolation of oval cells by centrifugal elutriation and comparison with other cell types purified from normal and preneoplastic livers. *Cancer Res.*, **44**, 324–331

42. Scarpelli, D. G. (1985). Multipotent developmental capacity of cells in the adult animal. *Lab. Invest.*, **52**, 331–333

43. Bannasch, P. (1985). Sequential cellular changes during chemical carcinogenesis. *J. Cancer Res. Clin. Oncol.*, **108**, 11–22

44. Tatematsu, M., Kaku, T., Medline, A. and Farber, E. (1985). Intestinal metaplasia as a common option of oval cells in relation to cholangiofibrosis in liver of rats exposed to 2-acetylaminofluorene. *Lab. Invest.*, **52**, 354–362

45. Grisham. J. W. (1980). Cell types in long-term propagable cultures of rat liver. *Ann. NY Acad. Sci.*, **349**, 128–137

46. Ishikawa, T., Shimamine, T. and Takayama, S. (1975). Histologic and electron microscopy observations on diethylnitrosamine-induced hepatomas in small aquarium fish (*Oryzias latipes*). *J. Natl. Cancer Inst.*, **55**, 909–916

47. Scarpelli, D. G. (1967). Ultrastructural and biochemical observations on trout hepatoma. In Halver, J. E. and Mitchell, I. A. (eds.) *Trout Hepatoma Research Conference Papers*, pp. 60–71. (Washington: U.S. Fish and Wildlife Service)

48. Aoki, K. and Matsudaira, H. (1977). Induction of hepatic tumors in a teleost (*Oryzias latipes*) after treatment with methylazoxymethanol acetate: brief communication. *J. Natl. Cancer Inst.*, **59**, 1747–1749

49. Sinnhuber, R. O., Hendricks, J. D., Wales, J. H. and Putnam, G. B. (1977). Neoplasms in rainbow trout, a sensitive animal model for environmental carcinogenesis. *Ann. NY Acad. Sci.*, **298**, 389–462

13

The elasmobranch liver. A model for chemical carcinogenesis studies in a 'naturally resistant' vertebrate

W. C. HAMLETT

INTRODUCTION

The elasmobranch fishes include the sharks, skates and stingrays. These important vertebrates occupy a pivotal position evolutionarily. They diverged some 350 million years ago from their sister group, the holocephalans (Chimaeras). Contemporary elasmobranchs are usually considered primitive and this is certainly true of many of their morphological characters, some of which have been conserved with very little change. There has recently been a renewed interest in the basic biology of this group, as well as in the use of them as models in biomedical research. The elasmobranchs may serve as valuable experimental models in which basic developmental and functional mechanisms of higher vertebrates may be elucidated. Apart from their importance as laboratory animals, they have a special relevance in comparative studies and evolutionary biology.

There is a dearth of information in the literature relating to the microscopic anatomy and ultrastructure of the elasmobranch liver. Indeed, few comprehensive studies have been undertaken to define and describe this important organ. This chapter represents the only description of the ultrastructure of the elasmobranch liver aside from previously published freeze-fracture accounts of the tight junctions in skate liver bile canaliculi[1-3].

Much remains unknown regarding the ultrastructural organization, physiology and biochemistry of almost every major organ in fishes. However, comparative fish histology and pathology are of increasing importance today. Recent efforts to utilize fish as sentinel organisms for monitoring environmental pollutants and carcinogens have met with success. The study of neoplasia in poikilothermic vertebrates will add to the basic understanding of neoplasia in general and, presumably, in homoeothermic vertebrates, including man. Of particular interest is the apparent 'natural resistance' of elasmobranchs to liver tumours. It has long been considered that the phylogenetic point at which neoplasms first occurred was in the class Pisces[4,5]. However, this view has been challenged and the phylogenetic point of neoplastic transformation may instead reside in invertebrates[6-9]. Few instances of neoplasia in elasmobranchs have been reported. A very important fact is that only one report

of a tumour in the elasmobranch liver has ever been reported[10] (a benign adenoma), whereas virtually hundreds of liver tumours in teleost fish have been described. The liver is known to be highly susceptible to the induction of cancer by experimental chemical agents.

Hamlett and Stoner[11] have proposed the use of both adult and embryonic elasmobranchs in chemical carcinogenesis studies. Their efforts represent a combined biochemical and whole-animal experimental protocol. It has been demonstrated that the potent chemical carcinogen, aflatoxin B_1 (AFB_1) exerts its carcinogenic effect most often in the liver. This has been demonstrated very clearly in the rainbow trout embryo[12]. The covalent binding of activated metabolite(s) of a carcinogen to cellular DNA is thought to be an essential step in the initiation of carcinogenesis[13] and it has recently been demonstrated[11,14] that AFB_1 is capable of binding to skate liver DNA. Considering the recent interest in the elasmobranch liver, the presentation of an ultrastructural description of this organ would seem desirable.

EMBRYONIC ORIGIN AND OVERALL ORGANIZATION OF THE ELASMOBRANCH LIVER

The liver rudiment initially appears as a midventral evagination of the developing duodenum that branches into the primordia of the gallbladder and the right and left lobes of the liver[15]. The vitelline veins then become surrounded by the developing liver. During this process, fenestrations appear in the vitelline veins and sinusoids which connect the right and left vitelline (i.e. hepatic) veins are thus produced.

Posterior to the developing liver, the right and left vitelline veins become closely associated with the duodenum. The right portion persists as the hepatic portal vein which receives blood from the intestine, stomach and pancreas[15]. The hepatic portal vein is formed by the union of the posterior intestinal, anterior intestinal and gastric veins. Near the liver, the hepatic portal divides, sending a major branch to each of the liver lobes. These, in turn, form a vascular network. Blood is thus distributed to the liver by both the hepatic artery and the hepatic portal vein and is collected by the hepatic veins for return to the heart.

Evolutionarily, the liver was originally a tubular exocrine gland. This is still evident in the ammocoetes larvae and in the adult hagfish[16]. The secretory component of the liver is delivered to the biliary system and, hence, to the gut. The purely tubular nature of the gland was replaced evolutionarily by a meshwork of parenchymal cells and sinusoids.

Amongst the elasmobranchs, the liver consists of a right and left lobe with a smaller caudate lobe between. The gallbladder is most often located in the caudate lobe. A bile duct connects it to the duodenum. The main lobes of the liver are typically extremely large and frequently extend the entire length of the abdominal cavity. In large sharks, this can amount to several metres. In the large shark (*Cetorhinus*), five barrels of oil have been obtained from a single specimen[17].

MICROANATOMY

Histologically, the elasmobranch liver, not unlike the teleost liver, is less definitively organized into lobules than in higher vertebrates. Hepatic arterioles are often quite a distance removed from their associated vein and bile duct. Central veins are irregularly dispersed between continuous masses of cells called muralia (one to two-cell plates) of laminae[18]. The laminae are very irregular compared with higher vertebrates.

The space between plates of hepatic cells is occupied by hepatic sinusoids (Figures 1 and 2). Portal areas are indistinct. When present, the portal area contains branches of the portal vein, hepatic artery and bile duct. Prominent granulated cells with pale cytoplasm are intermingled with the hepatocytes. As briefly outlined here, the microanatomy of the liver does not emerge clearly in histological sections. The anatomical unit of the mammalian liver, the hepatic lobule, is seen very clearly in the pig liver but is less obvious in man and rat. In the latter species, adjacent hepatic lobules merge and a regular distribution of portal areas is not evident at the periphery of the lobule.

Reticuloendothelial cells of von Kupffer may line the sinusoids and help in the removal of destroyed red blood cells[19]. However, no von Kupffer cells were identified by this author in the skate, *Raja erinacea*, or the shark, *Rhizoprionodon terraenovae*, using light and electron microscopy. Their presence must be confirmed by experimental methods before this controversy can be settled.

Conspicuous patches of pigment, i.e. lipofuscin, are frequently present in the liver of many lower vertebrates. This is also true of the elasmobranchs. Lipochrome pigment is rare in young animals. It is considered to be accumulations of indigestible residues, not completely degraded by lysosomal hydrolases. Additionally, melanocyte-type cells also occur.

Hepatocytes

The hepatocytes of elasmobranchs are similar morphologically to those of higher vertebrates. They are roughly polyhedral and their cytoplasm contains mitochondria, glycogen, rough endoplasmic reticulum and a Golgi complex (Figures 3, 10 and 19). They appear to differ only in that they contain abundant lipid deposits (Figures 1, 5 and 7). The cells form desmosomal junctions with adjacent hepatocytes and they are morphologically and functionally polarized. Where adjacent hepatocytes abut each other, desmosomal junctions function to adhere them (Figure 5). The plasmalemma of adjacent hepatocytes form bile canaliculi (Figures 3, 4, 9 and 10). The plasmalemma of each hepatocyte produces infoldings with microvilli extending into the lumen of the canaliculi. Freeze-fracture studies[1-3] reveal that the basic structural units of the tight junctions (zonula occludentes) of the bile canaliculi of the skate closely resemble those of rat liver and that these elements have thus been conserved evolutionarily. The tight-junction type has been described as 'leaky'[3]. This is similar to 'leaky junctions' in other epithelia[20]. Electron-microscopic studies have demonstrated that ionic lanthanum traverses tight junctions[3]. These junctional complexes form a semipermeable blood–bile barrier. Both the strand number and depth of the tight junctions are heterogeneous. Consequently, permeability could vary at multiple points along a single hepatocyte. In elasmobranchs, bile alcohols form the major solute in bile rather than bile acids[21]. Otherwise, the bile composition is qualitatively similar to mammalian bile[22].

Elasmobranchs do not form definitive adipose deposits[23]. Instead, the liver serves as a principal site for lipid storage. The lipid component of the elasmobranch liver is frequently higher than that seen in other vertebrate groups[24], and some lipids that are absent or sparingly represented in other vertebrates may be major constituents in elasmobranchs. Alkyldiacylglycerols form a major part of the hepatic lipid in sharks of the suborder Squaloidea[25-27]. The hydrocarbon, squalene, constitutes a large part (39–96%) of the hepatic lipid in some deep-sea sharks[28]. Both these substances have been demonstrated to provide hydrostatic lift to the shark, thus helping it to achieve a near-neutral buoyancy[29]. Cholesterol, free fatty acid and phospholipid are also present in the liver[24]. The large accumulation of low-density lipids (e.g. hydrocarbons and alkyldiacylglycerols) in the liver of elasmobranchs may have evolved as an analogue of the teleost swim bladder[24].

Another function of liver lipid is in embryonic development and fetal nutrition. In oviparous elasmobranchs, lipid in the liver is transferred to the growing oocyte in the form of a specific lipoprotein, vitellogenin, a yolk granule precursor. Following fertilization, the embryo grows at the expense of the yolk sequestered in its yolk sac[30].

In viviparous species that develop yolk-sac placentae, yolk is initially deposited in the same manner as in oviparous species. The process of yolk utilization has recently been elucidated in the Atlantic sharpnose shark, *Rhizoprionodon terraenovae*[31]. As development proceeds and the yolk stores are depleted, the yolk sac becomes developmentally modified into a yolk-sac placenta which fulfils the nutrient requirements of the growing fetus until parturition[32-35]. Based on experimental ultrastructural studies of the shark yolk-sac placenta[32-34], it has been proposed that the maternal liver continues to elaborate yolk precursor molecules into the circulating plasma and that these cross the placenta to supply nutrients to the developing young. An unusual maternal–fetal relation-

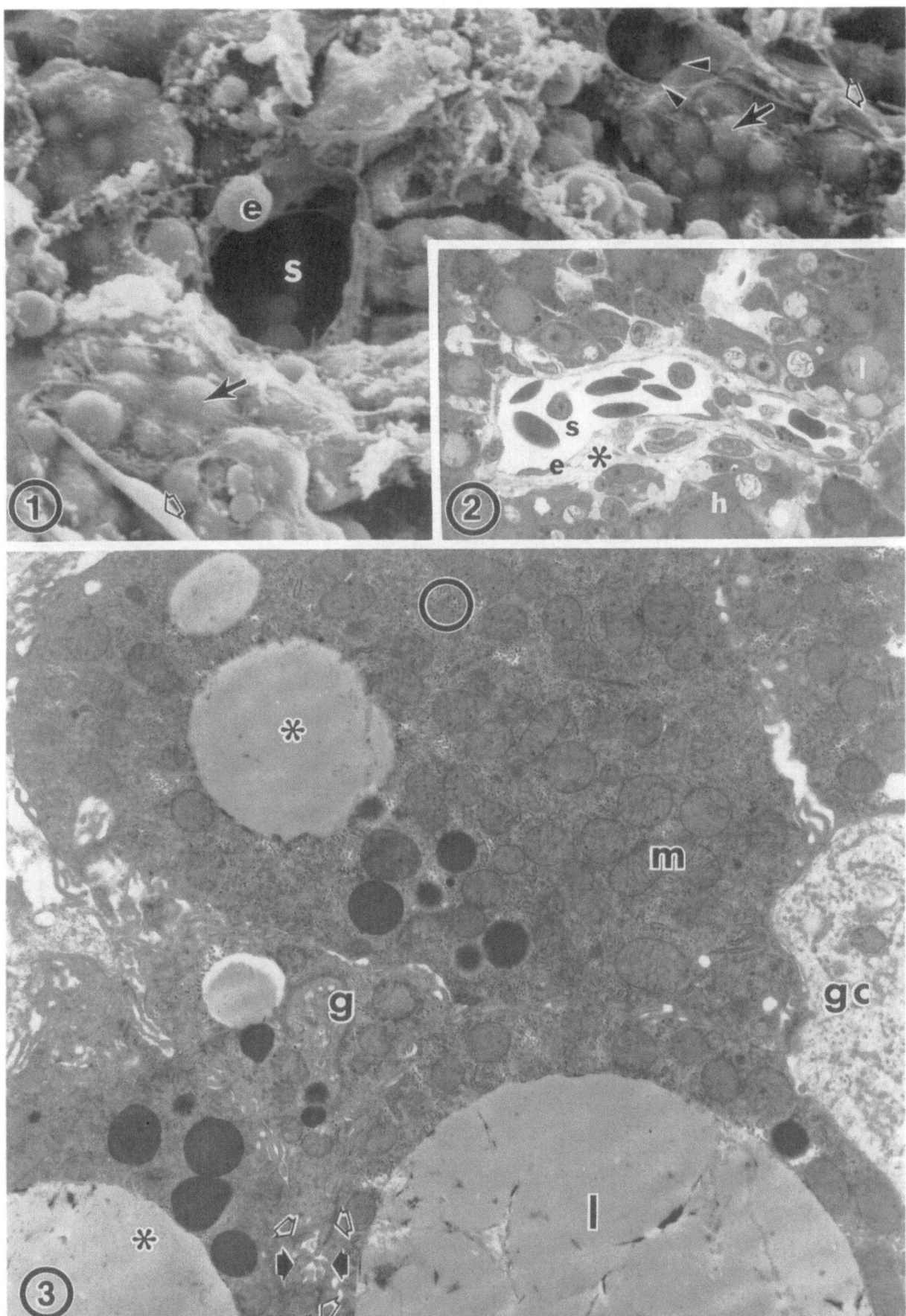

Figure 1 Scanning electron micrograph of *Raja erinacea* liver. Intracellular lipid deposits produce prominent bulging of the walls of hepatocytes (arrows). Erythrocytes (e) occupy a sinusoid (s). Fibrillar connective tissue elements occupy the space between hepatocytes (open arrows). Sinusoidal fenestrae are evident (arrow-heads). × 1430

Figure 2 Toluidine blue-stained 2 μm section of *Raja erinacea* liver. A small vessel (s) is central in the micrograph. The endothelium (e) is adjacent to the space of Disse (asterisk). l = lipid droplets; h = hepatocytes. × 1000

Figure 3 A very large lipid deposit (l) nearly fills the cytoplasm of one hepatocyte. Smaller lipid droplets occupy the cytoplasm of other hepatocytes (asterisks). Elements of the Golgi complex (g), glycogen (circle) and mitochondria (m) dominate the hepatocyte cytoplasm. A bile canaliculus (solid arrows) seen in transverse section has microvilli projecting into its lumen. A cell process from a granulocytic cell is seen at the right of the micrograph (gc). 'Leaky' tight junctions (open arrows) occur at the bile canalicular lumen. × 11 000

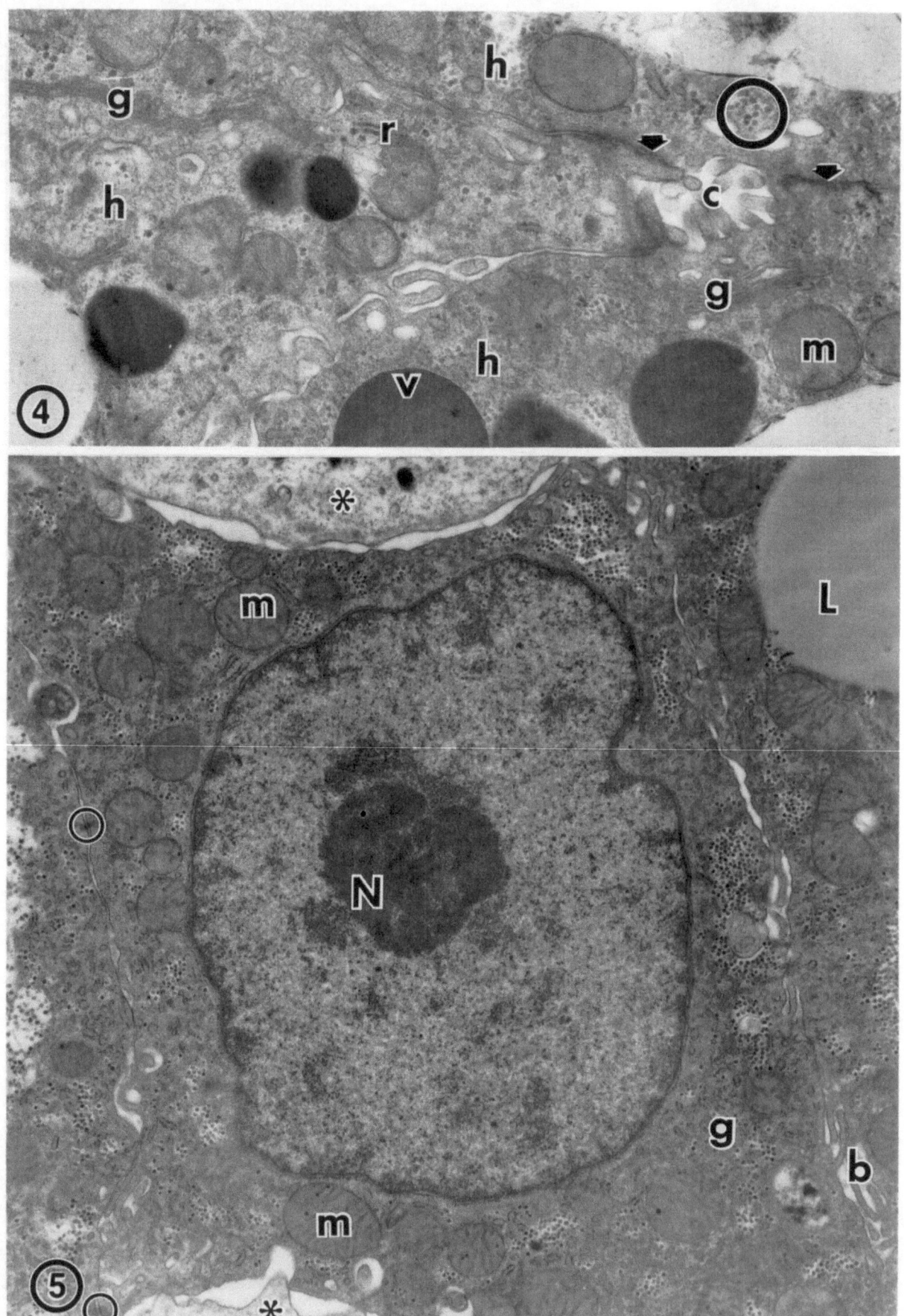

Figure 4 Several hepatocytes (h) contribute to the formation of a bile canaliculus (c). Tight junctions (arrows) seal the canaliculus. Mitochondria (m), glycogen (circle), rough endoplasmic reticulum (r) and elements of the Golgi complex (g) occupy the cytoplasm. Membrane limited vesicles (v) that may be lysosomes or peroxisomes are also evident. × 29 040

Figure 5 Electron micrograph of shark liver. Three contiguous hepatocytes are depicted. The large nucleus with a prominent nucleolus (N) occupies the central region. The cytoplasm is rich in mitochondria (m), glycogen (g) and lipid droplets (L). A bile canaliculus (b) is seen in longitudinal section between two adjacent hepatocytes. Desmosomes (circles) join adjacent hepatocytes. Asterisks indicate granulated cells. × 12 540

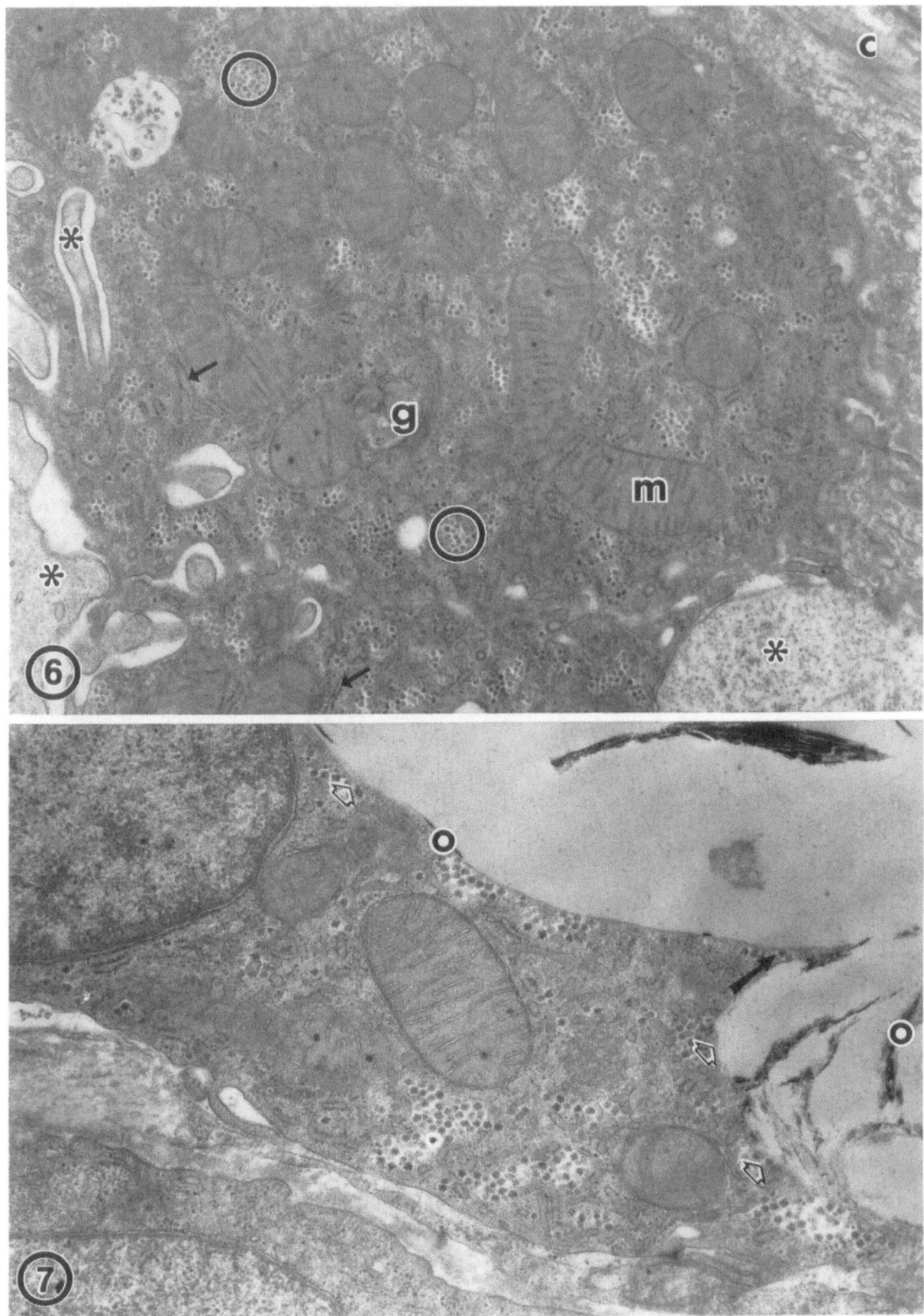

Figure 6 The hepatocyte cytoplasm is populated with mitochondria (m) in the normal configuration. Large amounts of glycogen (circles) fill the cytosol. Elements of the Golgi complex (g) and rough endoplasmic reticulum (arrows) also occur. Collagen (c) fills the interstices between cells. Pale-staining processes from granulated cells are evident (asterisks). × 21 080

Figure 7 Lipid inclusions of hepatocytes show angularity at their periphery (arrow). Osmiophilic material frequently adheres to the lipid (○). The lipid is somewhat soluble and, at points, blends into the cytoplasm (open arrows). × 21 250

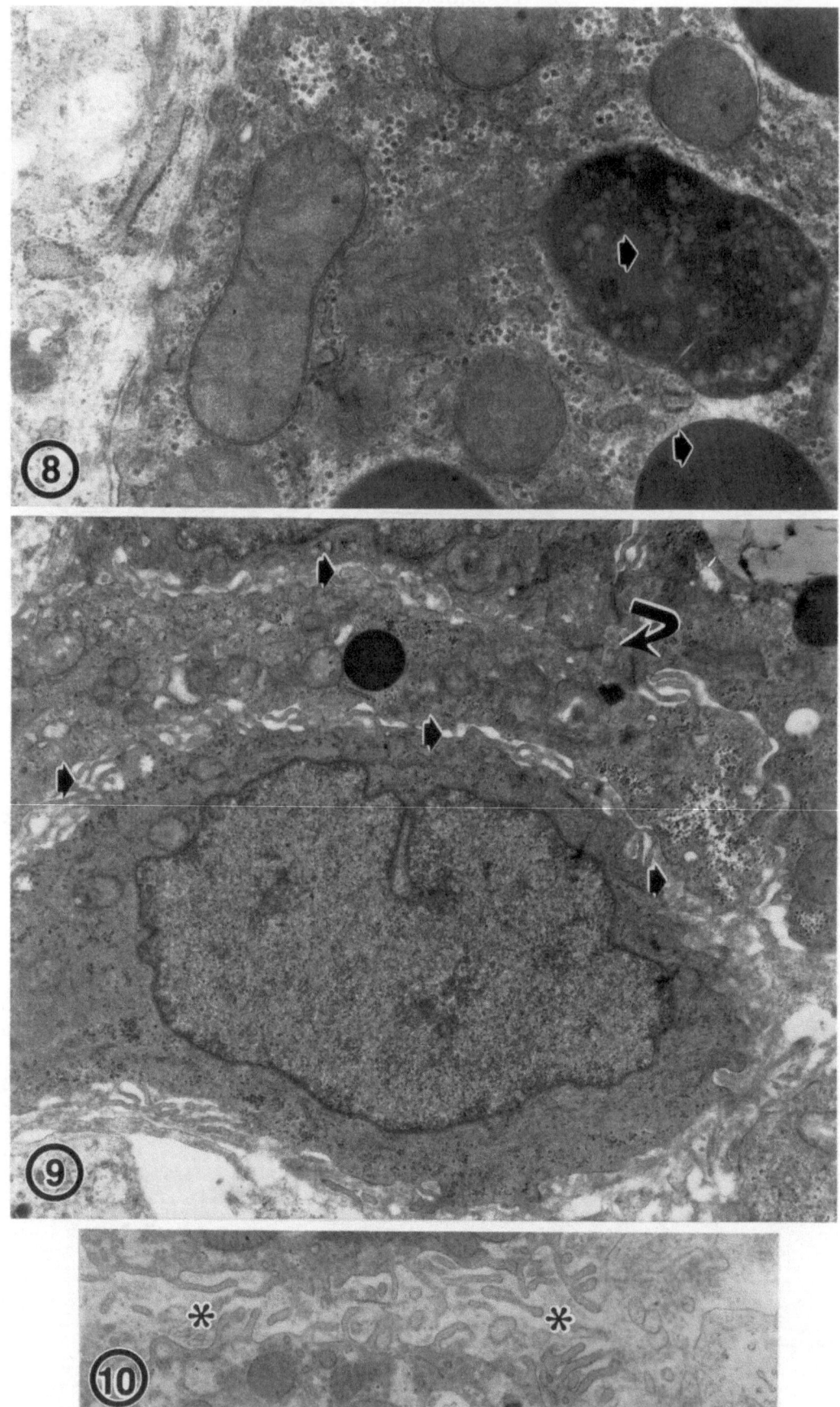

Figure 8 Heterogeneous organelles are often seen in the hepatocyte cytoplasm (arrows). These are most likely to be lysosomes, although specific histochemical tests have yet to be performed to confirm this. Early on, hepatic lysosomes were termed 'peribiliary dense granules'. Hepatic lysosomes are related to the digestion and lytic functions of hepatic cells. They are involved in bile formation, urea synthesis, detoxification and inactivation of chemicals. × 23 000

Figure 9 This low-power transmission electron micrograph shows several bile canaliculi in longitudinal section (arrows). Three canaliculi seem to converge and are shown contributing to a single bile canaliculus (curved arrow) seen in transverse section. × 7500

Figure 10 Microvilli from adjacent hepatocytes contribute to a bile canaliculus (asterisks). × 9120

ship is evident in the sharks, *Scoliodon sorrakowah*[36,37] and *S. laticaudus*[38]. The oocyte is only 1 mm in diameter and a specialized placenta is established very soon after implantation. There is, essentially, no prolonged yolk-dependent developmental period prior to the establishment of a functional placenta. It would be very interesting to know the relationship between the functional activity of the liver and the amount of nutrient transfer in these animals. To date, no experimental or quantitative data exist for these species.

The lipid inclusions often present heterogeneous profiles with angular incuttings at the periphery. Granular osmiophilic material is frequently adherent to the periphery of the inclusions. A similar finding has been reported for chick yolk platelets[39,40] and intracellular yolk drops in the endoderm of the shark yolk sac[14].

Granulocytes

Much controversy exists regarding the leukocytes of fish, especially in the elasmobranchs. Various methodologies, including light and electron microscopy, have been employed to describe the elements of elasmobranch blood[41–47]. Considerable confusion abounds regarding the terminology referring to elasmobranch leukocytes. With the advent of electron microscopy, Pica *et al.*[48] described two types of granulocytes in the electric ray and Hyder *et al.*[45] similarly described two types of granulocytes in the peripheral blood of the nurse shark. Other investigators, using electron microscopy, have described four different types of granulocytes in the dogfish, *Scyliorhinus canicula*[43,46,41]. There is currently considerable interest in the immune system of elasmobranchs since it is highly effective and shows a substantial resistance to natural infection[45]. Of more interest is the origin of these blood cells since elasmobranchs do not possess either bone marrow or lymph nodes. Instead, elasmobranchs have both lymphoid (lymphocyte-producing tissues) and myeloid (bone marrow-like tissue) mixed to form 'lymphomyeloid' structures[49].

Transmission electron micrographs of peripheral blood leukocytes within liver sinusoids of the Atlantic sharpnose shark, *Rhizoprionodon terraenovae*, show some cells to be similar to the peripheral blood granulocyte described by Hyder *et al.*[45] (Figures 11, 14 and 19). The same cell type is also interspersed with liver hepatocytes and has been seen in the process of diapedesis (Figure 12). Hyder *et al.*[45] demonstrated that these granulocytes are capable of phagocytosis. To date, no experimental studies have been undertaken to test whether the granulocytes residing in the elasmobranch liver also possess the ability to phagocytose exogenous material. The presence of granulated cells, which may be phagocytic leukocytes, in the liver poses an interesting question. What function are they performing? In this investigation, using both light and transmission electron microscopy, I have been unable to identify von Kupffer cells in either the shark or skate liver. No experimental uptake studies, however, have yet been performed to substantiate this observation.

The liver granulocyte has a pale cytoplasm and does not form junctional complexes with hepatocytes (Figure 14). The nucleus is ovoid and slightly indented. There is a reduced Golgi complex, scant rough endoplasmic reticulum and few mitochondria. Prominent granules with a periodic fibrillar substructure characterize the granulocyte. These granules are similar to those previously described by Hyder *et al.*[45] in the granulocyte of the nurse shark.

Sinusoids and space of Disse

Hepatic sinusoids are a modified capillary bed with fenestrations (Figures 15 and 19). The sinusoids are composed of ordinary endothelium with no basal lamina. They show pinocytotic activity. No von Kupffer cells were observed. The endothelial cells are separated from the underlying hepatocytes by the space of Disse. Villous projections of the hepatocytes extend into the space which is continuous with the sinusoidal lumen via the fenestrae. Electron-dense flocculent material fills the interstices between the endothelium and the hepatocytes. No perisinusoidal fat-storing cells of Ito were observed.

Capsule

The elasmobranch liver is enveloped by a mesothelium and connective tissue which is equivalent to Glisson's capsule of higher vertebrates (Figures 16 and 19). This mesothelial covering is composed of squamous cells with surface microvilli. The nucleus is lobate and the cytoplasm displays rough endoplasmic reticulum and a sparse Golgi complex. Zonulae occludens, zonulae adherens and desmosomes connect cells at the luminal surface. Unusual spherical vesicles occur at the apex of these cells, subjacent to the microvilli. They are electron dense and have a more dense core. Their function is unknown. The mesothelial cells rest upon a prominent and undulating basal lamina. Collagen fibres and profiles resembling elastin fill the space between the basal lamina and the hepatocytes.

Biliary system

Bile is emptied into bile canaliculi. These communicate with small bile preductules. The latter have a small lumen surrounded by cuboidal epithelial cells but do not have a striate border. The bile preductules merge to form larger bile ducts. Cells of the bile duct are columnar to pyramidal (Figures 17 and 19). Connective tissue elements envelop the ducts circumferentially. Occludens junctions seal the apex of neighbouring cells. The apices of these cells have microvilli. Subjacent to this is a population of pale-staining vesicles. The nucleus is basal and there is a prominent supranuclear Golgi complex. A large population of normal mitochondria populate the apical cytoplasm. Lateral cell membranes elaborate extensive projections that extend into the intercellular space.

CONCLUSIONS AND FUTURE DIRECTIONS

The elasmobranch fishes constitute a provocative vertebrate group. Aside from the innate interest in their natural history and their assumed potential threat to man, much can be learned from these primitive vertebrates. They have remained virtually unchanged for millions of years and they successfully inhabit widely divergent ecological niches. From a purely comparative point of view, elasmobranchs are widely used as laboratory

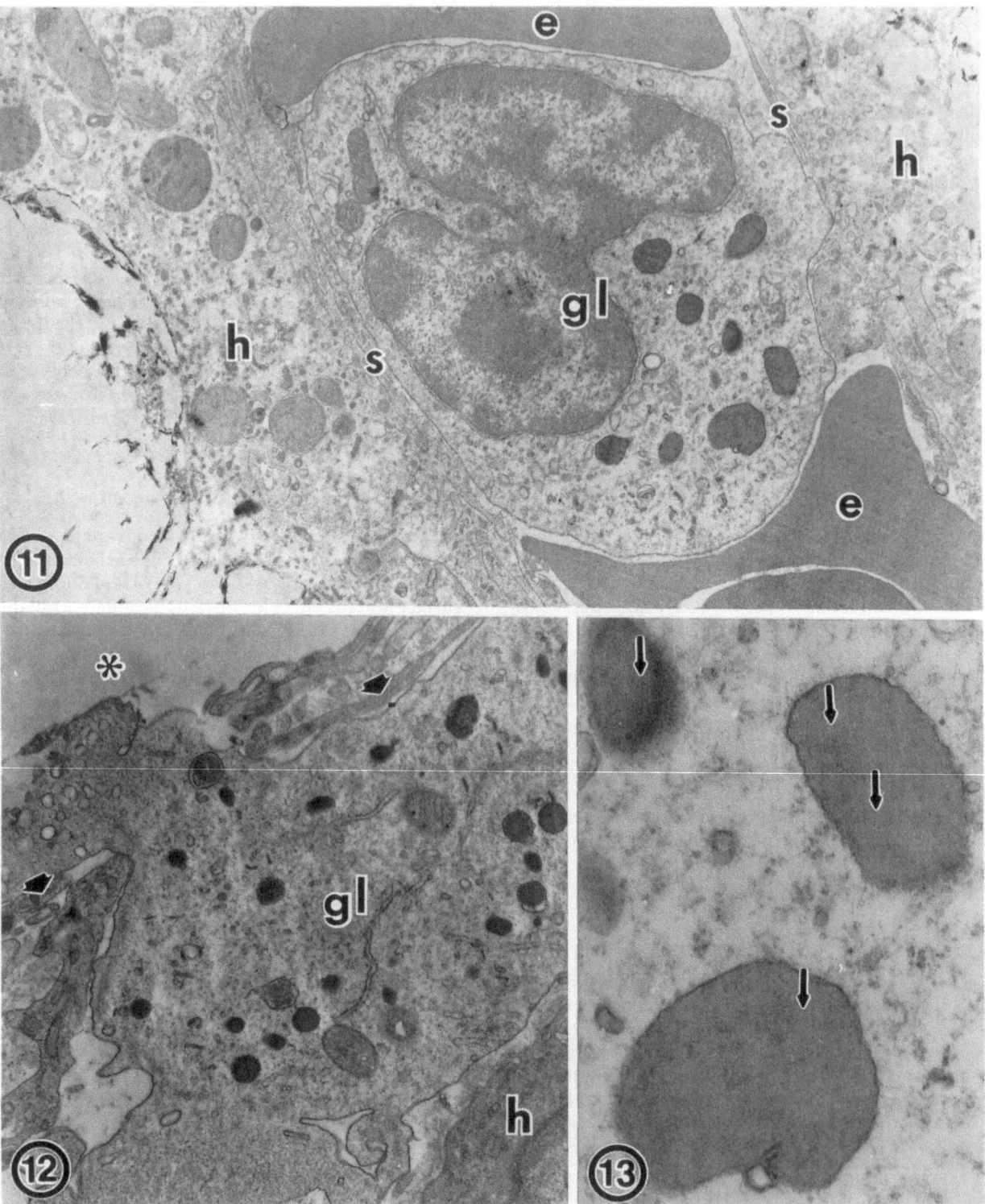

Figure 11   A peripheral blood granulated leukocyte (gl) and nucleated erythrocytes (e) are seen in a liver sinusoid. Hepatocytes (h) are in close proximity to the very thin sinusoidal endothelium (s). × 8800

Figure 12   A granulated leukocyte (gl) is seen in the process of diapedesis. The sinusoidal lumen is at the upper left (asterisk) of the micrograph. The granulated cell has entered the space of Disse. Note the sinusoidal endothelium (arrows) and adjacent hepatocyte (h). × 15 500

Figure 13   The granules of a peripheral leukocyte show periodic fibrillar substructure (arrows). These are virtually identical to inclusions present within the granulated cells seen in the liver. × 46 200

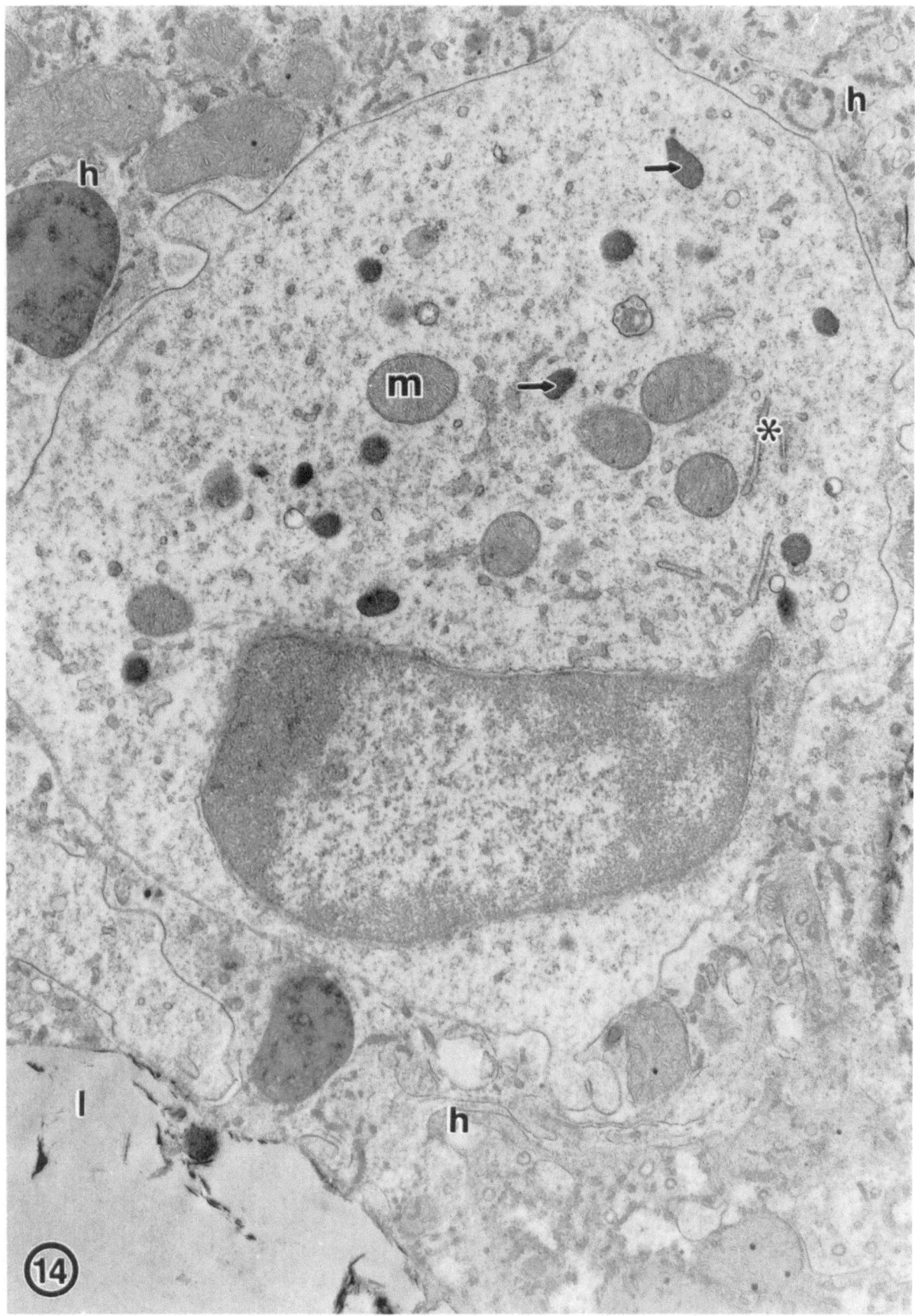

Figure 14 Hepatocytes (h) with large lipid droplets (l) surround a granulated cell. The indented nucleus of the granulated cell is eccentric. The cytoplasm contains scant endoplasmic reticulum (asterisk), mitochondria (m) and fibrillar granules (arrows). The function and phagocytic potential of this cell type has yet to be established. × 15 840

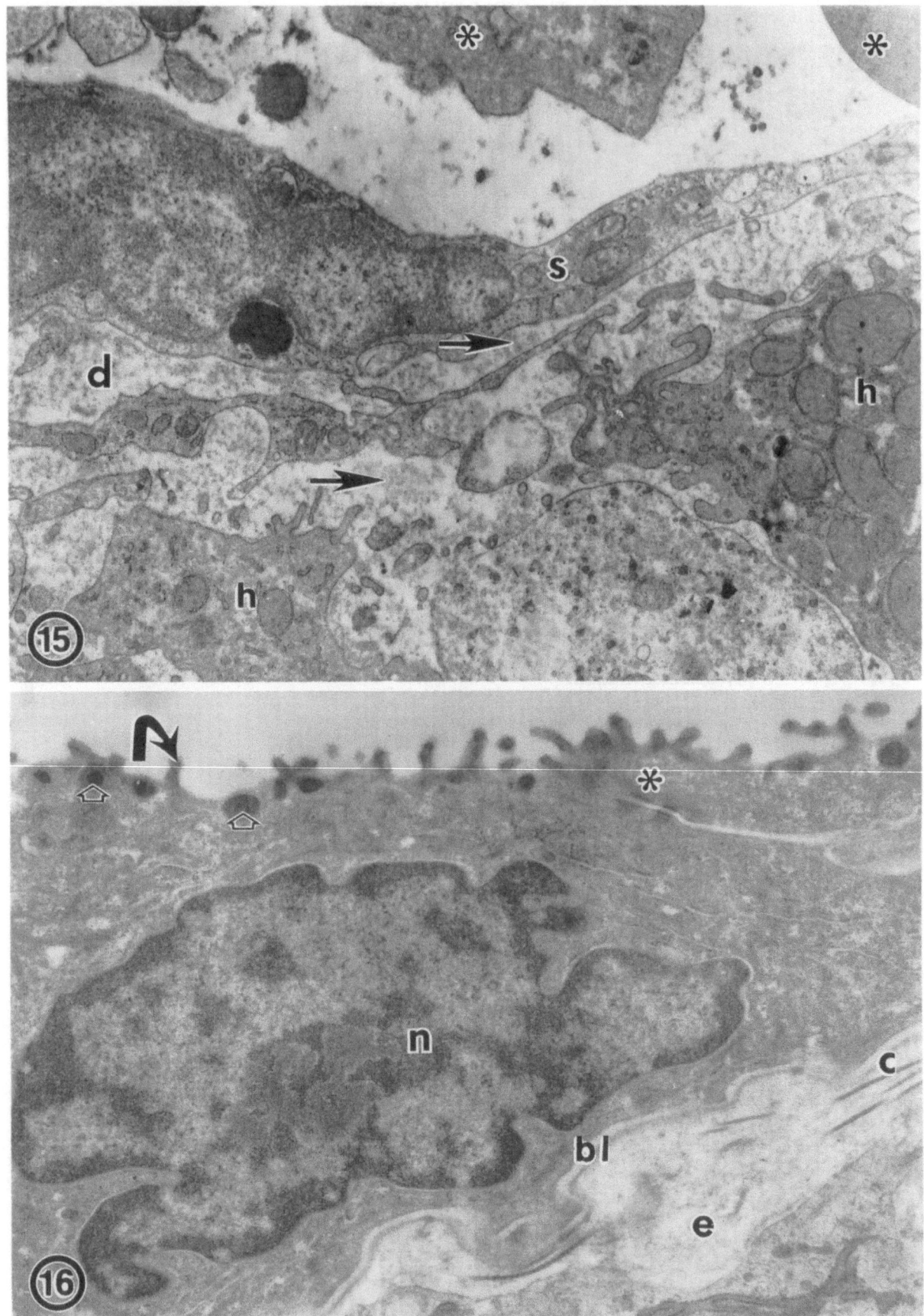

Figure 15 The sinusoidal endothelium (s) is flattened. Several peripheral blood cells are seen in the sinusoidal lumen (asterisks). The space of Disse (d) is filled with electron-dense flocculent material (arrows). Hepatocytes are evident (h) (and no perisinusoidal fat-storing cells of Ito are observed. The failure to observe these may be related to either their absence or rarity). × 15 840

Figure 16 The capsule covering the liver is equivalent to Glisson's capsule. The epithelium is a typical mesothelium. The cells are joined by zonulae occludens, zonulae adherens and desmosomes (asterisk). Microvilli (curved arrow) adorn the surface and the epithelium rests on a prominent basal lamina (bl). Unusual apical inclusions with a dense core (open arrows) are seen. Their functional significance is unknown. The space between the mesothelium and the hepatocytes is occupied by collagen (c) and what appears to be tangentially sectioned elastic fibres (e). The nucleus (n) is lobate. × 17 000

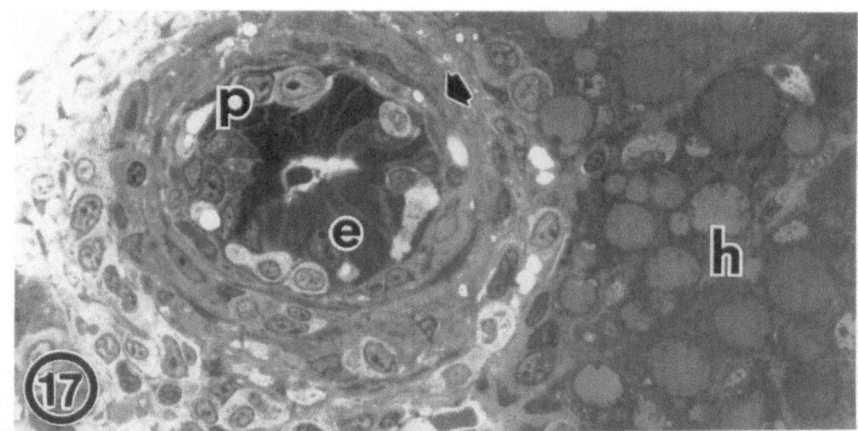

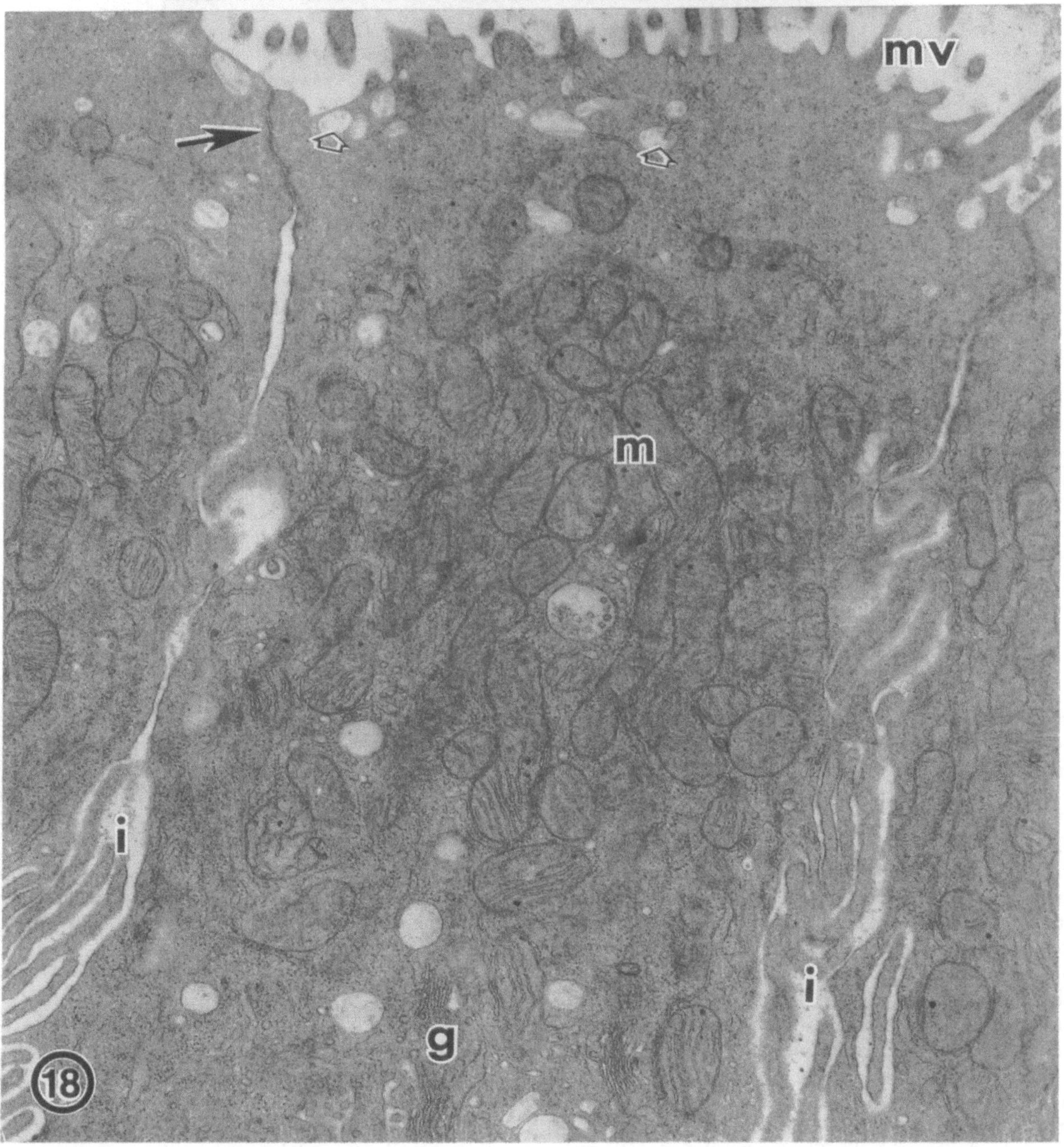

Figure 17   Epithelial cells of a bile duct are columnar to pyramidal (e). Pale-staining granulocytes (p) are located in a peripheral position. Connective tissue envelops the duct (arrow). Adjacent hepatocytes (h) are filled with lipid. × 1000
Figure 18   The columnar epithelium of the bile duct has microvilli (mv). The apical lateral membranes fuse to form occludens junctions (arrow). The remainder of the lateral membrane forms an elaborate series of complex interdigitations (i) with neighbouring cells. The cytoplasm is filled with abundant apical mitochondria (m) and a prominent Golgi complex (g). Clear vesicles occur at the cell apex (open arrows). × 24 800